**PERIPHERAL NEURONS
IN NOCICEPTION :
PHYSIO-PHARMACOLOGICAL
ASPECTS**

British Library Cataloguing in Publication Data
A catalogue record for this book is available from the British Library.

ISBN 2-7420-0081-X

Éditions John Libbey Eurotext
127, avenue de la République, 92120 Montrouge, France.
Tél.: (1) 46.73.06.60.

John Libbey & Company Ltd
13, Smiths Yard, Summerley Street, London SW 18 4HR, England.
Tel.: (01) 947.27.77.

John Libbey CIC
Via L. Spallanzani, 11, 00161 Rome, Italy. Tel.: (06) 862.289.

© John Libbey Eurotext, 1994, Paris

Il est interdit de reproduire intégralement ou partiellement le présent ouvrage — loi du 11 mars 1957 — sans autorisation de l'éditeur ou du Centre français du Copyright, 6 bis, rue Gabriel–Laumain, 75010 Paris.

PERIPHERAL NEURONS IN NOCICEPTION : PHYSIO-PHARMACOLOGICAL ASPECTS

J.M. BESSON
G. GUILBAUD
H. OLLAT

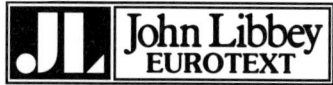

Illustration de couverture :
Edvard Munch, le cri, 1893;
Photo Bridgeman-Giraudon, ADAGP, Paris, 1995

Contents

List of contributors	VII
Preface	IX

1. **Nociceptors in animals**
   H.O. Handwerker, P.W. Reeh 1

2. **Mechanically evoked secondary hyperalgesia in the primate**
   R.H. LaMotte 13

3. **On visceral nociceptors**
   G.F. Gebhart, J.N. Sengupta 23

4. **Communications from the uterus (and other tissues)**
   K.J. Berkley 39

5. **Chemical activation and sensitization of nociceptors**
   A. Dray 49

6. **Capsaicin sensitivity of primary sensory neurones and its regulation**
   G. Jancsó, A. Ambrus 71

7. **A new site of coupling between sympathetic neurones and afferent neurones following peripheral nerve lesions**
   W. Jänig, M. Devor, E.M. McLachlan, M. Michaelis 89

8. **Capsaicin and pharmacology of nociceptors**
   J. Szolcsányi, R. Pórszász, G. Pethö 109

9. **Studies on the release of CGRP into the skin blister base**
   T.H.M. Mirzai, T.L. Yaksh 125

10. **Peripheral aspects of opioid activity : studies in animals**
    V. Kayser, G. Guilbaud 137

11. **Peripheral opioid analgesia : mechanisms and therapeutic applications**
    C. Stein 157

12. **Strategies for the design of a peripherally acting analgesic drug**
    R.G. Hill 167

13. Presynaptic control of thin primary afferents : an ultrastructural analysis
    S.M. Carlton 185

14. A possible relation between neuropathic pain and central sensory sprouting following peripheral nerve lesions
    R.E. Coggeshall 201

15. Deafferentation-induced alterations in the adult rat dorsal horn
    C.C. LaMotte 209

16. Plasticity of sensory transmission and modulation following peripheral nerve lesion with special emphasis on peptidergic, nitric oxidergic, α_2 adrenergic and opioidergic systems
    X.J. Xu, Z. Wiesenfeld-Hallin 225

17. The release of neuropeptides in the spinal cord following peripheral stimuli : *in vivo* studies
    A.W. Duggan 241

18. Pharmacological and physiological modulations of the release of peptides from nociceptors
    F. Cesselin, E. Collin, S. Bourgoin, M. Pohl, A. Mauborgne, J.J. Benoliel, M. Hamon 255

List of contributors

Ambrus A., Department of Physiology, Albert Szent-Giörgyi Medical University, Dom tér 10, H-6720 Szeged, Hungary.
Benoliel J.J., INSERM U 288, Neurobiologie Cellulaire et Fonctionnelle, Faculté de Médecine Pitié-Salpêtrière, 91, Bd de l'Hôpital, 75634 Paris Cedex 13, France.
Berkley K.J., Department of Psychology (R-54), Florida State University, Tallahassee, Florida 32306-1051, USA.
Bourgoin S., INSERM U 288, Neurobiologie Cellulaire et Fonctionnelle, Faculté de Médecine Pitié-Salpêtrière, 91, Bd de l'Hôpital, 75634 Paris Cedex 13, France.
Carlton S.M., Department of Anatomy and Neuroscience, and Marine Biomedical Institute, University of Texas Medical Branch, Galveston, Texas 77555-0843, USA.
Cesselin F., INSERM U 288, Neurobiologie Cellulaire et Fonctionnelle, Faculté de Médecine Pitié-Salpêtrière, 91, Bd de l'Hôpital, 75634 Paris Cedex 13, France.
Coggeshall R.E., Department of Anatomy and Neuroscience, and Marine Biomedical Institute, University of Texas Medical Branch, Galveston, Texas 77555-0843, USA.
Collin E., INSERM U 288, Neurobiologie Cellulaire et Fonctionnelle, Faculté de Médecine Pitié-Salpêtrière, 91, Bd de l'Hôpital, 75634 Paris Cedex 13, France.
Devor M., Department of Cell and Animal Biology, Institute of Life Sciences, Hebrew University of Jerusalem, Jerusalem 91904, Israël.
Dray A., Sandoz Institute for Medical Research, 5 Gower Place, London WC1E5BN, UK.
Duggan A.W., Department of Preclinical Veterinary Sciences, University of Edinburgh, Summerhall, Edinburgh, EH9 1QH, UK.
Gebhart G.F., Department of Pharmacology, The University of Iowa, Bowen Science Building, Iowa City, IA52242, USA.
Guilbaud G., Unité de Recherches de Physiopharmacologie du Système Nerveux, INSERM U 161, 12, rue d'Alésia, 75014 Paris, France.
Hamon M., INSERM U 288, Neurobiologie Cellulaire et Fonctionnelle, Faculté de Médecine Pitié-Salpêtrière, 91, Bd de l'Hôpital, 75634 Paris Cedex 13, France.
Handwerker H.O., Department of Physiology and Biokybernetics, University of Erlangen/Nürnberg, Universitätsstr. 17, D-91054 Erlangen, Germany.
Hill R.G., Merck, Sharp and Dohme Research Laboratories, Neuroscience Research Centre, Terlings Park, Harlow, UK.
Jancsó G., Department of Physiology, Albert Szent-Giörgyi Medical University, Dom tér 10, H-6720 Szeged, Hungary.
Jänig W., Physiologisches Institut, Christian-Albrechts-Universität zu Kiel, Olshausenstr. 40, 24098 Kiel, Germany.
Kayser V., Unité de Recherches de Physiopharmacologie du Système Nerveux, INSERM U 161, 12, rue d'Alésia, 75014 Paris, France.
LaMotte C.C., Section of Neurosurgery, Yale University School of Medicine, New Haven, CT 06510, USA.
LaMotte R.H., Department of Anesthesiology, Yale University School of Medicine,

333 Cedar St, New Haven CT06510, USA.
Mauborgne A., INSERM U 288, Neurobiologie Cellulaire et Fonctionnelle, Faculté de Médecine Pitié-Salpêtrière, 91, Bd de l'Hôpital, 75634 Paris Cedex 13, France.
McLachlan E.M., Prince of Wales Medical Research Institute, Randwick, NSW 2031, Australia.
Michaelis M., Physiologisches Institut, Christian-Albrechts-Universität zu Kiel, Olshausenstr. 40, 24098 Kiel, Germany.
Mirzai T.H.M., Department of Anesthesiology, University of California, San Diego LaJolla, CA 92093, USA.
Pethö G., Department of Pharmacology, University Medical School of Pécs, H-7643 Pécs, Szigeti ut 12, Hungary.
Pohl M., INSERM U 288, Neurobiologie Cellulaire et Fonctionnelle, Faculté de Médecine Pitié-Salpêtrière, 91, Bd de l'Hôpital, 75634 Paris Cedex 13, France.
Pórszász R., Department of Pharmacology, University Medical School of Pécs, H-7643 Pécs, Szigeti ut 12, Hungary.
Reeh P.W., Department of Physiology and Biokybernetics, University of Erlangen /Nürnberg, Universitätsstr. 17, D-91054 Erlangen, Germany.
Sengupta J.N., Department of Pharmacology, The University of Iowa, Bowen Science Building, Iowa City, IA52242, USA.
Stein C., Department of Anesthesiology and Critical Care Medicine, John Hopkins University, Baltimore, Maryland 21287-5354, USA.
Szolcsányi J., Department of Pharmacology, University Medical School of Pécs, H-7643 Pécs, Szigeti ut 12, Hungary.
Wiesenfeld-Hallin Z., Department of Clinical Physiology, Section of Clinical Neurophysiology, Karolinska Institute, Huddinge University Hospital, S-141 86 Huddinge, Sweden.
Xu X.J., Department of Clinical Physiology, Section of Clinical Neurophysiology, Karolinska Institute, Huddinge University Hospital, S-141 86 Huddinge, Sweden.
Yaksh T.L., Department of Anesthesiology, University of California, San Diego LaJolla, CA 92093, USA.

Preface

Over the last two decades, there has been an explosion in research on pharmacology of pain. Several tens of strategies for the design of new molecules have been developped. Unfortunately, the clinicians are still waiting for the ideal analgesic and their therapeutic to relieve pain is still limited to a large number of non steroid anti-inflammatory drugs (NSAIDs) and to morphine (or derivatives), with, in addition, tricyclic anti-depressive and anticonvulsant agents for some specific pain syndromes.

The importance of spinal and supraspinal mechanisms in integrative processes of pain is beyond doubt, but, for many groups, the first neurone in the pathways seems to be a favoured target for the design and development of effective analgesics, lacking the side effects often seen with substances acting at supraspinal levels.

At this first peripheral stage, the different processes are already extremely complex. However, recent multiple studies have provided some clues for a better understanding of pain processing not only at the periphery itself but also in the central nervous system.

No doubt that the expansion of electrophysiological recordings of peripheral afferent fibers of different types supplying the skin (in animals and humans), the joints, the muscles, or different viscera in various species, is of major interest. The clear demonstration of the involvement of the sympathetic system in pain, in some pathological conditions, using different experiments including electrophysiological recordings of efferent fibers in animal and man, is also an important step. From a general point of view, the development of experimental models of clinical pain is surely, although with obvious limitations, one of the most hopeful directions to take. In parallel, many pharmacological investigations, based on electrophysiological, behavioural, neurochemical and molecular methods, have been undertaken, in order to design new compounds acting at the periphery.

Despite the accumulation of data obtained with relatively consistent methodological approaches, researchers have to face multiple complex factors : the physico-chemical surrounding of the afferent terminals in the different tissues (pH, various ions, pCO_2, pO_2...), the sympathetic tone, the myriad chemicals (the "peripheral soup"), which all interact directly or indirectly, with the excitability of the afferent fibers, the multiple receptors, a problem confounded by the colocalisation and corelease of various chemicals. Finally, this complexity is repeated and becomes even more complete at afferent fiber terminal sites in the spinal dorsal horn or in the trigeminal complex.

This book dealing with the "Pharmacological aspects of peripheral neurones involved in nociception", and written by leading expert in the field, obviously covers these problems, but it is not a simple catalogue, and its originality is to consider both the basic aspects together with reflections on the possible directions of research for the design of new molecules with analgesic properties.

J.M. Besson, G. Guilbaud, H. Ollat

1

Nociceptors in animals

H.O. HANDWERKER, P.W.REEH

Institut für Physiologie und Biokybernetik, University of Erlangen/Nürnberg, Germany.

It had been presumed that nociceptors consist mainly of slowly conducting nerve fibers even before the rise of electrophysiological single unit recording techniques (for a review, *see* [34]). Yngve Zotterman was first to record multi-unit activity of slowly conducting nerve fibers in the cat [87] and Ainsley Iggo published the first record from a single unmyelinated nociceptor unit excited by heating the skin to noxious levels [41]. The thermal thresholds of these nociceptors were similar to the threshold of heat pain in man and of nocifensive reflexes in other mammalian species which had been studied before, *e.g.* by Hardy and co-workers [37]. Decades have passed since these pioneering studies and subsequent research has lead to classification of different types of afferent units with presumed nociceptive functions by thorough assessment of their receptive characteristics.

Nociceptor types in the skin

Bessou and Perl recording from unmyelinated afferent units from the cat's hairy skin found a class of units responding maximally to noxious heat, but also to "moderate to intense" mechanical stimuli and to irritant chemicals (acids). They coined the term "polymodal nociceptor" [5]. Synonymously, the more descriptive term "CMH units" has been used meaning mechano- and heat responsive C-fibers. CMH units have frequently been encountered in the hairy and glabrous skin of cat [3], monkey [54], rat [23, 58] and rabbit [57]. They were also frequently found in microneurography experiments on skin nerves of human subjects (*see* contribution by Torebjörk in this volume).

Myelinated nociceptive afferents have also been found in cat [3, 9], rat [58], rabbit [21] and monkey [10-13, 43, 65, 68], mainly among those fibers having slow conduction velocities (A-delta units). However, in primates some myelinated nociceptors have been encountered with conduction velocities in the range of fast conducting A-alpha/beta units [26, 27]. Thus, some laboratories prefer to refer to "A" instead of "A-delta" nociceptors. Since many pain studies, in particular those analysing evoked potentials, have relied on electrical stimulation of A-delta units, one has to keep in mind that the proportion of non-nociceptive elements among the A-delta units is generally higher than among C-units. Sensitive warmth, cold [18, 19, 39, 42] and mechanoreceptors [6-8, 10, 86] have frequently been found in the A-delta range of conduction velocities.

Two types of myelinated nociceptor units have been described : one sort of units being heat and mechano-receptive (AMH) is driven by mechanical stimuli, by noxious heating and also by algogenic chemicals similarly to polymodal C-fibers [1, 13, 69]. Another type of units found in subprimate mammals is usually not excited by noxious heating stimuli up to 60°C and rather insensitive to chemical stimuli, but responds to strong mechanical stimulation. These units have been named HTM A-delta fibers (high threshold mechanoceptive) [30, 58, 60, 71, 81]. In the monkey skin a type of AMH unit has been described that responds to strong mechanical stimulation and to heating stimuli above 50°C after long delay. These units were named "AMH I" to distinguish them from the AMH II having moderate heat thresholds comparable to those of CMH [11, 13, 64, 65, 69]. Most AMH I having thresholds above 53°C when first tested were found in glabrous skin of the monkey. Thresholds may drop, however, upon repetitive testing and hence these units may contribute to heat hyperalgesia [11, 65].

We have suggested a new nomenclature since this one seems to be confusing : AMH II could be renamed AMH_m where the suffix "m" stands for "moderate threshold, close to pain threshold" and AMH I could be renamed AMH_h , "h" standing for "high thresholds, several degrees centigrade above pain threshold, and long utilization times" [34].

Physical stimulation of nociceptors

In order to characterize nociceptors it is insufficient to search for primary afferent units that are characterized by high thresholds for certain stimuli, since the particular form of stimulation might just be inadequate for the respective unit. Nociceptor activity should be related to pain in man or to nocifensive reactions in other animals in several respects, in particular, nociceptors should encode the intensity of pain inducing stimuli about as well as they are reflected in the magnitude of pain reactions. Furthermore, nociceptor discharges and pain sensations should be modulated in parallel, *e.g.* in inflammation. Interestingly, another possible criterion cannot be applied : it has been shown in experiments on human subjects that adaptation rates of nociceptor discharges and of pain sensations during prolonged noxious stimulation are quite different pointing to a modulating role of central nervous processing [2].

But even the application of the first two criteria meets some problems: *e.g.* though it is clear from differential nerve blocks that at least in the hairy skin of human subjects heat pain is related to unmyelinated afferent units (for a review, *see* [34]), heat thresholds of single CMH units vary over a wide range between 40° and 50°C in the hairy and glabrous skin of man and other mammalian species [3, 17, 23, 35, 54, 58]. More importantly, in experiments on human subjects the thresholds of individual CMHs were often somewhat lower than the pain thresholds [82]. Using radiant heat for stimulation, van Hees tried to quantify the rate of impulses in CMH units that is necessary to evoke thermal pain sensations. For this purpose he calculated the mean impulse frequencies of single CMH units during periods of skin heating for up to 15 sec, and compared them with the pain reports of the subjects. Mean impulse rates below 0.3/sec were reported as non-painful, whereas discharge frequencies exceeding 0.4/sec were mostly accompanied by pain. Discharges exceeding 1.5/sec were invariably associated with strong pain [83, 84]. It can be conluded from these findings that summation of nociceptor impulses at central synapses is required to induce pain reactions. Probably, somewhat lower nociceptor thresholds compared to pain thresholds are explained by the functioning of central gating mechanisms. For this reason, the response characteristics in the noxious range provide a better criterion for the function of a presumed nociceptor unit than the identity of thresholds [29, 74].

Recently, it has been discussed whether very low firing rates in CMH units may have trophic functions rather than transmit sensory information, since the release of vasoactive substances from the endings seems to occur already at very low discharge rates [59, 80].

Often, mechanical stimuli exceeding the threshold of a particular CMH or AMH unit studied in microneurography experiments on human subjects are not painful. Indeed, the mismatch between nociceptor and pain thresholds is greater for mechanical than for heat stimulation though in some early studies pin prick stimuli were found to induce the highest discharge rates to mechanical stimuli in AMHs and CMHs [5, 9]. Von Frey hair stimulation at strengths inducing vigorous discharge rates in CMH units of human skin (which have thresholds similar to those of other mammals) were often assessed as non-painful by the experimental subjects even when discharge rates were exceeded, which in case of heat stimuli were always correlated with pain reports [84]. This mismatch has been explained by the different amount of total input to the CNS from the two types of stimuli and with differential central processing : v. Frey hairs apparently stimulate a smaller area than most heat stimuli, providing much less spatial summation, and, in addition, they also excite low threshold mechanoreceptors that may modulate the nociceptor input in the CNS [2].

Chemical stimulation of nociceptors

Since most CMH and AMH_m units are sensitive to chemical stimulation with pain producing substances, in contrast to sensitive mechanoreceptors, chemical stimuli can be used to characterize nociceptors. Of particular interest are substances that are released from inflamed tissues and contribute to inflammation and inflammatory pain states. Several of these agents have been shown to excite nociceptors when injected intra-arterially in animal experiments, amongst them serotonin (5-HT) and bradykinin [4, 22].

These and other endogenous chemical stimuli also cause pain when applied intra- or subcutaneously as reviewed in a classical monograph [45]. In the classical experiments on the cantharidine blister base in man, pain thresholds below 10^{-7} M were found for bradykinin and somewhat higher thresholds for 5-HT and acetylcholine (in the range of 10^{-7} - 10^{-5} g/ml). H^+ ions induced pain when applied in isotonic solution to a blister base at a pH of about 3.0, whereas intracutaneous injections induce pain at a pH of 6.2. K^+ ions, which are increased in inflammatory exudates, are effective at the blister base at 8-16 mE/l (for a review, see [34]). These threshold concentrations for pain perception are difficult to compare with the thresholds of polymodal nociceptors studied *in vivo* due to technical problems. Animal experiments have been performed either with close arterial injection or with local application of the agents to the receptive fields and under both conditions the concentration of the substances at the nerve endings cannot be assessed properly.

However, these experiments have lead to insights regarding the excitability spectrum of nociceptive afferent units. For the identification of nociceptors in deep body structures, *e.g.* in muscle, joints and viscera, chemical stimulation, mainly with 5-HT and bradykinin, was particularly important [24, 25, 38, 40, 44, 47, 61-63, 67, 76, 77].

In vitro preparations for chemical stimulation of nociceptors

The understanding of the chemical excitability of nociceptors has been boosted by the development of *in vitro* techniques that allow a much better control of the chemical environment of the nerve endings than *in vivo* experiments where in addition uncontrolled vascular reactions have to be taken into account [14, 15, 63, 70]. In our laboratory a superfused rat skin-nerve preparation has been used for studying cutaneous nociceptors ; it allows to treat their receptive fields directly with chemicals in controlled concentrations. The following data result from a number of studies on this preparation using the single fiber recording method.

We have tested a number of endogenous chemicals involved in inflammations and investigated their interactions in exciting and sensitizing nociceptors. Herein, we have focused on the most numerous subpopulation of the CMH nociceptor that proved to provide the widest spectrum of chemosensitivity. In terms of prevalence, *i.e.* number of units excited, bradykinin (10^{-5}M) and H$^+$ ions (pH = 6.1) are the most effective agents each driving about 60% of the CMH units [55, 78]. At equal and pathophysiologically relevant concentration (10^{-6}M), however, the hydrogen ions were more potent than bradykinin or a combination of other inflammatory mediators including bradykinin [36, 46, 78]. In addition, low pH induces significantly higher discharge rates and produces long-lasting non-adapting activity while the inflammmatory mediators lose their excitatory action due to tachyphylaxis upon repeated or continuous application. However, combining low pH with bradykinin, histamine, serotonin and prostaglandin E$_2$ (10^{-6}M) in one "inflammatory soup" prevents the tachyphylaxis and has a higher algogenic potency than individual agents. This combination has also been used to recruit part of the mechanically and thermally insensitive ("sleeping") nociceptors that were recently described *in vivo* [20, 33] and *in vitro* [51].

In the rat skin-nerve preparation, serotonin (5-HT) alone excites only a small proportion of CMH units, but reliably increases their responsiveness to bradykinin [31, 55]. 5-HT can emerge in inflamed or injured tissue through degranulation of mast cells (*e.g.* in rat and in the human respiratory tract) and of blood platelets, the latter being activated, *e.g.* by collagen. Platelet superfusion of nociceptive nerve endings, however, is more potent than 5-HT application in exciting nociceptors. This turned out from recent experiments when cutaneous receptive fields were first incubated with human "platelet rich plasma", ineffective by itself, that was then activated with 10^{-5} M ADP, again ineffective by itself. Within 2-4 min, about 70 % of the nociceptive nerve terminals developed ongoing activity that could not be precluded by different 5-HT antagonists or by previous treatment of the blood donor with acetylsalicylic acid [73]. This finding bears consequences as to the interpretation of previous results from work done *in vivo*. Chemicals known to activate thrombocytes, such as noradrenalin, prostaglandin E$_2$, serotonin etc., may affect nociceptors indirectly. In addition, blood platelets coming into contact with collagen may contribute to the sustained nociceptor discharge following cutaneous injury [71]. In leukocytic inflammation (carrageenin induced), the "platelet activating factor" secreted may assist to explain the ongoing nociceptor acitivity found [71].

In previous *in vivo* [77] and *in vitro* [66] studies on subcutaneous nociceptor preparations, potentiation of the bradykinin effect was also reported to follow prostaglandin E$_2$ administration. In the knee joint of the cat, even an excitatory and mechanically sensitizing effect of prostaglandins in high dosage was accomplished [67]. In the skin *in vitro*, prostaglandin E$_2$ failed to excite or sensitize nociceptors to physical stimulation, and its amplification of the bradykinin responsiveness was inconsistent [55]. Accordingly, inhibition of prostaglandin synthesis has a limited effect on cutaneous nociceptor sensitization [16]. Recent experiments took into account that bradykinin can stimulate endogenous prostaglandin release. Even so, during cyclo-oxygenase block with flurbiprofen, nociceptor responses to combined inflammatory mediators (10^{-6}M) did not depend on presence or absence of PGE_2 in the superfusate [72].

Another key substance in inflammation seems to be histamine as released from mast cells or from basophilic leukocytes. This substance apparently plays an important role in cutaneous sensation, in that it produces marked itching when brought into the superficial skin layers. However, histamine excites only a small fraction of CMH units in human microneurography experiments [32]. In rat skin *in vitro*, likewise, only a small proportion of CMH units is weakly excited by histamine [55]. Many more nociceptor units are recruited, however, when histamine stimuli are conditioned with bradykinin. Following bradykinin pretreatment 75 % of the nociceptors respond to histamine [55]. Accordingly, in human skin infiltrated with a very low concentration of bradykinin (10^{-7}M), histamine iontophoresis no longer produced itch but a sensation of burning pain [49]. However, in a combination of inflammatory mediators applied to the rat skin-nerve preparation, histamine does not increase the excitatory effect.

Acetylcholine also was found to activate nociceptors *in vivo* [22] and to activate a considerable proportion of CMHs *in vitro* at physiological concentrations but to leave them with a marked desensitization to mechanical stimulation [79]. Interestingly, it has been recently published that keratinocytes are endowed with the enzymes to synthesize and to degrade acetylcholine and with the capability to release it in relevant amounts [28]. Nothing is yet known about the conditions of this release.

In view of the multiplicity of agents affecting nociceptors it might be interesting to recognize a number of substances that play a role in inflammatory processes but are largely ineffective in exciting nociceptors. Among them is substance P that is released, together with CGRP and NKA, from activated nociceptive nerve endings. This neuropeptide has been assumed to cause "neurogenic inflammation", *i.e.* vasodilatation and plasma extravasation [56]. Substance P does not excite nociceptors nor sensitize them to physical stimulation but it has a conditioning, sensitizing effect on their responsiveness to inflammatory mediators [46]. This effect has only been encountered in the very beginning of the response and disappeared when the "inflammatory soup" had built up an ongoing nociceptor discharge. This agrees well with the assumption that neuropeptides are the first mediators to be released early after cutaneous injury.

In contrast, oxygen radicals are secreted during a later stage of inflammatory processes by invading macrophages and neutrophilic leukocytes. They are assumed to contribute to tissue destruction. Nociceptors are only weakly activated by highest concentrations (>1mM) of hydrogen peroxide but afterwards left with complete desensitization to natural stimuli [50]. These results may explain the limited efficacy of superoxide dismutase in the therapy of painful arthritis.

Another chemical radical, nitric oxide (NO•), has recently gained major scientific interest as a short distance messenger, released *e.g.* from macrophages in inflamed tissue. In preliminary experiments, gaseous NO• (0.126 % in N_2) dissolved in the superfusate over receptive fields in an estimated nanomolar concentration caused a mild but significant activation and sensitization of nociceptors [52].

High osmotic pressure is a frequent constituent of inflammatory exsudates [75], and hyperosmolar solutions are known from clinical experience to be painful when injected into human tissue. However, pure osmotic stimuli per se, such as sucrose solutions or distilled water, are but weakly exciting a small proportion of nociceptors while producing a marked desensitization to mechanical stimulation in a larger population [85]. Yet, when hyperosmolarity was created with salt solutions, in particular with sodium chloride, a strong and dose-dependent excitation of 82 % of all nociceptors resulted, again followed by marked transient desensitization. Osmotic effects from either source are unspecific in that they affect not only nociceptive but also sensitive mechanoreceptive primary afferents with rapidly conducting fibers.

Sensitization and hyperalgesia

Chemical excitation of nociceptors inducing ongoing, though usually low-frequent discharges, may contribute to ongoing pain under resting conditions (together with central nervous modulations). To most patients in pain, however, the hyperalgesia to physical stimuli seems to be more of a problem. The underlying neurobiological mechanisms relate to sensitization of primary afferent units and of secondary neurons in the CNS (for a review, *see* [34]). The biophysical and biochemical mechanisms of primary afferent sensitization are complex, and the relative weights of its constituents are not yet known. Bradykinin, for example, produces a pronounced nociceptor sensitization to heat by which the threshold temperature for nociceptor excitation may drop as low as into the range of body temperature [48]. In contrast, bradykinin and even a combination of inflammatory agents [46] do not induce a measurable sensitization to mechanical stimuli in the rat skin. Only a small, specialized subpopulation of A-delta fibers, high-threshold mechanoreceptive nociceptors, has yet been shown to become sensitized to punctuate mechanical (v. Frey hair) stimulation, following injury to the skin, *in vivo* [71]. In CMH units *in vitro*, however, prolonged or repeated treatment of their receptive fields with H^+ ions effectively lowers their thresholds to mechanical stimulation [78].

Conclusions

In recent years, our understanding of nociceptor excitability has been boosted by the development of handy *in vitro* preparation techniques. A pattern of substances contributing to nociceptor excitation and sensitization is now emerging. However, the recording technique for studying nociceptors remained essentially the same since the days of Zotterman's and Iggo's basic discoveries. Modern techniques of membrane physiology, such as the patch clamp method cannot be applied to the tiny nociceptive terminals at present. Therefore, our understanding of membrane mechanisms is still derived from conjectures based on the study of other biological objects. Probably the future progress will depend on a careful comparison of quantitative data obtained from extracellular recordings in nociceptor preparations with membrane processes analysed in larger cellular models that could explain the excitability changes.

Acknowledgements

Experimental work of the authors reported in this review has been supported by the Deutsche Forschungsgemeinschaft, Sonderforschungsbereich 353.

References

1. Adriaensen H, Gybels J, Handwerker HO, Van Hees J. Response properties of thin myelinated (A-delta) fibers in human skin nerves. *J Neurophysiol* 1983 ; 49 : 111-22.
2. Adriaensen H, Gybels J, Handwerker HO, Van Hees J. Nociceptor discharges and sensations due to prolonged noxious mechanical stimulation--a paradox. *Hum Neurobiol* 1984 ; 3 : 53-8.
3. Beck PW, Handwerker HO, Zimmermann M. Nervous outflow from the cat's foot during noxious radiant heat stimulation. *Brain Res* 1974 ; 67 : 373-86.
4. Beck PW, Handwerker HO. Bradykinin and serotonin effects on various types of cutaneous nerve fibers. *Pflugers Arch* 1974 ; 347 : 209-22.
5. Bessou P, Perl ER. Responses of cutaneous sensory units with unmyelinated fibers to noxious stimuli. *J Neurophysiol* 1969 ; 32 : 1025-43.
6. Brown AG, Iggo A, Miller S. Myelinated afferent nerve fibers from the skin of the rabbit ear. *Exp Neurol* 1967 ; 18 : 338-49.
7. Burgess PR, Petit D, Warren RM. Receptor types in cat hairy skin supplied by myelinated fibers. *J Neurophysiol* 1968 ; 31 : 833-48.
8. Burgess PR, Howe JF, Lessler MJ, Whitehorn D. Cutaneous receptors supplied by myelinated fibers in the cat. II. Number of mechanoreceptors excited by a local stimulus. *J Neurophysiol* 1974 ; 37 : 1373-86.
9. Burgess PR, Perl ER. Myelinated afferent fibers responding specifically to noxious stimulation of the skin. *J Physiol Lond* 1967 ; 190 : 541-62.
10. Burgess PR, Perl ER. Cutaneous mechanoreceptors and nociceptors. In : Iggo A, ed. *Handbook of sensory physiology.* Vol 2. Heidelberg, Berlin, New York : Springer, 1973 : 29-78.
11. Campbell JN, Meyer RA, Lamotte RH. Sensitization of myelinated nociceptive afferents that innervate monkey hand. *J Neurophysiol* 1979 ; 42 : 1669-79.
12. Campbell JN, Raja SN, Meyer RA, Mackinnon SE. Myelinated afferents signal the hyperalgesia associated with nerve injury. *Pain* 1988 ; 32 : 89-94.
13. Campbell JN, Raja SN, Cohen RH, Manning DC, Khan AA, Meyer RA. Peripheral neural mechanisms of nociception. In : Wall PD, Melzack R, eds. *Textbook of pain.* Edinburgh, London, Melbourne : Churchill Livingstone, 1989 : 22-45.
14. Cervero F, Sann H. Mechanically evoked responses of afferent fibers innervating the guinea-pigs ureter, an *in vitro* study. *J Physiol Lond* 1989 ; 412 : 245-66.
15. Cohen RH, Perl ER. Chemical factors in the sensitization of cutaneous nociceptors. *Prog Brain Res* 1988 ; 74 : 201-6.
16. Cohen RH, Perl ER. Contributions of arachidonic acid derivatives and substance P to the

sensitization of cutaneous nociceptors. *J Neurophysiol* 1990 ; 64 : 457-64.
17. Croze S, Duclaux R, Kenshalo DR. The thermal sensitivity of the polymodal nociceptors in the monkey. *J Physiol Lond* 1976 ; 263 : 539-62.
18. Darian-Smith I, Johnson KO, Dykes R. Cold fiber population innervating palmar and digital skin of the monkey : responses to cooling pulses. *J Neurophysiol* 1973 ; 36 : 325-46.
19. Darian-Smith I, Johnson KO, Lamotte CC, Kenins P, Shigenaga Y, Ming VC. Coding of incremental changes in skin temperature by single warm fibers in the monkey. *J Neurophysiol* 1979 ; 42 : 1316-31.
20. Davis KD, Meyer RA, Campbell JN. Chemosensitivity and sensitization of nociceptive afferents that innervate the hairy skin of monkey. *J Neurophysiol* 1993 ; 69 : 1071-81.
21. Fitzgerald M, Lynn B. The sensitization of high threshold mechanoreceptors with myelinated axons by repeated heating. *J Physiol Lond* 1977 ; 365 : 549-63.
22. Fjällbrant N, Iggo A. The effect of histamine, 5-hydroxytryptamine and acetylcholine on cutaneous afferent fibers. *J Physiol Lond* 1961 ; 156 : 578-90.
23. Fleischer E, Handwerker HO, Joukhadar S. Unmyelinated nociceptive units in two skin areas of the rat. *Brain Res* 1983 ; 267 : 81-92.
24. Fock S, Mense S. Excitatory effects of 5-hydroxytryptamine, histamine and potassium ions on muscular group IV afferent units: a comparison with bradykinin. *Brain Res* 1976 ; 105 : 459-69.
25. Franz M, Mense S. Muscle receptors with group IV afferent fibers responding to application of bradykinin. *Brain Res* 1975 ; 92 : 369-83.
26. Georgopoulos AP. Functional properties of primary afferent units probably related to pain mechanisms of primate glabrous skin. *J Neurophysiol* 1976 ; 39 : 71-84.
27. Georgopoulos AP. Stimulus-response relations in high-threshold mechanothermal fibers innervating primate glabrous skin. *Brain Res* 1977 ; 128 : 547-53.
28. Grando SA, Kist DA, Qi M, Dahl MV. Human keratinocytes synthesize, secrete and degrade acetylcholine. *J Invest Dermatol* 1993 ; 101 : 32-6.
29. Gybels J, Handwerker HO, Van Hees J. A comparison between the discharges of human nociceptive nerve fibers and the subject's ratings of his sensations. *J Physiol Lond* 1979 ; 292 : 193-206.
30. Handwerker HO, Anton F, Reeh PW. Discharge patterns of afferent cutaneous nerve fibers from the rat's tail during prolonged noxious mechanical stimulation. *Exp Brain Res* 1987 ; 65 : 493-504.
31. Handwerker HO, Reeh PW, Steen KH. Effects of 5HT on nociceptors. In : Besson JM, ed. *Serotonin and pain*. Amsterdam : Elsevier Science, 1990 : 1-15.
32. Handwerker HO, Forster C, Kirchhoff C. Discharge patterns of human C-fibers induced by itching and burning stimuli. *J Neurophysiol* 1991 ; 66 : 307-15.
33. Handwerker HO, Kilo S, Reeh PW. Unresponsive afferent nerve-fibers in the sural nerve of the rat. *J Physiol Lond* 1991 ; 435 : 229-42.
34. Handwerker HO, Kobal G. Psychophysiology of experimentally induced pain. *Physiol Rev* 1993 ; 73 : 639-71.
35. Handwerker HO, Neher KD. Characteristics of C-fiber receptors in the cat's foot responding to stepwise increase of skin temperature ot noxious levels. *Pflugers Arch* 1976 ; 365 : 221-9.
36. Handwerker HO, Reeh PW. Pain and inflammation. In : Bond MR, Charlton JE, Woolf CJ, eds. Proceedings of the VIth World Congress on Pain. Amsterdam : Elsevier Science Publishers BV (Biomedical Division), 1991 : 59-69.
37. Hardy JD, Wolff HG, Goodell H. *Pain sensations and reactions*. Baltimore : Williams & Wilkins, 1952.
38. Haupt P, Janig W, Kohler W. Response pattern of visceral afferent fibers, supplying the colon, upon chemical and mechanical stimuli. *Pflugers Arch* 1983 ; 398 : 41-7.

39. Hensel H, Iggo A. Analysis of cutaneous warm and cold fibers in primates. *Pflugers Arch* 1971 ; 329 : 1-8.
40. Hiss E, Mense S. Evidence for the existence of different receptor sites for algesic agents at the endings of muscular group IV afferent units. *Pflugers Arch* 1976 ; 362 : 141-6.
41. Iggo A. Cutaneous heat and cold receptors with slowly conducting (C) afferent fibers. *Q J Exp Physiol* 1959 ; 44 : 362-70.
42. Iggo A. Cutaneous thermoreceptors in primates and subprimates. *J Physiol Lond* 1969 ; 200 : 402-30.
43. Iggo A, Ogawa H. Primate cutaneous thermal nociceptors. *J Physiol Lond* 1971 ; 216 : 77-8.
44. Janig W, Morrison JF. Functional properties of spinal visceral afferents supplying abdominal and pelvic organs, with special emphasis on visceral nociception. *Prog Brain Res* 1986 ; 67 : 87-114.
45. Keele CA, Armstrong D. *Substances producing pain and itch*. London : Edward Arnold, 1964.
46. Kessler W, Kirchhoff C, Reeh PW, Handwerker HO. Excitation of cutaneous afferent nerve-endings *in vitro* by a combination of inflammatory mediators and conditioning effect of substance-P. *Exp Brain Res* 1992 ; 91 : 467-76.
47. Kniffki KD, Mense S, Schmidt RF. Responses of group IV afferent units from skeletal muscle to stretch, contraction and chemical stimulation. *Exp Brain Res* 1978 ; 31 : 511-22.
48. Koltzenburg M, Kress M, Reeh PW. The nociceptor sensitization by bradykinin does not depend on sympathetic neurons. *Neuroscience* 1992 ; 46 : 465-73.
49. Koppert W, Reeh PW, Handwerker HO. Conditioning of histamine by bradykinin alters responses of rat nociceptor and human itch sensation. *Neurosci Lett* 1993 ; 152 : 117-20.
50. Kress M, Koltzenburg M, Reeh PW, Handwerker HO. Responsiveness and functional attributes of electrically localized terminals of cutaneous C-fibers *in vivo* and *in vitro*. *J Neurophysiol* 1992 ; 68 : 581-95.
51. Kress M, Riedl B, Reeh PW. Reactive oxygen species do not play a major role in acute hyperalgesia. *Soc Neurosci Abstr* 1992 ; 18 : 134.
52. Kress M, Riedl B, Reeh PW. Nitric oxide causes mild activation and mechanical sensitization of nociceptive C-fibers in the rat skin, *in vitro*. Abstr 7th World Congr Pain 1993 : 140.
53. Kumazawa T, Mizumura K. Temperature dependency of the chemical responses of the polymodal receptor units *in vitro*. *Brain Res* 1983 ; 278 : 305-7.
54. Kumazawa T, Perl ER. Primate cutaneous sensory units with unmyelinated (C) afferent fibers. *J Neurophysiol* 1977 ; 40 : 1325-39.
55. Lang E, Novak A, Reeh PW, Handwerker HO. Chemosensitivity of fine afferents from rat skin *in vitro*. *J Neurophysiol* 1990 ; 63 : 887-901.
56. Lembeck F. Sir Thomas Lewis nocifensor system, histamine and substance-P-containing primary afferent nerves. *Trends Neurosci* 1983 ; 6 : 106-8.
57. Lynn B. The heat sensitization of polymodal nociceptors in the rabbit and its independence of the local blood flow. *J Physiol Lond* 1979 ; 287 : 493-507.
58. Lynn B, Carpenter SE. Primary afferent units from the hairy skin of the rat hind limb. *Brain Res* 1982 ; 238 : 29-43.
59. Lynn B, Shakhanbeh J. Neurogenic inflammation in the skin of the rabbit. *Agents Actions* 1988 ; 25 : 228-30.
60. Lynn B, Shakhanbeh J. Properties of A delta high threshold mechanoreceptors in the rat hairy and glabrous skin and their response to heat. *Neurosci Lett* 1988 ; 85 : 71-6.
61. Mense S. Nervous outflow from skeletal muscle following chemical noxious stimulation. *J Physiol Lond* 1977 ; 267 : 75-88.
62. Mense S. Sensitization of group IV muscle receptors to bradykinin by 5-hydroxytryptamine and prostaglandin E_2. *Brain Res* 1981 ; 225 : 95-105.
63. Mense S, Schmidt RF. Activation of group IV afferent units from muscle by algesic agents. *Brain*

Res 1974 ; 72 : 305-10.
64. Meyer RA, Campbell JN, Raja SN. Peripheral neural mechanisms of cutaneous hyperalgesia. In : Fields HL, Dubner R, Cervero F, eds. *Advances in pain research and therapy.* Vol.9. New York : Raven Press, 1985 : 53-71.
65. Meyer RA, Campbell JN. Myelinated nociceptive afferents account for the hyperalgesia that follows a burn to the hand. *Science* 1981 ; 213 : 1527-9.
66. Mizumura K, Sato J, Kumazawa T. Effects of prostaglandins and other putative chemical intermediaries on the activity of canine testicular polymodal receptors studied *in vitro*. *Pflugers Arch* 1987 ; 408 : 565-72.
67. Neugebauer V, Schaible HG, Schmidt RF. Sensitization of articular afferents to mechanical stimuli by bradykinin. *Pflugers Arch* 1989 ; 415, 330-335.
68. Perl ER. Myelinated afferent fibers innervating the primate skin and their response to noxious stimuli. *J Physiol Lond* 1968 ; 197 : 593-615.
69. Raja SN, Meyer RA, Campbell JN. Peripheral mechanisms of somatic pain. *Anesthesiology* 1988 ; 68 : 571-90.
70. Reeh PW. Sensory receptors in mammalian skin in an *in vitro* preparation. *Neurosci Lett* 1986 ; 66 : 141-7.
71. Reeh PW, Bayer J, Kocher L, Handwerker HO. Sensitization of nociceptive cutaneous nerve fibers from the rat's tail by noxious mechanical stimulation. *Exp Brain Res* 1987 ; 65 : 505-12.
72. Reeh PW, Brehm S. Nociceptor excitation by inflammatory mediators and by mechanical stimulation in rat skin is neither enhanced by PGE_2 nor suppressed by flurbiprofen. *Soc Neurosci Abstr* 1993 ; 19 : 234.
73. Ringkamp M, Schmelz M, Kress M, Alwang M, Ogilvie A, Reeh P.W. Human platelets acitvated with adenosine diphsophate (ADP) can excite nociceptors in rat skin, *in vitro*. Abstr 7th World Congr Pain 1993 : 21.
74. Robinson CJ, Torebjork HE, Lamotte RH. Psychophysical detection and pain ratings of incremental thermal stimuli : a comparison with nociceptor responses in humans. *Brain Res* 1983 ; 274 : 87-106.
75. Schade H. *Die physikalische Chemie in der inneren Medizin.* Dresden, Leipzig : Th. Steinkopff, 1923.
76. Schaible HG, Schmidt RF. Discharge characteristics of receptors with fine afferents from normal and inflamed joints : influence of analgesics and prostaglandins. *Agents Actions (Suppl.)* 1986 ; 19 : 99-117.
77. Schaible HG, Schmidt RF. Excitation and sensitization of fine articular afferents from cat's knee joint by prostaglandin E_2. *J Physiol Lond* 1988 ; 403 : 91-104.
78. Steen KH, Reeh PW, Anton F, Handwerker HO. Protons selectively induce lasting excitation and sensitization to mechanical stimulation of nociceptors in rat skin, in vitro. *J Neurosci* 1992 ; 12 : 86-95.
79. Steen KH, Reeh PW. Actions of cholinergic agonists and antagonists on sensory nerve endings in rat skin. *J Neurophysiol* 1993 ; 154 : 103-16.
80. Szolcsanyi J. Antidromic vasodilatation and neurogenic inflammation. *Agents Actions* 1988 ; 23 : 4-11.
81. Szolcsanyi J, Anton F, Reeh PW, Handwerker HO. Selective excitation by capsaicin of mechano-heat sensitive nociceptors in rat skin. *Brain Res* 1988 ; 446 : 262-8.
82. Torebjork HE, Lamotte RH, Robinson CJ. Peripheral neural correlates of magnitude of cutaneous pain and hyperalgesia : simultaneous recordings in humans of sensory judgments of pain and evoked responses in nociceptors with C-fibers. *J Neurophysiol* 1984 ; 51 : 325-39.
83. Van Hees J. Human C fiber input during painful and nonpainful stimulation with radiant heat. In : Bonica JJ, Albe-Fessard D, eds. *Advances in pain research and therapy.* Vol 1. New York :

Raven Press, 1976.
84. Van Hees J, Gybels J. C nociceptor activity in human nerve during painful and non painful skin stimulation. *J Neurol Neurosurg Psychiatry* 1981 ; 44 : 600-7.
85. Wedekind C, Reeh PW. The effects of osmotically anisotonic solutions on sensory nerve endings in rat skin, *in vitro*. *Pflugers Arch* 1992 ; 420 (1) : R 52.
86. Whitehorn D, Howe JF, Lessler MJ, Burgess PR. Cutaneous receptors supplied by myelinated fibers in the cat. I. Number of receptors innervated by a single nerve. *J Neurophysiol* 1974 ; 37 : 1361-72.
87. Zotterman Y. Studies in the peripheral nervous mechanism of pain. *Acta Med Scand* 1933 ; 80 : 185-242.

2

Mechanically evoked secondary hyperalgesia in the primate

R. H. LAMOTTE

Department of Anesthesiology, Yale University School of Medicine, New Haven, USA.

A local cutaneous injury can result in a lowered pain threshold and enhanced pain to normally painful stimuli in the skin surrounding the injury (secondary, 2º, hyperalgesia). Two kinds of mechanical stimuli were used to measure the magnitude and spatial extent of 2º hyperalgesia surrounding an intradermal injection of capsaicin into the forearms of human subjects :
 - stroking the skin with innocuous, textured surfaces that, for normal skin, evoked differing sensations of roughness but not pain,
 - indenting the skin with punctate stimuli that normally elicited a sensation of pricking pain.
 After the capsaicin injection, all the textured surfaces evoked pain to differing degrees in the surrounding skin and the punctate stimuli evoked a greater than normal magnitude and duration of pain. "Punctate" hyperalgesia occupied a greater area of skin, in relation to "stroking" hyperalgesia, lasted longer and, once fully developed, was less dependent on peripheral neuronal activity. Evidence from previous studies was cited to support the hypothesis that both types of mechanical hyperalgesia occur as a result of the "central sensitization" of spinothalamic tract neurons.

Normally, a sharp object such as a needle or the thorn of a rose bush, that lightly pricks the skin evokes a very transient sensation of pricking pain. Textured surfaces that do not contain sharp elements (unlike coarse sandpaper, for example) would not be expected to evoke a pain sensation when stroked across the skin. For example, the clothing we wear and most objects that we touch with the hand may elicit differing sensations of roughness or smoothness but are rarely abrasive enough to be painful. A quite different picture emerges, however, after the skin is injured. The skin becomes tender to the touch and a normally painful mechanical stimulus such as a needle elicits abnormally intense pain that has a longer than normal duration (hyperalgesia). Clothing brushed against the skin might elicit pain and still rougher surfaces would be expected to produce even greater amounts of pain even though they had not evoked pain before the injury. Thus, normally painful indentations of the hyperalgesic skin with a sharp object or stroking the skin with an innocuous textured surface evoke abnormal pain. Furthermore, not only is the injured skin hyperalgesic (primary hyperalgesia) but the apparently normal skin surrounding the injury may become so as well (secondary hyperalgesia) [3, 9].

The underlying neuronal mechanisms responsible for the development of secondary (2°) hyperalgesia have been the object of study in our laboratory. We have sought to characterize the changes in sensation evoked by two different types of mechanical stimulation after the development of 2° hyperalgesia : punctate indentation and laterally stroked textured surfaces. Studies of the peripheral and central neuronal mechanisms contributing to each type of mechanical hyperalgesia have been described in detail [1, 6-8, 12, 14] and will only be briefly summarized.

The method of producing the hyperalgesia was to deliver an intradermal injection of 10 μl of 100 μg of capsaicin in a vehicle of tween-80 saline. This produced an intense sensation of burning pain which decreased rapidly in magnitude and disappeared typically within 10-15 min. Immediately upon injection, the surrounding skin became hyperalgesic to gently stroking the skin with a cotton swab and to punctate stimulation with a Von Frey type nylon filament (Figure 1A). The cotton swab was attached to a flexible metal strip which, when slightly bent, delivered a bending force of approximately 100 mN. The nylon filament, referred to as our standard filament (0.58 mm diam.), exerted a bending force of 225 mN. The areas of hyperalgesia to each stimulus were mapped by applying each stimulus outside the hyperalgesic area and then shifting the locus in the direction of the injection site until the subject reported an abrupt change in sensation : tenderness and pain to the cotton swab (where there normally is only a tactile sensation) and, to the von Frey stimulus, an abnormally intense and longer than normal sensation of pricking pain. The injection site itself was analgesic to light pin pricks but exhibited only slightly reduced pain sensations in response to the standard filament which possibly disturbed surrounding skin. A small area of hyperalgesia to heat developed around the injection site (Figure 1A).

Within the area of punctate hyperalgesia, the magnitude of pain was measured at test sites located 0, 1, 2 and 3 cm away from the injection site. Using the method of magnitude estimation [13], the pain evoked by the standard Von Frey filament was found to increase by six fold over those obtained from uninjected skin (Figure 5A) [12]. By using Von Frey filaments of different diameters to produce different bending forces, it was found that the threshold for punctate pain for five subjects decreased approximately eight fold in comparison with thresholds obtained for uninjected skin [7].

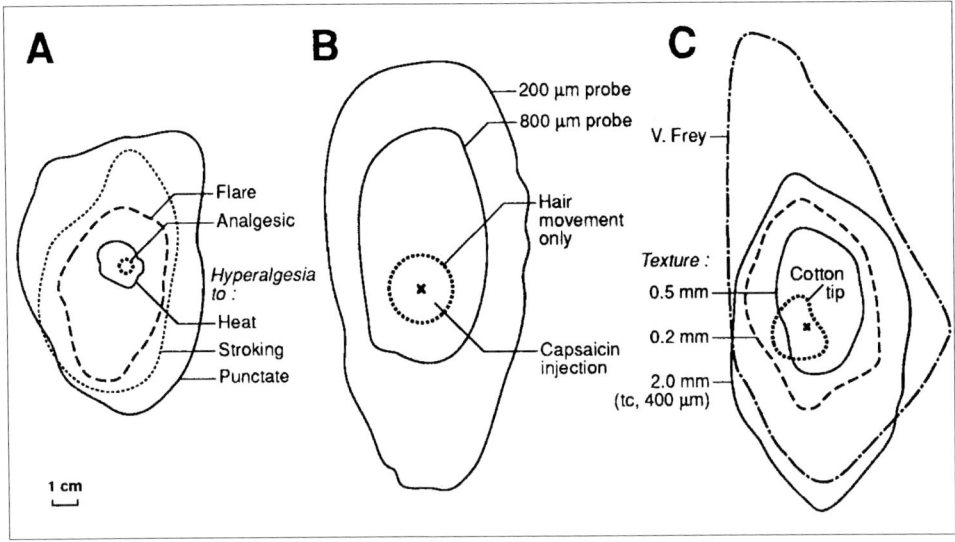

Figure 1. Areas of secondary (2°) hyperalgesia to different kinds of mechanical stimulation of the skin surrounding an injection of capsaicin into the volar forearm. Each panel presents the results of an experiment with a different subject. A : Areas of the flare and hyperalgesia to heat (38°C probe), stroking (cotton swab) and punctate stimuli ("standard" Von Frey, 225 mN -see text). (From [7].) B : Hyperalgesia to hair movement and to punctate stimuli consisting of Von Frey filaments with hemispherically shaped tips of 200 and 800 μm each applying the same force of 294 mN. C : Hyperalgesia to stroking the skin with textured surfaces of differing roughness. The textured surfaces and cotton swab were each applied with a compressional force of approximately 300 mN. The textures consisted of hexagonal arrays of raised elements that differed in center-to-center spacing. Two textures (0.5 and 2.0 mm spacing) had hemispherically shaped raised elements, 250 μm diam. and 165 μm high. The other texture (2.0 mm spacing) had truncated cones (tc) with 225 μm diam. tops and heights of 400 μm. The area produced by punctate stimulation with a Von Frey monofilament (225 mN) is also shown.

Since the Von Frey filaments confound force both with filament diameter and the uncertain geometry of the tip (cut flat but still of irregular shape), a pilot experiment was recently undertaken to determine the effects of tip shape on the area of hyperalgesia. Tip shape was defined as the radius of curvature of a hemispherically tipped cylinder that was attached to a nylon filament which, in turn, was calibrated, by length, to deliver a desired bending force. It was found that blunt tips with radii of 2 mm or more evoked little or no hyperalgesia (as is the case if the experimenter presses the hyperalgesic area with a finger or the flat eraser on a pencil). In contrast, very small radii of curvature of 50 μm resulted in the same area of hyperalgesia as that obtained with the standard filament. An example of a map obtained 30-40 min after injection using hemispherically tipped filaments of 200 and 800 μm diameter (force of 294 mN) is shown in Figure 1B. The area of hyperalgesia was significantly larger when mapped with the smaller tip diameter. Note also the still smaller area obtained in response to gentle movement of hairs. The sharp punctate stimuli activate nociceptors whereas moving hairs or gently stroking the skin with a cotton swab would be expected to activate low-threshold mechanoreceptors and few, if any, nociceptors. However, if textured surfaces other than the cotton swab were used in which the elements making up the texture were of sufficiently great height and small diameter one might expect a significant engagement of activity in nociceptors as well as low threshold mechanoreceptors.

In a pilot experiment designed to explore this possibility, textured surfaces were constructed consisting of a hexagonal pattern of hemispherically shaped raised elements each of the same diameter (250 μm) and height (165 μm). The center-to-center spacing between elements (within rows) was 0.5, 1.0, 1.5 and 2.0 mm. Each pattern was on 2 cm diameter plate that had tapered and was attached to the end of a long, flexible strip of metal. When the strip was held between the experimenter's fingers at a specified location and the plate pressed against the skin to produce a minimal amount bending in the strip, a force of approximately 300 mN was delivered as the texture was stroked across the skin. The textures were readily discriminated on the basis of perceived roughness which was ranked in order of increasing inter-element spacing from least (0.5 mm) to greatest (2.0 mm). Designated regions of skin within the anticipated area of 2º hyperalgesia were stroked with each texture a distance of 2-3 cm at about 1 cm/sec before and after the injection of capsaicin. A subject's magnitude estimates of pain produced by one stroke from each texture revealed that none of the textures were perceived as painful prior to the capsaicin but that after the injection, all evoked pain (Figure 2). The magnitude of pain increased with inter-element spacing. (A smooth, untextured plate was also used in the experiment and given a spacing of zero). Since the skin conforms better around each element as the spacing is increased, the amount of indentation and compressional and lateral forces exerted by the element would be expected to increase with spacing. This would be analogous to increasing the force applied by one of the hemispherically tipped Von Frey filaments.

The textured plates evoked different areas of hyperalgesia (Figure 1C). These areas were obtained approximately 45 min after the injection when the area of hyperalgesia to stroking with the cotton swab had shrunken from its maximal value. Progressively larger areas were obtained with textured plates with inter-element spacings of 0.5, 1.0 and 2.0 mm. A still larger area was obtained with a texture made up of raised truncated cones (diam of 250 μm diam. at the top, height of 400 μm and center-to-center spacing of 1.0 mm). The edge of the flat top of each conically shaped element was sharp, *i.e.* had a small radius of curvature, hence evoking more pain and a larger area of hyperalgesia. Although these anecdotal observations must be confirmed in a larger study, it seems reasonable to hypothesize that a greater ratio of activated nociceptors to activated low-threshold nociceptors will be engaged with probe tips or textural elements of progressively smaller radii of curvature. In any case, the preliminary results with textural elements and probes of different sizes or shapes underscore the importance of controlling the microgeometrical properties of an object contacting the skin in determining the magnitude and area of enhanced pain in hyperalgesic skin.

In the following, each experiment used the cotton swab and the standard Von Frey filament which we believe engaged respectively low and high ratios of activated nociceptors to activated low-threshold mechanoreceptors. The results of these

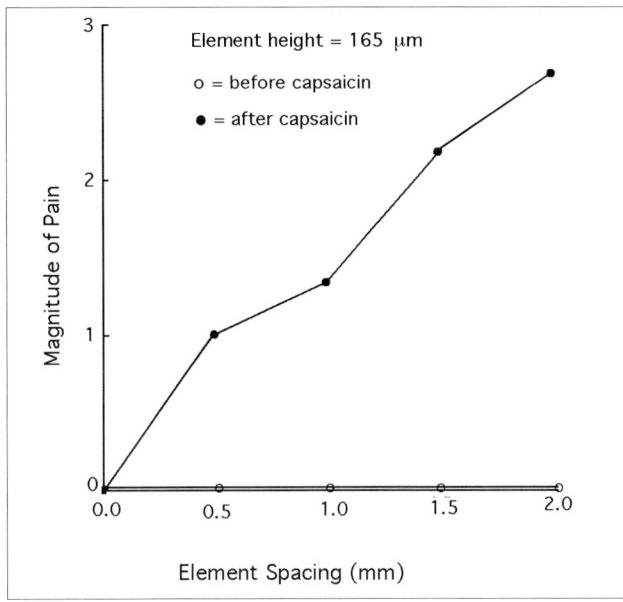

Figure 2. A subject's estimates of the magnitude of pain produced by stroking the skin with textured surfaces of differing roughness. Each texture consisted of a hexagonal pattern of hemispherically shaped elements each with a base diameter of 250 μm and a height of approximately 165 μm. The center-to center spacing between elements within rows was different for each texture (a smooth, untextured surface was assigned a spacing of zero). The same region of skin was stroked before (open circles) and after (closed circles) the development of 2° hyperalgesia produced by an injection of capsaicin.

experiments demonstrated important differences in the functional properties of the hyperalgesia elicited by each stimulus : the hyperalgesia to punctate stimulation had a larger area, lasted longer and was less dependent for its maintenance on primary afferent activity.

The maximal area of hyperalgesia was, on the average, 1.4 times greater for punctate that for stroking stimuli (Figure 1). Within the first 15 min after injection, the mean maximal areas of hyperalgesia, obtained from 20 subjects, were 54.9 and 37.6 cm^2 for the von Frey filament and the cotton swab, respectively [7].

The duration of hyperalgesia was greater for the punctate stimulus, lasting a median of 21 hours as opposed to a median of 2 hours for stroking [7].

Once fully developed, the areas of hyperalgesia to stroking and to the punctate stimulus differed as to the degree to which they were dependent on peripheral neuronal activity. This was demonstrated by cooling a 1-cm^2 area of skin centered on the injection site to 1°C for 2-5 min with a Peltier thermode [7]. The cooling, begun 15 min after the injection of capsaicin, rendered the skin under the thermode analgesic to pinpricks. The areas of hyperalgesia to stroking and to punctate stimulation were determined in 10 subjects before and during cooling and once more after the skin was rewarmed. During cooling, the area of stroking hyperalgesia decreased to a median of 26.7% of the original size (Figure 3). Rewarming for 2-5 min returned the area to approximately its original size. In contrast, cooling reduced the area of punctate hyperalgesia in only 4 of the 10 subjects and then only to a median of 74% the original size. In three of the subjects, magnitude estimates of pain produced by the standard filament were obtained and found to decrease during cooling to 66-80% of those obtained prior to cooling. This result suggested that punctate hyperalgesia was

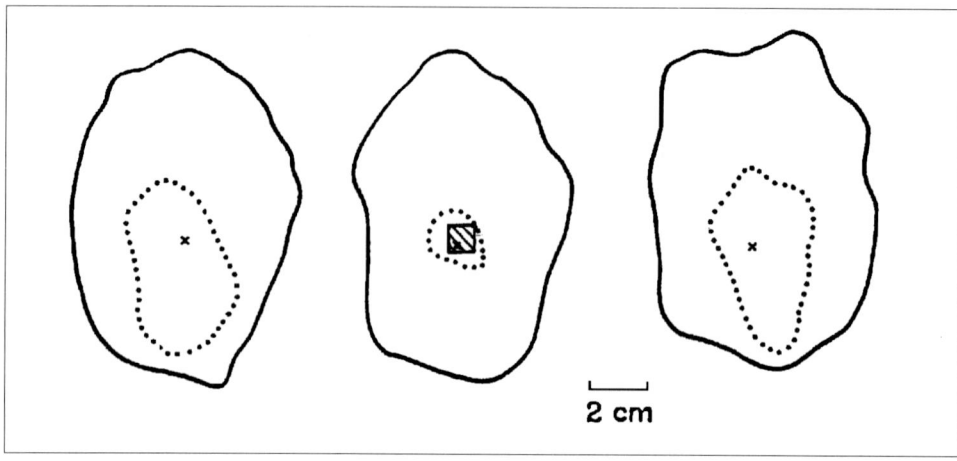

Figure 3. Demonstration that once 2° hyperalgesia has developed it is only partially dependent on input from peripheral sensory receptors. The skin was anesthetized by cooling it to 1°C by means of a contact thermode (hatched square in middle). During cooling, the area of hyperalgesia to stroking the skin with a cotton swab (...) was significantly reduced but not eliminated. In contrast, the area of hyperalgesia to punctate stimulation with a Von Frey filament was not changed even though the magnitude of pain elicited by each poke with the filament was reduced by approximately 30%. (From [7].)

dependent to some extent on primary afferent activity but to a much lesser degree than stroking hyperalgesia. A working hypothesis is that hyperalgesia to nociceptive stimuli (*e.g.* sharp, punctate stimuli) once developed is much less dependent on continued afferent activity than hyperalgesia to innocuous stimuli (*e.g.* cotton swab).

Although there is still controversy over which type or types of chemosensitive nociceptive afferent fibers are responsible for initiating the development of 2° hyperalgesia [6], all the available evidence points to the conclusion that the sensitized neurons are located in the central and not the peripheral nervous system. A survey of all the known types of primary afferent fibers in the monkey [1] and mechanoheat sensitive nociceptive C-fibers in the human [6] demonstrated the lack of any definitive sensitization (enhanced responsiveness or lowered response thresholds to mechanical stimulation of the skin) after an injection of capsaicin inside, adjacent to or outside the receptive field. If the injection of capsaicin was within or sufficiently close to the receptive field, the most common outcome was "desensitization" - that is, an elevation of response threshold or a decrease in responsiveness to cutaneous stimulation. This may be the reason why human subjects reported an analgesia to pinprick in the bleb produced by the capsaicin injection.

The most compelling sensory evidence for "central sensitization" was provided by experiments in which a peripheral nerve was infiltrated with a local anesthetic and capsaicin then injected into the anesthetic skin distal to the block [7]. The duration of the anesthesia in relation to the time of the capsaicin injection was varied. When recovery from the anesthetic occurred two or three hours after the injection, no

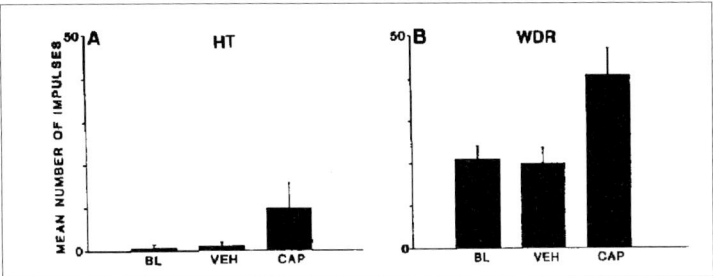

Figure 4. The sensitization of two classes of spinothalamic tract (STT) cells to gently stroking the skin after an injection of capsaicin into their cutaneous receptive fields. A : The mean number of impulses ± SE evoked in 7 high threshold (HT) STT cells by a single stroke with a cotton swab before (BL) and after injections of vehicle (VEH) and capsaicin (CAP). B : Mean number of impulses evoked in 12 wide dynamic range (WDR) STT cells (same format as in panel A). (From [12].)

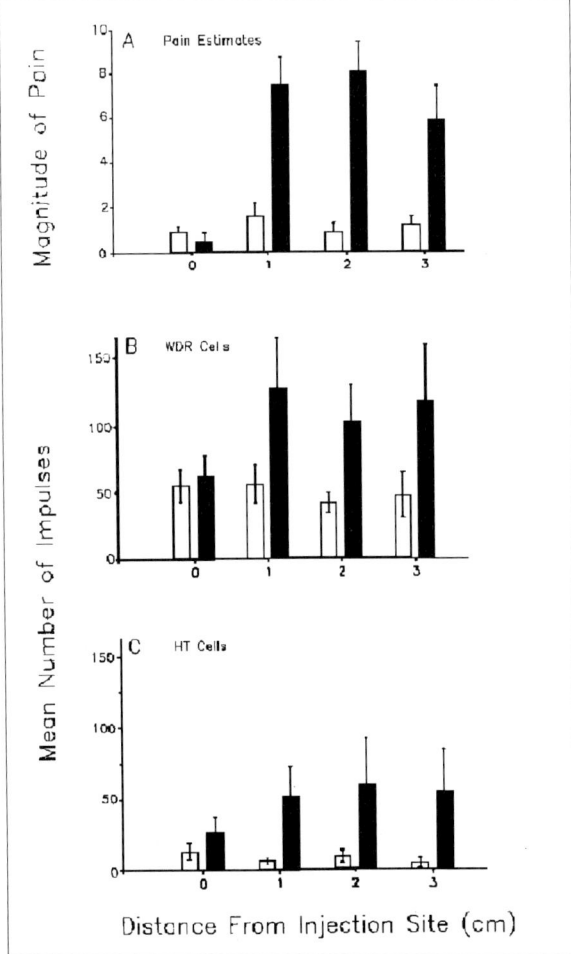

Figure 5. The correspondence between the development of 2° hyperalgesia to punctate stimulation of the skin in humans after an injection of capsaicin and the sensitization of spinothalamic tract cells in monkeys after an injection of capsaicin. A : Mean normalized magnitude estimates of pain to the standard Von Frey filament applied on or 1, 2 and 3 cm away from the injection site before (open bars) and after (solid bars) an injection of capsaicin on the forearm. B : Mean number of impulses evoked in 8 WDR neurons by the standard filament applied on or 1, 2 and 3 cm away from the injection site before (open bars) and after (solid bars) capsaicin injection. C : Mean number of impulses evoked in 7 HT cells (same format as in B). (From [12].)

hyperalgesia was present nor did it develop later. If the anesthetic lasted only 0.5 - 1.5 hours, the hyperalgesia was considerably reduced in area in comparison to that produced by a control injection of capsaicin, without a prior nerve block, on the other arm. Thus, the nerve block prevented capsaicin-activated nerve impulses from reaching the central nervous system (CNS) and sensitizing neurons that are responsive to mechanical stimulation of the skin.

Another set of experiments demonstrated that the hyperalgesia to stroking the skin resulted from a change in the processing of tactile information in the CNS [14]. An electrode inserted into a peripheral nerve delivered electrical pulses that evoked sensations of touch without pain in human subjects. The tactile sensation was referred to a small area on the skin. When capsaicin was injected 7 to 20 mm outside this area and the area became hyperalgesic to stroking the skin, the same intraneural electrical stimulus then evoked a sensation of pain, in addition to touch. This pain sensation, which had the same quality of "soreness" as that elicited by stroking the skin, disappeared as soon as the area to which it was referred was no longer hyperalgesic. At that moment, the electrical stimulus then elicited touch without pain. One hypothesis, based on the results of this experiment, is that nociceptive neurons in the CNS became sensitized to activity in low-threshold mechanoreceptive afferent fibers after the injection of capsaicin. That is, spinal neurons that received a convergent input from both low-threshold mechanoreceptive and nociceptive primary afferent fibers and which normally responded little or not at all to activity evoked by innocuous tactile stimulation of the skin were sensitized by activity in capsaicin activated chemonociceptive afferent fibers. The sensitized spinal neurons then responded vigorously to input from low-threshold, mechanoreceptive afferent fibers.

Support for this hypothesis came from experiments in which the responses of identified spinothalamic tract (STT) neurons were recorded before and after an injection of capsaicin into their cutaneous receptive fields [12]. Two types of STT cells were studied in the anesthetized monkey : high threshold (HT) cells that responded best to pinching with little or no response to innocuous stimulation of the skin, and wide-dynamic range (WDR) cells that responded in a graded manner to cutaneous stimuli of increasing intensity. The same stimuli used in the psychophysical experiments in humans, namely the cotton swab and the standard nylon filament, were applied to selected sites proximal and distal to the injection site before and about 5 min after capsaicin was injected into the center of the receptive field. Injection of the vehicle for capsaicin had little or no significant effect on the responses of either type of STT neuron to stroking or punctate stimuli. However, after capsaicin, the responses to stroking were increased approximately nine fold in HT cells and two fold in WDR cells (Figure 4). Similarly, capsaicin resulted in nine and 2.5 fold increases respectively in HT and WDR responses to the punctate stimulus delivered to test sites located 1-3 cm away from the injection site (Figure 5B and C). The sensitization to punctate stimulation correlates remarkably well with the six-fold enhanced magnitude estimates of punctate pain reported by the human observers (Figure 5A). There was no increase in response at the injection site which humans had reported was hypo - and not hyperalgesic - at least to pinprick. In addition, many STT cells exhibited an afterdischarge to punctate stimulation that may contribute to the finding that punctate stimulation of hyperalgesic skin in humans lasted longer than it did for stimulations of normal skin.

The enhanced responses of both types of STT cells to innocuous stroking and to normally painful punctate stimulation provide a basis for the $2°$ hyperalgesia to these stimuli after an injection of capsaicin. The underlying mechanism of central sensitization is under study in a number of laboratories. An equally important question is the identity and nature of the chemosensitive primary afferent fibers that are responsible for bringing about the sensitization. They are unlikely to be the garden variety polymodal nociceptors since these respond weakly to capsaicin in relation to other stimuli, such as equally painful heat stimuli that produce far less $2°$ hyperalgesia [7]. They are likely to branch widely in the skin (or, alternatively, have smaller receptive fields that are functionally coupled) because $2°$ hyperalgesia does not cross a narrow mediolateral strip of local anesthetic [7]. Similarly, an injection of capsaicin within the anesthetized skin after a proximal nerve block sometimes results in a transient region of hyperalgesia outside the anesthetized region several centimeters away [7]. There is preliminary evidence for the existence of chemonociceptors that are selective for noxious chemical stimuli such as capsaicin a few of which have widely separated receptive fields [2, 4, 10]. These fibers, if they prove to be the hypothesized fibers in question, may play an important role in the development and maintenance of chronic pain and cutaneous hyperalgesia particularly in patients with peripheral nerve injuries that result in abnormal increases in the sensitivities of nociceptors to endogenous chemical stimuli [11, 15].

Acknowledgments

Our research was supported by PMs grant NS 14624. We thank Mr AK Petersen for his assistance in constructing the textures and filaments.

References

1. Baumann TK, Simone DA, Shain CN, LaMotte RH. Neurogenic hyperalgesia : the search for the primary cutaneous afferent fibers that contribute to capsaicin-induced pain and hyperalgesia. *J Neurophysiol* 1991 ; 66 : 212-27.
2. Handwerker HO, Schmidt R, Forster C, Schmelz M, Traversa R, Torebjork HE. Microneurographic assessment of sensitive and insensitive C-fibers in a human skin nerve. *Soc Neurosci Abstr* 1993 ; 19 : 1404.
3. Hardy JD, Wolff HG, Goodell H. Experimental evidence on the nature of cutaneous hyperalgesia. *J Clin Invest* 1950 ; 29 : 115-40.
4. Kress M, Koltzenburg M, Reeh PW, Handwerker HO. Responsiveness and functional attributes of electrically localized terminals of cutaneous C-fibers *in vivo* and *in vitro*. *J Neurophysiol* 1992 ; 58 : 581-95.

5. LaMotte RH. Subpopulations of "nocifensor neurons" contributing to pain and allodynia, itch and alloknesis. *APS J* 1992 ; 1(2) : 115-26.
6. LaMotte RH, Lundberg LER, Torebjork HE. Pain, hyperalgesia and activity in nociceptive C units in humans after intradermal injection of capsaicin. *J Physiol* 1992 ; 448 : 749-64.
7. LaMotte RH, Shain CN, Simone DA, Tsai E. Neurogenic hyperalgesia : psychophysical studies of underlying mechanisms. *J Neurophysiol* 1991 ; 66 : 190-211.
8. LaMotte RH. 1993.
9. Lewis T. Experiments relating to cutaneous hyperalgesia and its spread through somatic nerves. *Clin Sci* 1936 ; 2 : 373-421.
10. Meyer RA, Davis KD, Cohen RH, Treede RD, Campbell JN. Mechanically insensitive afferents (MIAs) in cutaneous nerves of monkey. *Brain Res* 1991 ; 561 : 252-61.
11. Sato J, Perl ER. Adrenergic excitation of cutaneous pain receptors induced by peripheral nerve injury. *Science* 1991 ; 251 : 1608-10.
12. Simone DA, Oh U, Sorkin LS, Owens C, Chung JM, LaMotte RH, WillisWD. Neurogenic hyperalgesia : central neural correlates in responses of spinothalamic tract neurons. *J Neurophysiol* 1991 ; 66 : 228-46.
13. Stevens S. *Psychophysics introduction to its perceptual, neural, and social prospects.* New York : Wiley, 1975.
14. Torebjork HE, Lundberg LER, LaMotte RH. Central changes in processing of mechanoreceptive input in capsaicin-induced secondary hyperalgesia in humans. *J Physiol* 1992 ; 448 : 763-80.
15. Wall PD, Gutnick M. Ongoing activity in peripheral nerves : the physiology and pharmacology of impulses originating from a neuroma. *Exp Neurol* 1974 ; 45 : 580-93.

3

On visceral nociceptors

G.F. GEBHART, J.N. SENGUPTA

Department of Pharmacology, The University of Iowa, College of Medicine, Iowa City, IA 52242, USA.

The term "nociceptor" was introduced by Sherrington [53] to describe sensory receptors sensitive to stimuli which threatened or caused tissue damage. Nociceptors were first documented in skin and have been widely studied (*see* [55] for general overview). Nociceptors in skin are exteroceptive receptors which inform the organism about the location, intensity and duration of their adequate mechanical, thermal and/or chemical stimuli. They are thus important for protection against potential or actual hazards in the external environment and essential to normal life. Mechanically and chemically sensitive nociceptors from joints and muscle have also been documented (*see* [36, 47] for recent reviews) and one might reasonably expect that identical or analogous receptors sensitive to threatening or damaging stimuli applied to visceral tissue also exist. However, that the viscera are innervated by nociceptors has not been clearly established.

Visceral pain

Background

Early investigators concluded that injury to visceral organs did not produce pain [31, 54]. Lennander [31] examined the sensitivity of the human colon and reported it to be insensitive to mechanical stimuli of any intensity, including presumably noxious stimuli (*e.g.* cutting). These observations supported his belief that visceral organs were devoid of sensory innervation. He suggested that visceral pain arose from the parietal peritoneum, through adhesions, by stretch of the parietal wall or by traction on the mesentery. Similarly, Mackenzie [33] considered the viscera to be insensate. He studied abdominal wall muscle rigidity and contractions in visceral disease states, suggesting that painful muscle rigidity was a "viscero-motor" reflex initiated from a viscus. Mackenzie postulated that visceral pain resulted from non-painful visceral input which produced an "irritable focus" in the spinal gray matter. The irritable focus activated somatic sensory and other spinal neurons, leading to (1) referral of the visceral sensation to cutaneous sites (a widely appreciated characteristic of visceral pain) and (2) viscero-motor and viscero-sensory reflexes and the development of deep and superficial tenderness (hyperalgesia), respectively. Mackenzie's well-known model of "convergence-facilitation" of visceral sensation is illustrated in Figure 1.

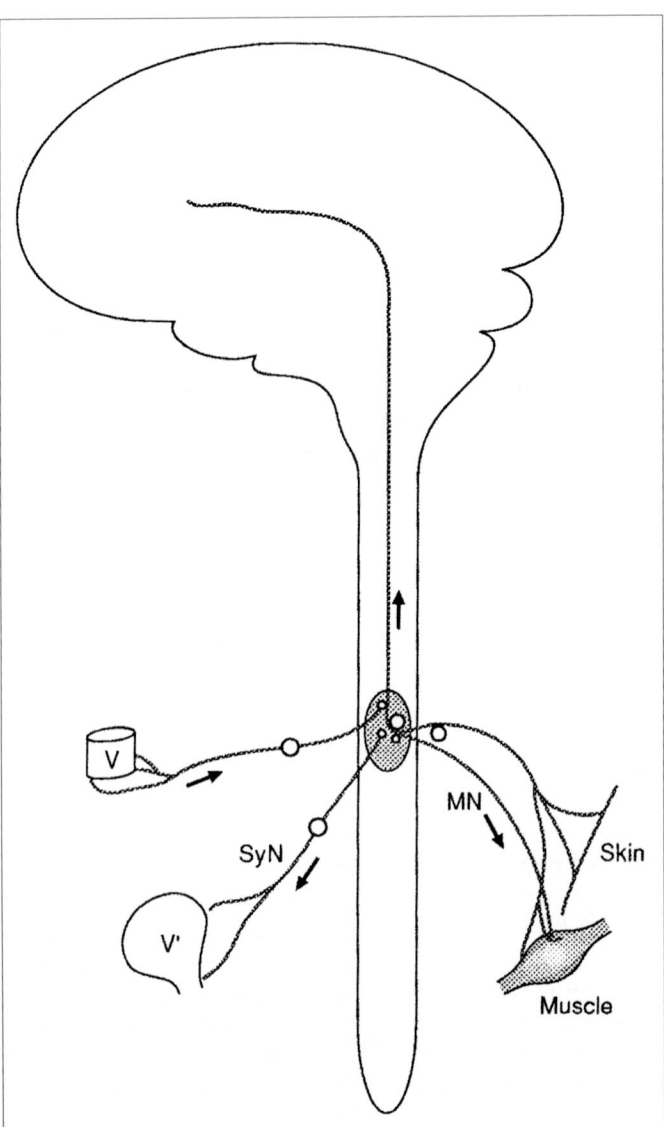

Figure 1. Mackenzie's representation of visceral pain mechanisms and its referral to cutaneous sites. Non-painful input from a viscus (V) initiates an irritable focus in the spinal grey matter, leading to activation of motor nerves (MN) that produce muscle rigidity and contractions and activation of sympathetic nerves (SyN) that produce viscero-visceral reflexes. The irritable focus (shaded area) also leads to the development of cutaneous hyperalgesia and persistent muscle activation. (Modified from [33].)

Other investigators subsequently and successfully demonstrated that sensations did arise directly from the viscera [24, 25, 46]. The principal sensation studied was pain, and early studies focused on the afferent pathways that conveyed the information to the central nervous system [2, 32, 39, 44]. It also became clear that the condition of the viscus contributed significantly to conscious sensation. Studies in humans of the appendix and the stomach in normal and inflamed conditions established that mechanical probing was generally not sensed unless the viscus was inflamed, and then the dominant sensation was pain [30, 56]. In light of the recent discovery of "silent nociceptors" (*see* below), the altered visceral sensations associated with inflammation suggest the presence of at least one type of nociceptor innervating the viscera.

Mechanisms of visceral pain

The theories that have been advanced to account for visceral pain follow predictably from those advanced earlier to explain somatic pain (*e.g.* specificity, intensity and pattern theories). The weight of experimental evidence accumulated over the past 25-30 years best supports the theory of specificity to account for somatic pain. Because visceral nociceptors have yet to be unequivocally documented, however, models and mechanisms of visceral pain continue to be advanced and argued. One theory of visceral pain proposes that pain results from the spatial and temporal summation of information and the frequency of discharge generated in non-specific sensory afferent fibers innervating the viscera (*e.g. see* [29], for arguments and discussion). This theory posits that the reflexes, regulations and sensations associated with a viscus are produced by activation of a functionally homogeneous (*i.e.* non-specific) population of visceral sensory fibers. An opposing theory argues that specific nociceptors innervate the viscera and mediate visceral pain. These nociceptors comprise a group of afferent fibers with thresholds for response to mechanical stimulation at or above intensities considered to be noxious.

The former view dominated thinking until it was documented experimentally that populations of low- and high-threshold visceral afferent fibers could be clearly distinguished among fibers innervating organs such as the esophagus, gall bladder, urinary bladder and colon. Consequently, Cervero and Jänig [6] recently suggested that :
  - different proportions of low- and high-threshold afferent fibers in different viscera mediate acute visceral sensation, including brief pain,
  - activation of "silent nociceptors" by prolonged visceral stimulation such as leads to inflammation sensitizes high threshold afferent fibers which, together with low threshold and silent afferent fibers, contribute to persistent visceral pain.

As reviewed below, high threshold visceral afferent fibers appear to constitute approximately 30% of the population of visceral sensory fibers that respond to mechanical stimulation (with the notable exception of the ureter) and mechanically-insensitive afferent fibers (so-called silent nociceptors) may comprise an even greater proportion of the spinal visceral afferent fiber population.

High threshold visceral afferent fibers

A number of studies have documented the presence of clearly different populations of low- and high-threshold mechanosensitive afferent fibers innervating the viscera. Cervero [4] first documented the presence of fibers with high thresholds for response in a study of splanchnic nerve afferent fibers innervating the gall bladder and biliary duct of the ferret. The larger group of fibers (65%) responded to innocuous intensities (2-5 mmHg) of gall bladder distension; a smaller proportion (32%) of the sample of 31 fibers had high thresholds and responded only to distending pressures >20 mmHg, a pressure which also produced pseudaffective responses in the anesthetized ferret. Because pain is the only conscious sensation that arises from the gall bladder, Cervero suggested that these high threshold fibers subserved nociception and were important to sharp, localized pain. In the esophagus of the American opossum, Sengupta et al. [52] also documented the presence of high threshold mechanosensitive afferent fibers in the thoracic sympathetic chain and splanchnic nerve. Most fibers responded at low pressures of esophageal distension (63%), but 37% of the 91 fibers studied responded first at a mean distending pressure of 33 mmHg. This latter group of fibers have been suggested to represent specific nociceptors in the esophagus [6].

In a study of afferent fibers in the lumbar colonic nerve of the cat, Blumberg et al. [3] reported that 32% of 75 fibers studied first responded to colonic distension at intensities ≥ 25 mmHg (7 fibers had apparent thresholds >50 mmHg). These results were not interpreted by the authors to represent a separate population of high threshold fibers, but rather were considered to be the tail at the high end of a normal distribution of afferent fibers with a mean threshold for response in the physiological range [27]. In a subsequent examination of mechanosensitive properties of pelvic nerve afferent fibers in the S_2 dorsal root of the cat supplying the colon, all units that responded to distension of the colon were reported to have thresholds for response in the innocuous range (mean ≈ 21 mmHg; [30]). In a recent study in the rat [49], however, we found that 22% of 44 pelvic nerve afferent fibers in the S_1 dorsal root that responded to colorectal distension had high thresholds for response ranging between 28-38 mmHg (mean 33 mmHg). Two of these high threshold fibers were Aδ-fibers and eight were C-fibers. The same colorectal stimulus in awake rats at comparable intensities of distension produces cardiovascular and motor pseudaffective reflexes and acquisition of an avoidance behavior, confirming the behavioral relevance of the stimulus [40, 43]. The remaining proportion of the sample of pelvic nerve afferent fibers all responded at colorectal distending pressures ≤10 mmHg (mean: 2.9 mmHg ; Figure 2).

High threshold afferent fibers innervating the urinary bladder and the uterus/cervix have also been documented. Häbler et al. [21] recorded 7 unmyelinated afferent fibers in the S_2 dorsal root of the cat that responded to 30-50 mmHg distension of the urinary bladder, an intensity they presumed to be noxious. The proportion of high threshold afferent fibers in this sample of 297 C-fibers (2.4%) is likely an underestimation because fibers were identified by electrical stimulation of the pelvic nerve, which innervates (primarily) the urinary bladder and colon, and colonic distension was not

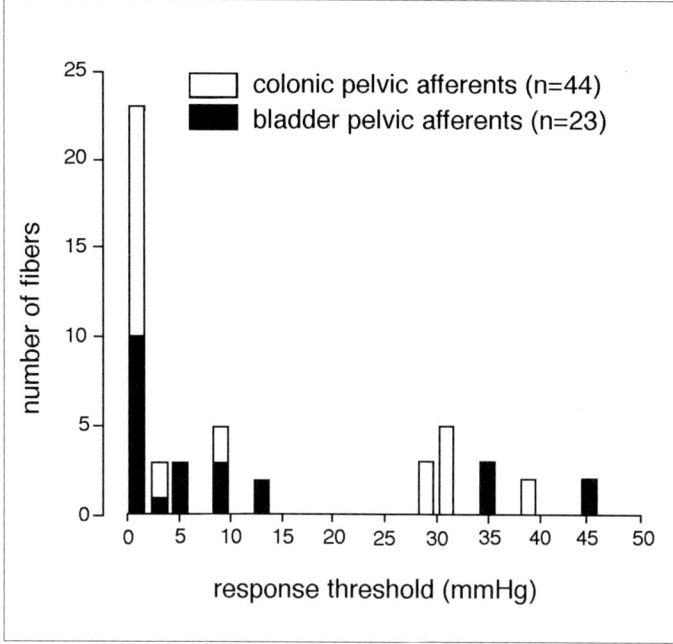

Figure 2. Frequency histogram of thresholds for response to urinary bladder distension (bladder pelvic afferents, $n=23$) or colorectal distension (colonic pelvic afferents, $n=44$) of pelvic nerve afferent fibers in the rat. (Data adapted from [18] and [50].)

tested. In a recent study of 329 unmyelinated and thinly myelinated pelvic nerve afferent fibers in the rat, distension of both the urinary bladder and colon were tested; 44% of the sample responded to distension of the bladder, 16% responded to colorectal distension and 6% responded to mechanical stimulation of the anal mucosa [49]. Five of 23 afferent fibers studied to date with graded bladder distension had response thresholds ≥35 mmHg (Sengupta and Gebhart, unpublished). An example is given in Figure 3 (see also Figure 2 for distribution of response thresholds).

Berkley et al. [1] and Hong et al. [26] reported the presence of high threshold afferent fibers in the hypogastric nerve of the rat and cat, respectively. Berkley and coworkers did not quantitatively determine thresholds for response, but noted that about 75% of the hypogastric nerve fibers studied only responded to intensities of mechanical stimulation that produced transient ischemia at the tip of the probe, concluding that the effective stimulus was not mechanical per se. Three units responded to von Frey filament pressures >5 gm. Because the search stimulus in their study was gentle probing of the wall of the uterus and surrounding ligaments with a blunt glass rod, it is unlikely that the full range of mechanically sensitive afferent fibers were sampled. In a study of hypogastric nerve afferent fibers in the cat, Hong et al. ([26] reported that 16/52 fibers (31%) had von Frey thresholds for response >30 mN, 9 of which had response thresholds ranging from 140 to >176 mN. Interestingly, in neither of these two studies was uterine distension found to be an effective stimulus.

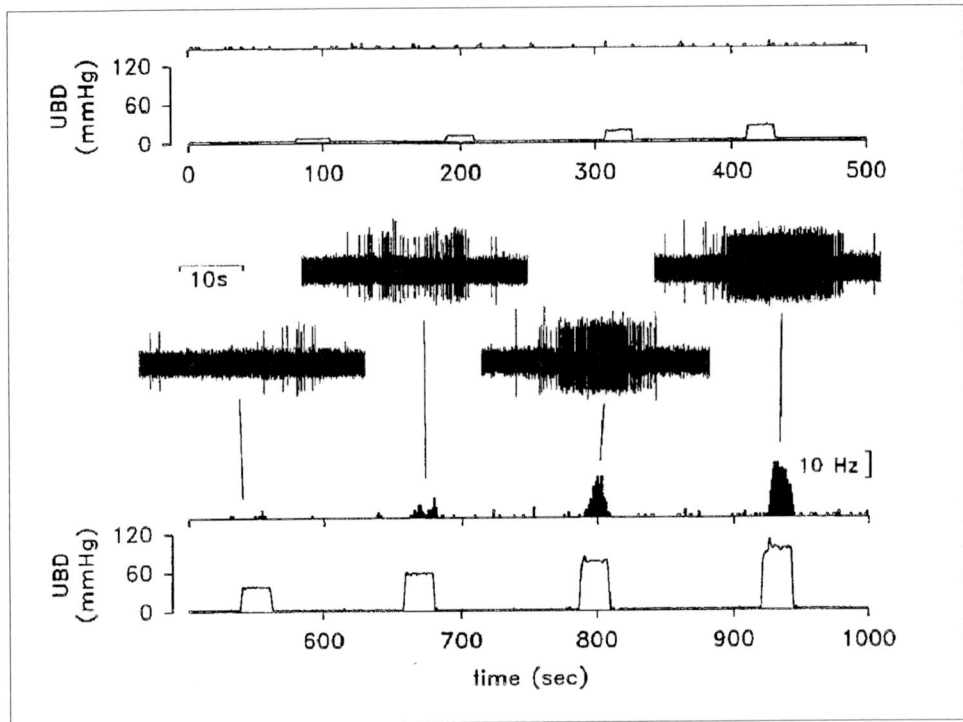

Figure 3. Example of a high threshold pelvic nerve afferent fiber innervating the urinary bladder in the rat. Responses are illustrated as peristimulus time histograms (1 sec bin width) to graded urinary bladder distension (UBD; 5-100 mmHg); the record is continuous left to right, top to bottom. Inset between the continuous histogram records are corresponding unit recordings, each 35 sec long. (From Sengupta and Gebhart (unpublished).)

In an *in vitro* study, Cervero and Sann [7] found that 76% of 46 afferent fibers recorded in the ureteric nerve innervating the ureter of the guinea pig had thresholds for response ≥25 mmHg; 24% of the sample had low thresholds for response (≤8 mmHg) and also responded during contraction of the ureter. This is the only study known to us in which the proportion of high threshold afferent fibers found exceeded the proportion of low threshold fibers. Thus, the ureter appears to be unique among the viscera studied to date. Typically, when high threshold fibers are identified in a sample, they constitute on average about 30% of the mechanically sensitive fibers studied.

There is also evidence for the existence of high threshold gastric afferent fibers in the vagus nerve. Davison and Clarke [12] reported that afferent fibers in the vagus nerve of the rat had a wide range of thresholds for response to gastric distension; 16 fibers had response thresholds considered to be low (≤8 mmHg) and 5 fibers were considered to be high threshold fibers, responding at pressures >10-16 mmHg. We have also recorded from vagal afferent fibers in the rat which have high thresholds for response to gastric distension; an example is given in Figure 4. In preliminary behavioral studies, gastric distension at intensities of 60 mmHg in awake rats leads to acquisition of an avoidance behavior (Sengupta and Gebhart, unpublished).

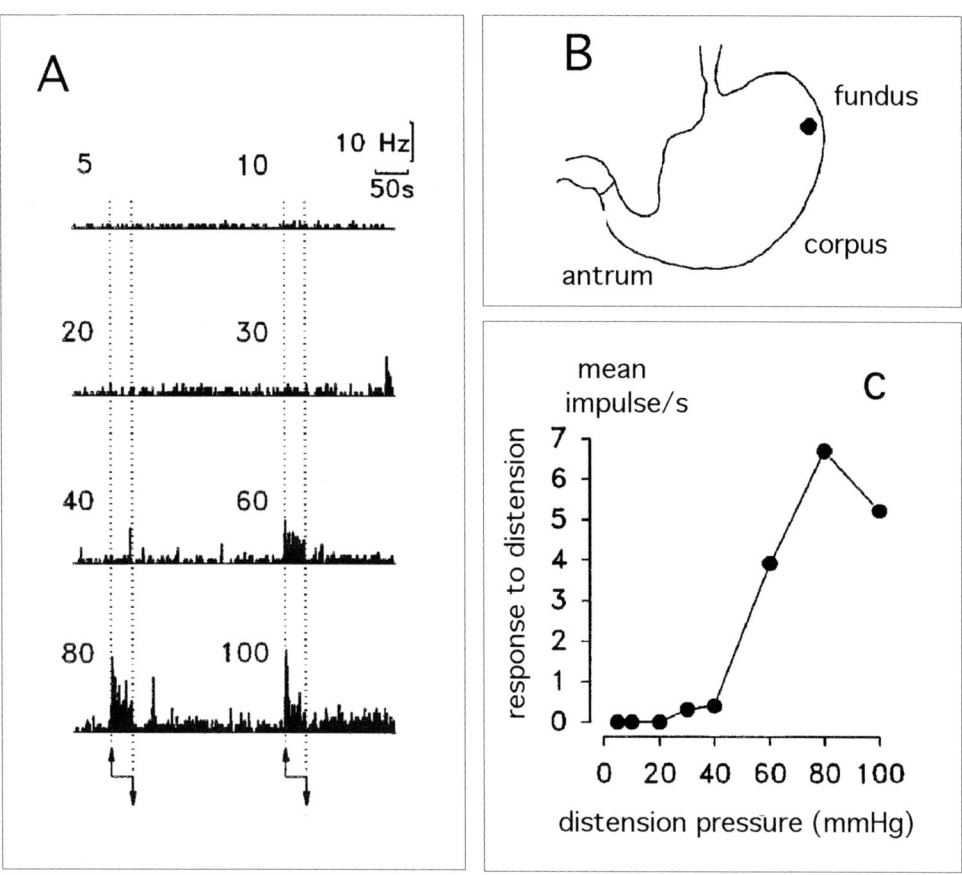

Figure 4. Example of a high threshold vagal afferent fiber innervating the stomach in the rat. A : Responses are illustrated as peristimulus time histograms (1 sec bin width) to graded intensities (5-100 mmHg) of gastric distension; the record is continuous left to right, top to bottom. The data in A are presented in C as a stimulus-response function; the receptive field is illustrated in B. (From Sengupta, Hummel and Gebhart, unpublished.)

These and other studies provide convincing evidence that there exists separate populations of low- and high-threshold afferent fibers that innervate many viscera. The low threshold afferent fibers are assumed to mediate sympatho-sympathetic or sympatho-vagal regulatory reflexes which, under normal physiological conditions, are generally not sensed. Low threshold afferent fibers also likely play a role in non-painful sensations that arise from the urinary bladder and gastrointestinal tract (*e.g.* fullness, gas, nausea, etc.). High threshold afferent fibers are believed to mediate nociception, for example, in organs such as the gall bladder and ureter from which the only conscious sensation is pain. In addition, stimulation at or above intensities required to activate high threshold afferent fibers typically produces pseudaffective reflexes. It should be appreciated, however, that pseudaffective reflexes are produced at intensities of colonic distension which humans do not report as painful [42]. Thus, it cannot be assumed on the basis of production of a pressor response, for example, that the stimulus is noxious. It also cannot be assumed that intensities of hollow organ distension reported to be noxious in humans apply to non-human animals in the absence of behavioral studies in non-human animals. Unfortunately, information about the quality of most visceral stimuli used in non-human animal studies is limited (or cannot be obtained for some viscera). Studies in behaving animals, however, are required to complement reflex and electrophysiological studies and to allow direct correlation between response measures and behavior in the same specie (*see* [19], for discussion). Accordingly, that high threshold afferent fibers in the viscera are nociceptors remains to be proved.

While a high threshold for response may be necessary, it is not sufficient to characterize a visceral sensory fiber as nociceptive. The encoding properties of afferent fibers are important and may be more relevant than response threshold to understanding function. Quantitative examination of responses to graded distension of the colon, however, suggests that the encoding properties of pelvic nerve afferent fibers innervating the colon of the rat are not different for afferent fibers characterized as low threshold and high threshold [49]. The slopes of the stimulus-response functions were virtually identical and the response magnitudes of low threshold afferent fibers to all intensities of colorectal distension studied (to 100 mmHg) were greater than response magnitudes of high threshold fibers. Similarly, examination of stimulus-response functions of three classes of afferent fibers innervating the esophagus of the opossum reveals that low- and high-threshold spinal afferent fibers have identical slopes and response magnitudes to esophageal distension in the noxious range; all vagal afferent fibers studied had low thresholds for response and saturated at esophageal distending pressures ≥50 mmHg [51]. If high threshold visceral afferent fibers are not necessarily nociceptive-specific (*e.g.* they may be intensity receptors), it may be that so-called "silent nociceptors" are the afferent fibers that principally mediate visceral pain.

Mechanically intensitive afferent fibers

First characterized among the afferent fiber population innervating the knee joint of the cat [48], and named sleeping or silent nociceptors, mechanically insensitive afferent fibers have subsequently been found in cutaneous and visceral nerves [35]. Typically, a proportion of these mechanically insensitive afferent fibers develop activity ("respond") to applied inflammatory mediators or sensitizing soups (joint and cutaneous afferent fibers [23, 37, 48]) or to mucosal irritation with mustard oil, turpentine, etc. (urinary bladder and colon [21]), after which some also exhibit mechanical sensitivity.

Jänig's laboratory first documented the chemical sensitivity of mechanically insensitive afferent fibers in the pelvic nerve innervating the urinary bladder of the cat. In their first report [21], 11 of 95 (11%) unmyelinated, mechanically insensitive afferent fibers in the S_2 dorsal and ventral roots responded to instillation of mustard oil (1-2.5%) into the urinary bladder of the cat. These afferent fibers (7 in the dorsal root and 4 in the ventral root) had no spontaneous activity before treatment and did not respond to urinary bladder distension (75 mmHg), but were activated at a latency of less than 2 min after intravesical administration of mustard oil. Some ($n=3$) fibers that were tested after removal of mustard oil or turpentine from the urinary bladder were activated by increases in intravesical pressure, but did not encode the distending pressure. These afferent fibers were considered by the authors to be good candidates for "chemosensitive visceral nociceptors." On the basis of these results and consideration of the function of sensory innervation of the colon and urinary bladder, Jänig and Koltzenburg [27] suggested that the function of more than 90% of the unmyelinated afferent fibers in the pelvic nerves was obscure because they could not be activated by "extreme noxious pressure stimuli" (75 mmHg).

In a recent study of mechanosensitive myelinated afferent fibers in the S_2 dorsal and ventral roots of the cat, Häbler *et al.* [22] reported that 16 of 23 (69%) fibers were activated at short latency after instillation of mustard oil (1-2.5%) or turpentine (50%) into the urinary bladder. Twenty-one of the 23 fibers had response thresholds to urinary bladder distension <25 mmHg before application of the irritants and two fibers had thresholds for response >30 mmHg. None of the fibers displayed resting activity before irritation, but all subsequently developed ongoing activity after bladder irritation. Interestingly, turpentine, but not mustard oil, induced a sensitization to mechanical stimulation of the bladder. The slope of the stimulus-response function to graded increases in intravesical pressures was significantly greater when tested 50-60 min after intravesical administration of turpentine; there was no evidence of a change in response threshold. Because turpentine is believed to act by non-neurogenic mechanisms (and mustard oil has a direct excitatory effect ; *see* discussion in [22]), the results were interpreted to suggest that the sensitizing effects observed were the consequence of the release of endogenous inflammatory mediators.

In preliminary studies of pelvic nerve afferent fibers innervating the colon of the rat, we have similarly observed that mustard oil (2.5%) irritation of the colonic mucosa leads to activation of mechanically insensitive afferent fibers, which also subsequently exhibit mechanosensitivity (Figure 5). We estimate that ≈ 45% of pelvic nerve afferent fibers in the rat are mechanically insensitive (*i.e.* do not respond to either colorectal or urinary bladder distension [50]). Whether they are all sensitive to irritants such as mustard oil or turpentine remains to be determined, but the results of Häbler *et al.* [21] in studies of the urinary bladder suggest that only a relatively small fraction of the mechanically insensitive afferents will be affected by irritants applied to the colonic mucosa.

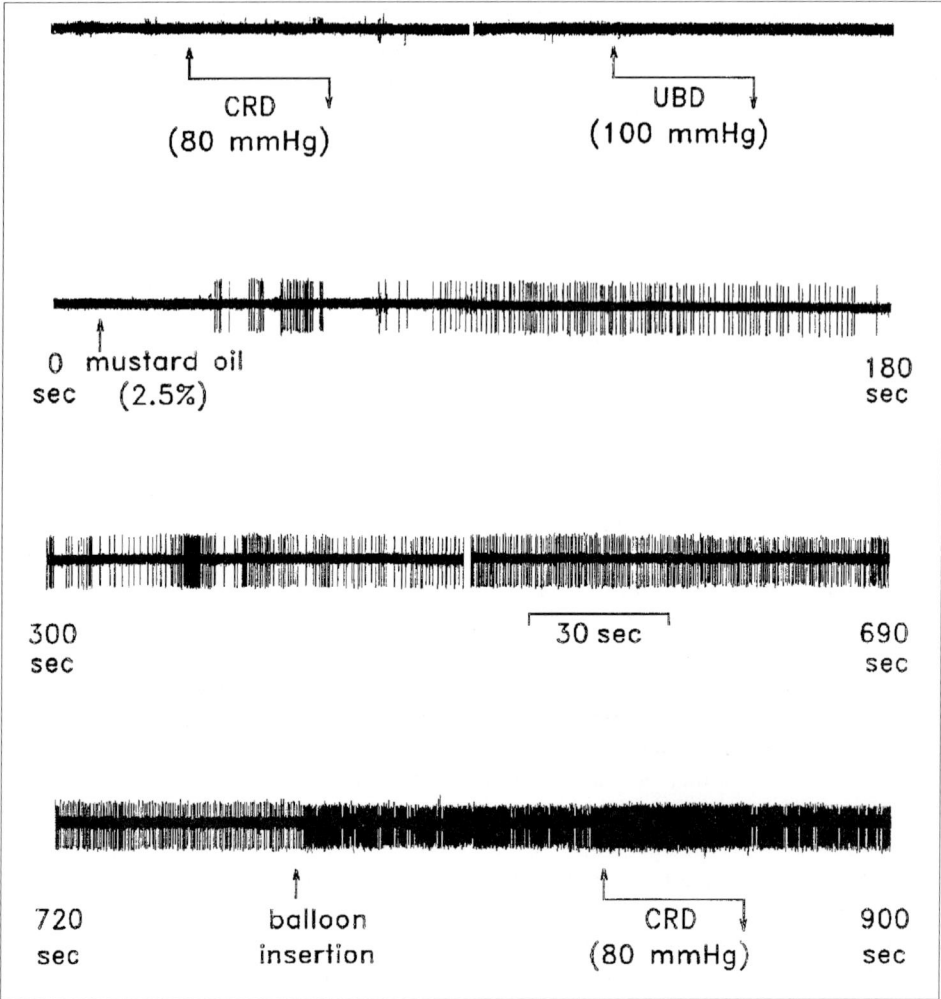

Figure 5. Example of a mechanically insensitive pelvic nerve afferent fiber in the rat. The fiber was identified by electrical stimulation of the pelvic nerve (1.0 m/sec conduction velocity) and did not respond to either colorectal distension (CRD) or urinary bladder distension (UBD). After instillation of mustard oil (2 ml, 5%) into the colon, the fiber developed spontaneous activity and sensitivity to mechanical stimulation. (From Sengupta and Gebhart, unpublished.)

Discussion

Several points merit consideration. Although considered at one time to be the tail of a normal distribution, it is now generally accepted that high threshold visceral afferent fibers are a clear and separate population of visceral sensory fibers (*e.g. see* Figure 2). Whether high threshold visceral afferent fibers are nociceptors or intensity receptors, however, is another question and cannot be resolved by the available evidence.

In the most recent discussion of visceral nociceptors [6], high threshold visceral afferents and those identified as silent (*i.e.* mechanically insensitive) are suggested to play important roles in acute and persistent visceral pain. Low threshold intensity encoding afferent fibers are considered responsible for regulatory reflexes and nonpainful sensations, but also contribute to painful sensations in circumstances where the excitability of central neurons has been increased by sensitization of afferent fibers. We agree that the 'silent,' mechanically insensitive afferent fibers are important to altered sensations that arise from the viscera, including persistent pain. Some of these mechanically insensitive afferent fibers may be visceral nociceptors or, as Häbler *et al.* [21] suggested, "chemosensitive visceral nociceptors." We have similarly suggested that the sensitization of visceral afferent fibers and subsequent central hyperexcitability contribute to a visceral hyperalgesia and, further, may be important to the maintenance of chronic, "functional" bowel disorders such as non-cardiac chest pain, non-ulcer dyspepsia and irritable bowel syndrome [17, 34].

We do not, however, consider that visceral afferent fibers with high thresholds for response to mechanical stimuli are necessarily visceral nociceptors. As reviewed above, these afferents encode mechanical stimuli in a manner indistinguishable from low threshold afferent fibers which, moreover, often exhibit greater magnitudes of response than high threshold afferent fibers. Thus, they would appear to be intensity receptors, probably located "in series" in visceral muscle layers, which function to provide information about the location, duration and intensity of conscious sensation from the viscera. Because of the low number of visceral sensory fibers and central convergence with somatic inputs, localization is poor, but duration and intensity can be accurately signaled.

Visceral afferent fibers terminate predominantly in laminae I and V of the spinal dorsal horn [4, 8] and central mechanisms are clearly important to visceral sensation, particularly if afferent inputs alter central neuron excitability. A significant proportion of high threshold visceral sensory fibers terminate in the superficial dorsal horn where we believe they contribute to conscious sensation, homeostatic processes, viscero-somatic and viscero-visceral reflexes, and behavior. As advanced by Craig [11] in his discussion of processing of afferent input in the superficial dorsal horn, inputs such as derived from visceral afferent fibers can lead to sensations that are typically poorly localized and display spatial summation, radiation and temporal persistence. It has long been appreciated that relatively long segments of the gut must be distended to produce conscious sensation (*see* [32]), emphasizing the role of spatial summation in visceral sensations.

Virtually all quantitative studies of visceral afferent fibers have employed mechanical stimuli and thresholds for response have been used to characterize the populations studied and, usually, to assign putative function. It must be acknowledged, however, that most gastrointestinal afferent fibers are mechanically insensitive; they respond to sugars, amino acids, hormones and changes in pH at the mucosal surface (*see* [49] for review). It is also overlooked that both low- and high-threshold mechanosensitive afferent fibers are often chemosensitive (e.g., to KCl, bradykinin, arachidonic acid metabolites, amines and/or other substances in addition to chemical irritants like mustard oil and turpentine). Because it is experimentally difficult to apply some stimuli in a quantitative fashion directly to a visceral receptor, we have yet to establish the adequate stimulus for most (for any?) visceral afferent fibers (notwithstanding the quantitative application of mechanical stimuli). Given the available evidence, it would be difficult to effectively argue against the assertion that visceral sensory fibers are generally polymodal.

There is also an underappreciated population of mechanically insensitive, thermosensitive afferent fibers that innervate the viscera. Thermosensitivity in the stomach has been demonstrated in the conscious human [56]. Temperatures between 18°C and 40°C produced no sensation, but outside this range stimuli were appropriately recognized as cool or warm. Thermosensitivity has also been documented in the rectum and anal canal of conscious humans [9, 38]. The anal canal of normal subjects was found to be sensitive to temperature changes of 0.5°C; the rectum was also thermosensitive, but significantly less so than the anal canal. In non-human animal studies, thermosensitive afferent fibers have been documented in the peritoneal cavity of the rabbit [45] and esophagus, stomach, duodenum, rectum and urinary bladder of the cat [10, 13-16, 20]. For example, thermosensitive vagal afferent fibers innervating the gastrointestinal tract of the cat were documented by El Ouazanni and Mei [14]. Later, they reported three types of thermosensitive C-fibers in the vagus nerve of the cat innervating the esophagus [15]. Because the thermoreceptive afferents did not respond to chemicals, esophageal distension or stroking of the serosa, they considered them to be thermospecific.

We have previously argued that the viscera should not be considered in a unitary fashion (*i.e.* the heart is not the colon [41]). Cervero and Jänig [6] suggest as much when they advance that the relative proportions of low- and high-threshold afferent fibers are important to the sensations that arise from a viscus. It was somewhat surprising to us, however, to find in fact that the proportion of high threshold afferent fibers innervating the esophagus, stomach, gall bladder and biliary duct, urinary bladder, colon and uterus/cervix is nearly the same (≈30%; the ureter is the exception). This argues against the position that acute pain arises from those viscera having disproportionate numbers of high threshold fiber innervation. These data suggest to us that high threshold afferent fibers in the viscera function principally as intensity receptors. Consideration of this issue, however, is argument in the absence of sufficient information. Mechanical distension of viscera is generally considered to reproduce a natural stimulus and is widely used in both human and non-human animal experimentation. Accordingly, classification of visceral sensory fibers as low- and high-threshold has been based on responses to mechanical stimulation. However, ischemia and inflammation are also natural visceral stimuli that can lead to conscious sensations and sugars, amino acids, hormones and pH are adequate stimuli for many gastrointestinal sensory fibers, although not usually associated with conscious sensation. Thermal stimuli are adequate for some visceral sensory fibers, producing both reflex responses (*e.g.* bladder cooling reflex ; *see* [16]) and conscious sensation (*e.g.* drinking a cold beverage on a empty stomach). Much has been made of "silent nociceptors," which are better termed mechanically insensitive, but the apparent adequate stimulus in the viscera (mucosal irritation) does not activate all of them. These afferent fibers have been characterized on the basis of what is not their adequate stimulus. Clearly, they are not all nociceptors.

Proposals to explain visceral pain mechanisms have important heuristic value. They generate discussion and, most important, stimulate experimental tests of hypotheses. The recent proposal by Cervero and Jänig [6], for example, presents several testable hypotheses. However, the focus heretofore on mechanosensitivity leaves unresolved a number of issues that need to be addressed before visceral pain mechanisms can be fully understood.

• The adequate stimulus for many, if not most, visceral afferent fibers is unknown and insufficient experimental attention has been given to this issue.
• Most visceral afferent fibers, including mechanosensitive high-threshold fibers, are non-specific in character; stimuli other than mechanical (*e.g.* chemical, thermal) are usually not tested.
• Only a small proportion of the so-called "silent nociceptor" population that innervate the viscera are nociceptors; most of these mechanically insensitive fibers likely have adequate stimuli unrelated to nociception.
• Visceral afferent fibers, in the presence of tissue injury and inflammation, can become sensitized, contribute to central hyperexcitability and lead to visceral hyperalgesia.

Acknowledgements

Supported by NIH grants NS 19912, HL 32295 and DA 02879 and an unrestricted pain research grant from Bristol-Myers Squibb Co. We thank Michael Burcham for preparation of the graphics and Marilynn Kirkpatrick for secretarial assistance.

References

1. Berkley KJ, Robbins A, Sato Y. Afferent fibers supplying the uterus in the rat. *J Neurophysiol* 1988 ; 59 : 142-63.
2. Bingham JR, Ingelfinger FJ, Smithwick RH. The effect of sympathectomy on abdominal pain in man. *Gastroenterol* 1950 ; 15 : 18-31.
3. Blumberg B, Haupt P, Jänig W, Köhler W. Encoding of visceral noxious stimuli in the discharge patterns of visceral afferent fibers from the colon. *Pflugers Arch* 1983 ; 398 : 33-40.
4. Cervero F. Afferent activity evoked by natural stimulation of the biliary system in the ferret. *Pain* 1982 ; 13 : 137-51.
5. Cervero F, Connell LA. Distribution of somatic and visceral primary afferent fibers within the thoracic spinal cord of the cat. *J Comp Neurol* 1984 ; 230 : 88-98.

6. Cervero F, Jänig W. Visceral nociceptors : a new world order ? *TINS* 1992 ; 10 : 374-8.
7. Cervero F, Sann H. Mechanically evoked responses of afferent fibers innervating the guinea-pig's ureter : an *in vitro* study. *J Physiol* 1989 ; 412 : 245-66.
8. Cervero F, Tattersall JEH. Somatic and visceral inputs to the thoracic spinal cord of the cat : marginal zone (lamina I) of the dorsal horn. *J Physiol* 1987 ; 388 : 383-95.
9. Cervero F, Miller R, Mortensen McC NJ. Temperature sensation in the anorectum of normal humans. *J Physiol* 1987 ; 387 : 52.
10. Clifton GL, Coggeshall RE, Vance WH, Willis WD. Receptive fields of unmyelinated ventral root afferent fibers. *J Physiol* 1976 ; 256 : 573-600.
11. Craig AD. Propriospinal input to thoracolumbar sympathetic nuclei from cervical and lumbar lamina I neurons in the cat and the monkey. *J Comp Neurol* 1993 ; 331 : 517-30.
12. Davison JS, Clarke GD. Mechanical properties and sensitivity to CCK of vagal gastric slowly adapting mechanoreceptors. *Am J Physiol* 1988 ; 255 : G55-G61.
13. El Ouazzani T. Thermoreceptors in the digestive tract and their role. *J Auton Nerv Syst* 1984 ; 10 : 346-254.
14. El Ouazzani T, Mei N. Mise en évidence électrophysiologique des thermorécepteurs vaguaux dans la région gastro-intestinale. Leur rôle dans la régulation de la motricité digestive. *Exp Brain Res* 1979 ; 34 : 419-34.
15. El Ouazzani T, Mei N. Electrophysiological properties and role of the vagal thermoreceptor of lower esophagus and stomach of the cat. *Gastroenterol* 1982 ; 83: 995-1002.
16. Fall M, Lindström S, Mazières L. A bladder-to-bladder cooling reflex in the cat. *J Physiol* 1990 ; 427 : 281-300.
17. Gebhart GF. Visceral pain mechanisms. In : Chapman R, Foley K, eds. *Current and emerging issues in cancer pain : research and practice*. New York : Raven Press, 1993.
18. Gebhart GF, Sengupta JN. Characterization of mechanosensitive pelvic nerve afferent fibers innervating the lower urinary tract. *Soc Neurosci* 1993 ; 214-4 : 512 (Abstract).
19. Gebhart GF, Meller ST, Euchner-Wamser I, Sengupta JN. Modeling visceral pain. In : Vecchiet L, Albe-Fessard D, Lindblom U, eds. *New trends in referred pain and hyperalgesia*. Amsterdam : Elsevier, 1993.
20. Gupta BN, Nier K, Hensel H. Cold-sensitive afferents from the abdomen. *Pflugers Arch* 1979 ; 380 : 203-4.
21. Häbler HJ, Jänig W, Koltzenburg M. Activation of unmyelinated afferent fibers by mechanical stimuli and inflammation of the urinary bladder in the cat. *J Physiol* 1990 ; 425 : 545-62.
22. Häbler HJ, Jänig W, Koltzenburg M. Receptive properties of myelinated primary afferents innervating the inflamed urinary bladder of the cat. *J Neurophysiol* 1993 ; 69 : 395-405.
23. Handwerker HO, Kilo S, Reeh PW. Unresponsive afferent nerve fibers in the sural nerve of the rat. *J Physiol* 1991 ; 435 : 229-42.
24. Head H. On distrubances of sensation with special reference to pain of visceral disease. *Brain* 1893 ; 16 : 1-132.
25. Hertz (Hurst) AF. The sensibility of the alimentary tract in health and disease. *Lancet* 1911 ; 1 : 1051-6.
26. Hong SK, Han HC, Yoon YW, Chung JM. Response properties of hypogastric afferent fibers supplying the uterus in the cat. *Brain Res* 1993 ; 622 : 215-25.
27. Jänig W, Koltzenburg M. On the function of spinal primary afferent fibers supplying colon and urinary bladder. *J Auton Nerv Syst* 1990 ; 30 : S89-S96.
28. Jänig W, Koltzenburg M. Receptive properties of sacral primary afferent neurons supplying the colon. *J Neurophysiol* 1991 ; 65 : 1067-77.
29. Jänig W, Morrison JFB. Functional properties of spinal visceral afferents supplying abdominal and pelvic organs, with special emphasis on visceral nociception. In : Cervero F, Morrison JFB,

eds. *Visceral sensation. Progress in brain research.* Amsterdam : Elsevier, 1986 ; 67 : 87-114.
30. Kinsella VJ. *The mechanism of abdominal pain.* Sydney : Australasian Medical Publishing Cpo, 1948.
31. Lennander KB. Uber die sensibilität der bauchhohle und über lokale und allgemeine anastehsie bei bruch und bauchoperationen. *Zentralbl Chir* 1901 ; 28 : 200-23.
32. Lewis T. *Pain.* London : McMillan, 1942 : 192p.
33. Mackenzie J. *Symptoms and their interpretation.* London : Shaw & Sons, 1909 : 297.
34. Mayer EM, Gebhart GF. Functional bowel disorders and the visceral hyperalgesia hypothesis. In : Mayer EM, Raybould H, eds. *Basic and clinical aspects of chronic abdominal pain.* Amsterdam : Elsevier, 1993.
35. McMahon SB, Koltzenburg M. Novel classes of nociceptors : beyond Sherrington. *TINS* 1990 ; 13 : 199-201.
36. Mense S. Nociception from muscle in relation to clinical muscle pain. *Pain* 1993 ; 54 : 241-89.
37. Meyer RA, Davis KD, Cohen RH., Treede RD, Campbell J. Mechanically insensitive afferents (MIAs) in cutaneous nerves of monkey. *Brain Res* 1991 ; 561 : 252-61.
38. Miller R, Bartolo DCC, Cervero F, Mortensen McC NJ. Anorectal temperature sensation : a comparison of normal and incontinent patients. *Br J Surg* 1987 ; 74 : 511-5.
39. Morley J. *Abdominal pain.* New York : William Wood and Co, 1931.
40. Ness TJ, Gebhart GF. Colorectal distension as noxious visceral stimulus : physiologic and pharmacologic characterization of pseudaffective reflexes in the rat. *Brain Res* 1988 ; 450 : 153-69.
41. Ness TJ, Gebhart GF. Visceral pain : a review of experimental studies. *Pain* 1990 ; 41 : 167-234.
42. Ness TJ, Metcalf AM, Gebhart GF. A psychophysical study in humans using phasic colonic distension as a noxious visceral stimulus. *Pain* 1990 ; 43 : 377-86.
43. Ness TJ, Randich A, Gebhart GF. Further evidence that colorectal distension is a noxious stimulus in rats. *Neurosci Lett* 1991 ; 131 : 113-6.
44. Ray BS, Neill CL. Abdominal visceral sensation in man. *Ann Surg* 1947 ; 126 : 709-24.
45. Riedel W. Warm receptors in the dorsal abdominal wall of the rabbit. *Pflugers Arch* 1976 ; 361 : 205-6.
46. Ross J. On the segmental distribution of sensory disorders. *Brain* 1888 ; 10 : 333-61.
47. Schaible HG, Grubb BD. Afferent and spinal mechanisms of joint pain. *Pain* 1993 ; 55 : 5-54.
48. Schaible HG, Schmidt RF. Effects of experimental arthritis on the sensory properties of fine articular afferent units. *J Neurophysiol* 1985 ; 54 : 1109-22.
49. Sengupta JN, Gebhart GF. Characterization of mechanosensitive pelvic nerve afferent fibers innervating the colon of the rat. *J Neurophysiol* 1994 ; in press.
50. Sengupta JN, Gebhart GF. Gastrointestinal afferent fibers and sensation. In : Jacobsen ED, Johnson LR, Christensen J, Alpers DH, Walsh JH, eds. *Physiology of the gastrointestinal tract.* New York : Raven Press, 1993.
51. Sengupta JN, Kauvar D, Goyal RK. Characteristics of vagal esophageal distension-sensitive afferent fibers in the opossum. *J Neurophysiol* 1989 ; 61 : 1001-10.
52. Sengupta JN, Saha JK, Goyal RK. Stimulus-response function studies of esophageal mechanosensitive nociceptor in sympathetic afferents of opossum. *J Neurophysiol* 1990 ; 64 : 796-812.
53. Sherrington CS. *The integrative action of the nervous system.* New Haven CT : Yale University Press, 1906 ; 411p.
54. Von Haller A. *Dissertation of the sensible and irritable parts of animals.* J Nourse, London 1755. Reprinted by the Johns Hopkins Press, Baltimore, MD, 1936.
55. Willis WD, Coggeshall RE. *Sensory mechanisms of the spinal cord.* 2nd edition. Plenum Press, 1991 : 575 p.
56. Wolf S. *The stomach.* Oxford University Press, 1965 : 321p.

4

Communications from the uterus (and other tissues)

K.J. BERKLEY

Department of Psychology, Florida State University, Tallahassee, Florida, USA.

Uterine afferent fibers in the hypogastric nerve of the virgin adult female rat normally require intense mechanical or chemical stimulation to be activated and can become sensitized under certain pathological conditions. Many other tissues throughout the body are also innervated by such insensitive, sensitizable afferent fibers. One possibility is that this rather large population of afferents serves more than one function by communicating information to the CNS in two ways. With propagated action potentials (a "fax" message), the fibers signal noxious events occurring in the tissues they innervate. With axonal transport of a varying complement of transsynaptically neuroactive molecules (a "postal" message), the fibers continually signal information about the ongoing status of the tissues they innervate.

Response properties of uterine afferent fibers in the rat in relation to escape behavior

The uterus of the rat is innervated by afferent fibers in the hypogastric nerve [3, 25, 28]. In adult nulliparous virgin rats, these afferent fibers have very low or no background levels of activity and can be activated primarily only by intense, abnormal stimuli such as ischemic levels of mechanical stimulation and high concentrations of chemical agents such as sodium cyanide, carbon dioxide, bradykinin and serotonin [3, 7]. As might be predicted from these results, conscious adult virgin rats will escape mechanical stimulation of the uterus only when the stimulus (distension) is intense enough to produce ischemia [5]. These results, as illustrated in Figure 1, suggest that information flow to the central nervous system from the uterus *via* action potentials does not normally occur in adult virgin rats.

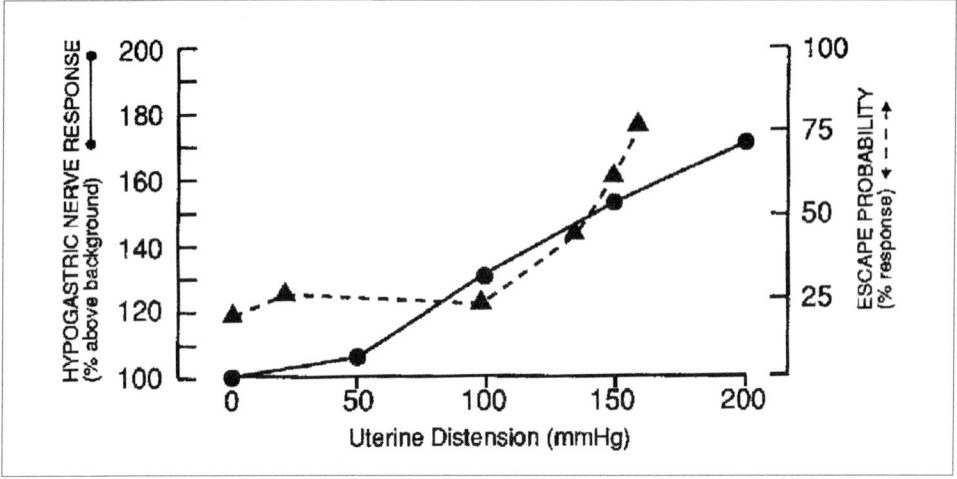

Figure 1. This figure, adapted from [5, 7], compares graphs of the probability of a conscious rat's escape responses to different amounts of uterine distension with responses of hypogastric nerve activity in an anesthetized rat to the same stimuli. Note that escape probability begins to rise at about the same pressure levels (>100mmHg) as do responses of fibers in the hypogastric nerve. Because these pressures are above the rat's normal blood pressure, it is likely the effective stimulus produces uterine ischemia.

Under different conditions, however, the situation can change. As shown in Figure 2, after the uterus has been irritated by vigorous manipulation for an hour or more with frequent applications of assorted mechanical stimuli, the background activity level of hypogastric nerve afferent fibers increases and fibers normally unresponsive to regularly-occurring gentle mechanical events such as uterine contractions begin to respond in association with them [3, 4, 7]. Similarly, conscious rats resist mechanical stimulation of their reproductive organs associated with mating and with obtaining vaginal smears under conditions in which the uterus has been inflamed with toxic bacterial agents ([31], Brown personal communication).

Classification of uterine afferent fibers and consideration of the information they convey to CNS

How do these data affect the concept of nociceptive afferent fibers or "nociceptive-specific afferents"? As noted above, the data indicate that, unless we have somehow missed finding a population of sensory afferents responsive to gentle or innocuous

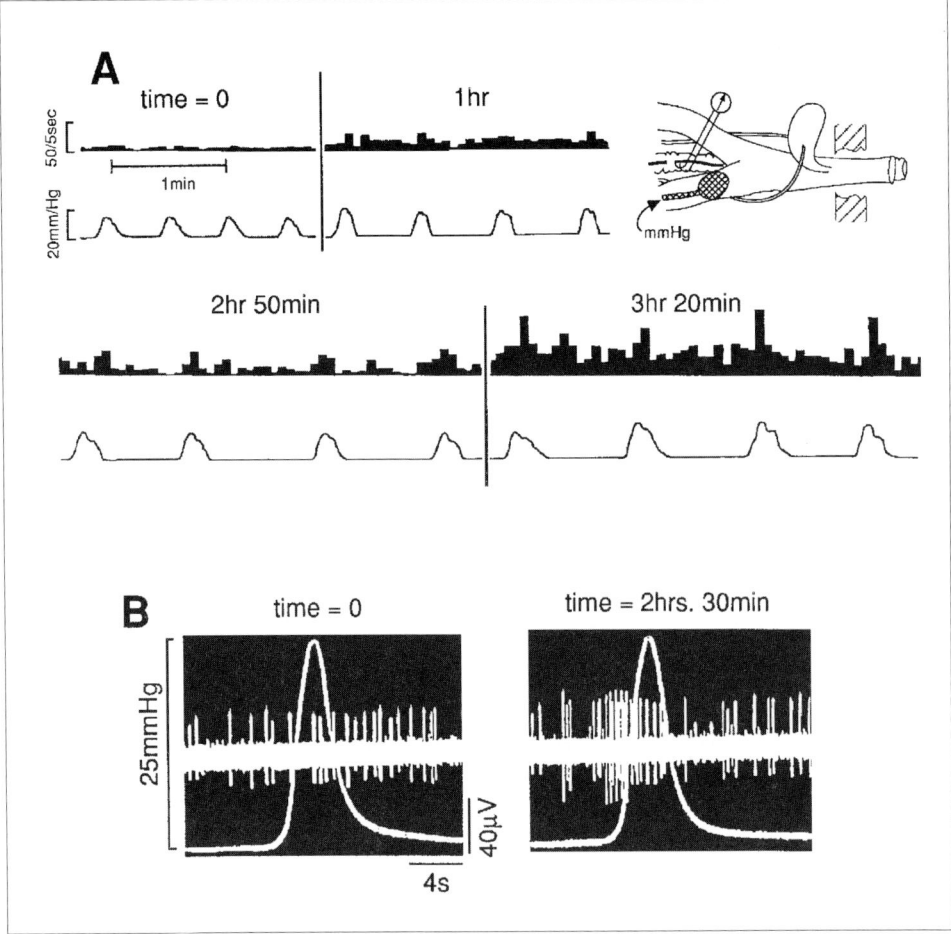

Figure 2. Responses of fibers in the hypogastric nerve in relation to uterine contractions. (Adapted from [4].) The diagram on the upper right of the figure illustrates the recording set up. Responses of fibers in a distal branch of the cut hypogastric nerve were recorded (recording electrode in diagram; upper histograms in A) together with pressure changes produced by uterine contractions as they moved across the part of the uterus containing the balloon (hatched item in diagram; lower records in A). Details of the recording procedures can be found in [3]. Part A shows that at the beginning of the recording session (time = 0), background activity levels were low and there were no obvious increases of activity in phase with uterine contractions. By the end of the recording session (during which time the uterus had been vigorously probed and stimulated), the magnitude of contractions had generally increased (amplitude and duration). In parallel, background levels of neural activity increased and additional activity was now evident in phase with the contractions. Part B makes use of the fact that variability of the individual contractions permitted comparison of neural activity in association with contractions of similar magnitude early and late in the experiment. As shown, such a comparison indicates that neural responses in phase with contractions near the end of the experiment do not depend upon the magnitude of the contraction. Such a result suggests that the irritation of the uterus by frequent stimulation during the course of the experiment had somehow produced a change in the sensitivity of the afferents.

mechanical or chemical stimuli, most or all of the peripheral sensory receptors supplying the uterus in the healthy adult virgin rat remain quiescent, sending virtually no information to the central nervous system *via* action potentials unless extraordinary circumstances, such as those that damage the organ or portend such damage, occur. Given this situation, is it appropriate to call these fibers "nociceptors" ?

In the Sherringtonian sense, these fibers fully qualify for such categorization because they appear to respond specifically to noxious stimulation. On the other hand, it seems unlikely that the extensive afferent innvervation of the uterus exists solely for conveying information about noxious events occurring in the uterus because such events occur so very rarely. It would seem more reasonable if those fibers could also convey information associated with ongoing reproductive events.

One answer to this argument might be that the response properties of the hypogastric afferent fibers makes them ideally suited for conveying useful information about the intense stimulus events that occur during parturition. Having an extensive innervation devoted to this important biological function would not seem so unlikely. It is then surprising that hypogastric neurectomies have no obvious effect on successful parturition [9] (*see* also reviews in [10] and [7]).

Given this situation, what sorts of purposes related to reproduction could the afferent fibers in the hypogastric nerve serve ? One purpose might be to communicate information continually to the spinal cord about the conditions of the uterine tissue during different stages of the estrous cycle. Another might be to communicate information continually from the spinal cord back to the uterine tissue about the status of neurons and glial cells near the spinal terminals of those afferents.

Mechanisms of communication by uterine afferent fibers : fast ("fax") and slow ("postal")

Since uterine afferent fibers in virgin adult rats are normally not producing action potentials, even in response to such normal uterine events as uterine contractions, how could communication take place ? The answer may lie in the fact that all neurons convey information over long distances in two main ways - one rapidly, *via* action potentials and another slowly, *via* axonal transport or diffusion processes.

Thus, it is possible that receptors in the hypogastric nerve innervating the uterus convey information appropriate to the function of that organ in these two ways. Action potentials would comprise an expensive and rarely or episodically used "fax" system, responsible centrally for initiating protective reflexes and having access to the neural systems associated with pain, and peripherally for releasing protective agents. Axonal transport or diffusion would comprise a continually active, but slower "postal" system responsible for helping the nervous system coordinate behavioral activities of the organism with events occurring in the reproductive organs.

For example, the "postal" axonal transport/diffusion system could be of importance for uterine afferent fibers to help coordinate appropriate evocation by vaginal or perineal cutaneous stimuli of lordosis and other behaviors necessary for successful conception during mating. It is well known that lordosis is more readily evoked by perineal and vaginal stimuli in certain stages of estrous than in others, and Pfaff's group has clearly shown that the ability of perineal stimulation to evoke lordosis in ovarectomized rats can be manipulated by the administration of estrogen [18]. Other data have shown, however, that removal of the uterus in addition to the ovaries enhances hormonally-induced lordosis responses as well as other reproductive behaviors (sexual receptivity and proceptivity and latency of induction of maternal behaviors [1]). While these "inhibitory effects" of the uterus could be due to the significant hormonal influences now thought to be exerted by substances released into the blood from the nonpregnant uterus [13], they could also be due in part to molecules that the uterine afferent fibers transport to the spinal cord (and that could vary with estrous stage and change after the uterus has been removed). In a similar vein, women who have had a hysterectomy (with ovaries conserved) report more severe climacteric symptoms than women who have not had their uterus removed [27]. Some of these effects too could be due to alterations in the composition of neuroactive agents normally released into the spinal cord by uterine afferent fibers. And finally, hypogastric neurectomies interfere with the steroidally-dependent effects of vaginocervical stimulation on responses to cutaneous stimulation [10], which could be interpreted as indicating that at least some of the influences on the effects of vaginocervical stimulation are due to changes in molecules transported by hypogastric afferent fibers.

Extending this concept of communication further, both the "postal" and the "fax" systems could work in consort for other aspects of reproduction, for example, pregnancy and parturition. Although as mentioned above, hypogastric neurectomies alone have no dramatic effects on parturition, their overall effects on reproductive events are significant when combined with pelvic neurectomies (*see* reviews in [6, 7, 10, 33]). Thus, as pregnancy advances, axons arising from the uterus, cervix and vagina could be transporting, *via* the pelvic as well as the hypogastric nerves, a changing mixture of various agents to the spinal cord. This changing input would alter peripheral and central excitability states in a manner appropriate for ensuring the effectiveness of the faster action potential messages from the uterus, cervix and vagina that would be elicited in fibers in both nerves by the intense stimuli occurring during parturition.

Dual modes of communication as a general property of all neurons

There is clear precedent for the idea of dual modes of sensory communication. Elegant experiments by McMahon, Devor, Fitzgerald, Woolf, Lewin and Wall and others (reviewed recently in [20, 21]) have demonstrated clearly that peripheral pathological events occurring in skin and muscle can exert longlasting effects on response properties of spinal neurons and that at least some of these effects on spinal neurons are due, not only (as is well known) to action potentials arriving in the spinal cord from peripheral axons, but also to changes in what the axons are transporting to the spinal cord. The simple extension of this concept presented here, which has been previously suggested by others, is that all fibers may convey information primarily and continuously by these slower means under all conditions, with some of them, particularly C-fibers, communicating their most important information primarily this way [30, 35, 36].

That such a situation may indeed exist not only for afferents arising from the uterus, and all other peripheral tissues, but also for CNS neurons is supported by a number of recent studies. These studies demonstrate :
- that there exists a surprisingly large population of afferents supplying skin, muscles and viscera that are normally electrically "silent" [11, 14, 19, 22, 24, 29],
- that there are dynamic changes in the axonal transport of a variety of potent molecules, including mRNAs and growth factors, by axons supplying peripheral organs [15, 16, 23],
- that axonal transport characteristics can be modified by neuroactive agents [32],
- that neuroactive agents and synaptic transmission can be modified by manipulations of axonal transport [17, 26],
- that release of large molecules (such as WGA-HRP) from sensory afferent fibers into the extracellular space of the spinal cord can be modified by certain pathological events occurring in the periphery [34],
- that some sort of transfer mechanism exists for transynaptic transport of molecules across sequences of synapses from the periphery and through pathways within the CNS [8].

Consequences of dual modes of communication for the concept of "nociceptors"

How does this concept of cooperating "postal" and "fax" communication systems affect our classification scheme for afferent fibers, particularly "nociceptors" ? For the future, it suggests that we may need to introduce a new classification scheme based not only on stimulus information coded by action potentials but also on the composition and dynamic characteristics of axonally transported molecules. For now, it suggests that at the very least we consider revising our current scheme to include the possibility that some receptors have more than one function. In other words, it might prove useful now to add to our current list of afferents a large class whose function under most circumstances is to convey information to the CNS *via* axonal transport or diffusion about the ongoing status of the tissue they innervate and whose function under other circumstances is to convey information *via* action potentials about abrupt, extraordinary changes occurring in that tissue. The utility of calling any of the fibers in this class "nociceptors" could then be debated.

Consequences for therapy

Whatever they might be called, recognition of a class of afferents which normally communicate much of their information *via* axonal transport or diffusion processes would have pharmacological consequences. It would bring into the realm of potential therapeutic pain-relieving agents compounds which either act on axonal transport processes or are themselves known to be transported, such as those now beginning to be considered for use experimentally [12] as well as clinically [2] for the treatment of peripheral neuropathies.

Acknowledgements

The experiments described in this paper carried out by the author and illustrated in the figures were supported by NIH grant NS 11892. I thank Mr. Richard Brunck for help with the figures.

References

1. Ahdieh HB. The role of the uterus in reproductive behavior. *Physiol Behav* 1984 ; 33 : 329-33.
2. Apfel SC, Arezzo JC, Lipson L, Kessler JA. Nerve growth factor prevents experimental cisplatin neuropathy. *Ann Neurol* 1992 ; 31 : 76-80.
3. Berkley KJ, Robbins A, Sato Y. Afferent fibers supplying the uterus in the rat. *J Neurophysiol* 1988 ; 59 : 142-63.
4. Berkley KJ, Robbins A, Sato Y. Sensory input from contractions of the uterus in the rat. *Soc Neurosci Abstr* 1988 ; 14 : 727.
5. Berkley KJ, Scofield S, Wood E. Uterine pain : the role of ischemia and the hypogastric nerve. *Soc Neurosci Abstr* 1990 ; 16 : 416.
6. Berkley KJ, Hotta H, Robbins A, Sato Y. Functional properties of afferent fibers supplying reproductive and other pelvic organs in pelvic nerve of female rat. *J Neurophysiol* 1990 ; 63 : 256-72.
7. Berkley KJ, Robbins A, Sato Y. Functional differences between afferent fibers in the hypogastric and pelvic nerves innervating female reproductive organs in the rat. *J Neurophysiol* 1993 ; 69 : 533-44.
8. Card JP, Rinaman L, Schwaber JS, Miselis RR, Whealy ME, Robbins AK, Enquist LW. Neurotropic properties of pseudorabies virus : uptake and transneuronal passage in the rat central nervous system. *J Neurosci* 1990 ; 10 : 1974-94.
9. Carlson RR, deFeo VJ. Role of the pelvic nerve vs. the abdominal sympathetic nerves in the reproductive function of the female rat. *Endocrinology* 1965 ; 77 : 1014-22.
10. Cunningham ST, Steinman JL, Whipple B, Mayer AD, Komisaruk BR. Differential roles of hypogastric and pelvic nerves in the analgesic and motoric effects of vaginocervical stimulation in rats. *Brain Res* 1991 ; 559 : 337-43.
11. Davis KD, Meyer RA, Campbell JN. Chemosensitivity and sensitization of nociceptive afferents that innervate the hairy skin of monkey. *J Neurophysiol* 1993 ; 69 : 1071-81.
12. Fitzgerald M, Wall PD, Goedert M, Emson L. Nerve growth factor counteracts the neurophysiological and neurochemical effects of chronic sciatic nerve section. *Brain Res* 1985 ; 332 : 131-41.

13. Freeman ME. The nonpregnant uterus as an endocrine organ. *News Physiol Sci* 1988 ; 3 : 31-2.
14. Häbler HJ, Jänig W, Koltzenburg M. A novel type of unmyelinated chemosensitive nociceptor in the acutely inflamed urinary bladder. *Agents Actions* 1988 ; 25 : 219-21.
15. Hansson HA, Rozell B, Skottner A. Rapid axoplasmic transport of insulin-like growth factor I in the sciatic nerve of adult rats. *Cell Tissue Res* 1987 ; 247 : 241-7.
16. Jirikowski GF, Sanna PP, Maciejewski-Lenoir D, Bloom FE. Reversal of diabetes insipidus in Brattleboro rats : intrahypothalamic injection of vasopressin mRNA. *Science* 1992 ; 255 : 996-8.
17. Kashiba H, Senba E, Kawai Y, Ueda Y, Tohyama M. Axonal blockade induces the expression of vasoactive intestinal polypeptide and galanin in rat dorsal root ganglion neurons. *Brain Res* 1992 ; 577 : 19-28.
18. Kow LM, Montgomery MO, Pfaff DW. Triggering of lordosis reflex in female rats with somatosensory stimulation : quantitative determination of stimulus parameters. *J Neurophysiol* 1979 ; 42 : 195-202.
19. Kress M, Koltzenburg M, Reeh PW, Handwerker HO. Responsiveness and functional attributes of electrically localized terminals of cutaneous C-fibers *in vivo* and *in vitro*. *J Neurophysiol* 1992 ; 68 : 581-95.
20. Lewin GR, McMahon SB. Dorsal horn plasticity following re-routeing of peripheral nerves : evidence for tissue-specific neurotrophic influences from the periphery. *Eur J Neurosci* 1991 ; 3 : 1112-22.
21. Lewin GR, Winter J, McMahon SB. Regulation of afferent connectivity in the adult spinal cord by nerve growth factor. *Eur J Neurosci* 1992 ; 4 : 700-7.
22. McMahon SB, Koltzenburg M. Novel classes of nociceptors : beyond Sherrington. *Trends Neurosci* 1990 ; 13 : 199-201.
23. Mercer JG, Lawrence CB, Copeland PA. Corticotropin-releasing factor binding sites undergo axonal transport in the rat vagus nerve. *J Neuroendocrinol* 1992 ; 4 : 281-5.
24. Meyer RA, Campbell JN. A novel electrophysiological technique for locating cutaneous nociceptive and chemospecific receptors. *Brain Res* 1988 ; 441 : 81-6.
25. Nance DM, Burns J, Klein CM, Burden HW. Afferent fibers in the reproductive system and pelvic viscera of female rats : anterograde tracing and immunocytochemical studies. *Brain Res Bull* 1988 ; 21 : 701-9.
26. Nguyen PV, Atwood HL. Maintenance of long-term adaptation of synaptic transmission requires axonal transport following induction in an identified crayfish motoneuron. *Exp Neurol* 1992 ; 115 : 414-22.
27. Oldenhave A, Jaszmann LJB, Everaerd WTAM, Haspels AA. Hysterectomized women with ovarian conservation report more severe climacteric complaints than do normal climacteric women of similar age. *Am J Obstet Gynecol* 1993 ; 168 : 765-71.
28. Peters LC, Kristal MB, Komisaruk BR. Sensory innervation of the external and internal genitalia of the female rat. *Brain Res* 1987 ; 408 : 199-204.
29. Schaible HG, Schmidt RF. Time course of mechanosensitivity changes in articular afferents during a developing experimental arthritis. *J Neurophysiol* 1988 ; 60 : 2180-95.
30. Schmitt FO. Molecular regulators of brain function : a new view. *Neuroscience* 1984 ; 13 : 991-1001.
31. Steiner DA, Brown MB. Impact of experimental genital mycoplasmosis on pregnancy outcome in Sprague-Dawley rats. *Infect Immun* 1993 ; 61 : 633-9.
32. Takenaka T, Kawakami T, Hikawa N, Bandou Y, Gotoh H. Effect of neurotransmitters on axoplasmic transport : acetylcholine effect on superior cervical ganglion cells. *Brain Res* 1992 ; 588 : 212-6.
33. Traurig HH, Papka RE, Rush ME. Effects of capsaicin on reproductive function in the female rat : role of peptide-containing primary afferent nerves innervating the uterine cervix in the neuroendocrine copulatory repsonse. *Cell Tissue Res* 1988 ; 253 : 573-81.

34. Valtschanoff JG, Weinberg RJ, Rustioni A. Peripheral injury and anterograde transport of wheat germ agglutinin-horse radish peroxidase to the spinal cord. *Neuroscience* 1992 ; 50 : 685-96.
35. Wall PD. Introduction. In : Wall PD, Melzack R, eds. *Textbook of pain.* Edinburgh : Churchill Livingstone, 1989 : 1-18.
36. Wall PD. The design of experimental studies in the future development of restorative neurology of altered sensation and pain. In : Dimitrijevic MR, Wall PD, Lindblom U, eds. *Recent achievements in restorative neurology,* Vol 3 : *Altered sensation and pain.* Basel : Karger, 1990 : 197-205.

5

Chemical activation and sensitization of nociceptors

A. DRAY

Sandoz Institute for Medical Research, London, UK.

Nociception begins with the generation of nerve impulses in fine afferent fibers and is followed by impulse propagation to the spinal cord and then signal transmission *via* the synaptic release of a variety of mediators in the spinal dorsal horn. Nociceptive afferent fibers are activated by potentially harmfull stimuli including pressure, heat and noxious chemicals. Particularly striking is their sensitivity to a variety of endogenous chemicals especially those produced during pathological changes induced by tissue injury, inflammation and anoxic insults. Of course fine afferent nerve terminals are affected by exogenous substances present in the environment or administered for medicinal or other reasons. Presently fine sensory neurons can also be classified according to whether they are sensitivity to the algogen, capsaicin [59] but there is a good deal of debate on the corresponding physiological classification of these capsaicin-sensitive neurons. It is clear that capsaicin-sensitive neurons exhibit afferent (nociceptor) activity as well as efferent properties associated with neurogenic inflamation, control of the microvasculature and neuroimmune-cell regulation [50, 60, 112]. Capsaicin-sensitive neurons thus appear to have the properties of "multifunctional neurons". However some of these may be unresponsive even to intense physiological stimuli and as such have been termed "silent or "sleeping" primary afferents.

The concept of "silent" nociceptors arose originally from the observations that a certain proportion of sensory nerves could not be excited by adequate natural stimuli despite their identification, using electrophysiological criteria, as fine primary afferent fibers. The lack of responsiveness was attributed to inadequate localization of a peripheral receptive field or the inadequate modalities of stimulation. The fact that many unmyelinated fibers in peripheral nerves may be preganglionic autonomic efferent fibers has also to be taken into consideration. However, under conditions of experimentally induced inflamation or following the administration of irritants, a larger number of fine sensory fibers (low and high threshold) exhibited spontaneous activity, became sensitized and responsive to mechanical stimulation. Such fibers have been observed in studies of joint afferents [77, 95], and in a smaller proportion of urinary bladder afferents [45] and skin afferents [47]. Silent-afferents may thus represent one extreme of the sensitivity range of sensory neurons. Under the influence of the appropriate environmental factors, they become sensitive to exogenous stimuli in much the same way as normally sensitive afferents become hypersensitive to exogenous stimuli.

Substances affecting afferent neurons

Chemical factors produced during pathophysiological conditions have received most attention with respect to the activation and sensitization of peripheral sensory neurons. There are also a number of other regulatory factors, some derived from target tissues, which are important for cell development and for maintaining the normal phenotype of afferent neurons. The amount of these substances increases following tissue damage, inflammation or nerve injury and these substances appear to have a major long term influence in altering the properties of sensory neurons and other associated neural and non-neural cells. Some of these physiological and pathophysiological factors have been summarized in Figure 1. These have been grouped according to their source or circumstances of production. A number of substances are produced or released following tissue injury, including bradykinin, serotonin, prostanoids, protons and potassium ions. During the activation of afferent nerve terminals, a number of neuropeptides (*e.g.* neurokinins, somatostatin, galanin, NPY) may be released. These peptides can either directly affect the excitability of sensory and postganglionic sympathetic nerves or produce indirect effects *via* the release of neuroactive substances from the vasculature or from immune cells. Immune cell (neutrophils, monocytes, macrophages, mast cells) also release or elaborate several active mediators including histamine, prostanoids and a number of cytokines, particularly IL1, IL6, IL8 and TNFα each of which produces mechanical hyperalgesia [22, 38]. Interestingly during inflammation, immune cells also synthesize a number of opioid peptides including endorphin and enkephalin [100].

A number of chemicals and cells are released from blood vessels following vascular injury. These may also "leak" from microvessels following the stimulation and contraction of vascular endothelial cells by neurogenic factors. Extravasation of plasma proteins and other low molecular weight substances from leaky vessels contribute to neurogenic inflammation. During inflammation, reflex or local chemical stimulation of sympathetic nerve fibers may release sympathetic transmitters as well as prostanoids [69]. Finally neurotrophic factors, such as nerve growth factor (NGF), are synthesised by target tissues normally innervated by afferent and sympathetic nerve terminals. This synthesis may be dramatically increased during inflammation in which these

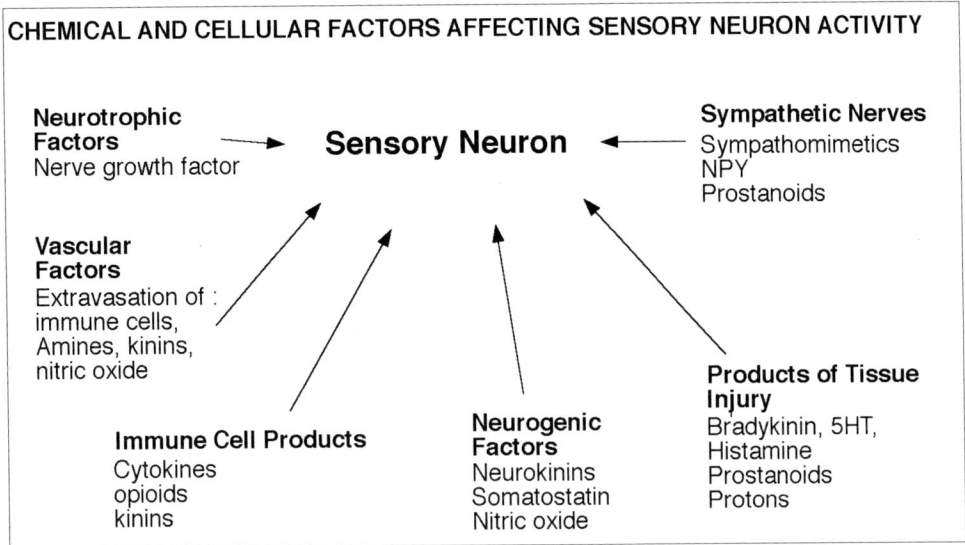

Figure 1. Pathophysiological factors which produce short and long lasting changes in the excitability and phenotype of sensory neurons.

circumstances these factors may also be synthesised by other types of reactive cells such as Schwann cells and keratinocytes.

The chemical agents mentioned above affect the excitability of sensory neurons either directly or indirectly *via* changes in the activity of surrounding tissues. This creates an environment in which signals can be amplified by different chemicals acting on common biochemical pathways, or by substances initiating cascades involving the simultaneous production of other mediators. In addition there is also a great potential for synergistic interactions and signal modulation between different substances and between neural and non-neural systems.

Steps in chemical transduction

A number of key events occur during the processing of chemical signals by afferent nerves. Thus sensory transduction and transmission in somatosensory neurons involves similar steps to those described for other sensory processes such as olfaction and gustation [98]. These mechanisms, shown in Figure 2, require a detector, usually a membrane receptor protein, which can be characterized pharmacologically or with molecular biological techniques. Facilitation and enhancement of signal generation can be produced by sensitization of afferent nerve terminals, making normally subthreshold stimuli effective. Ultimately signal generation is produced by chemically-induced changes in membrane ion permeability and depolarization of the peripheral nerve terminal. Additional activation of voltage gated cation channels leads to the propagation

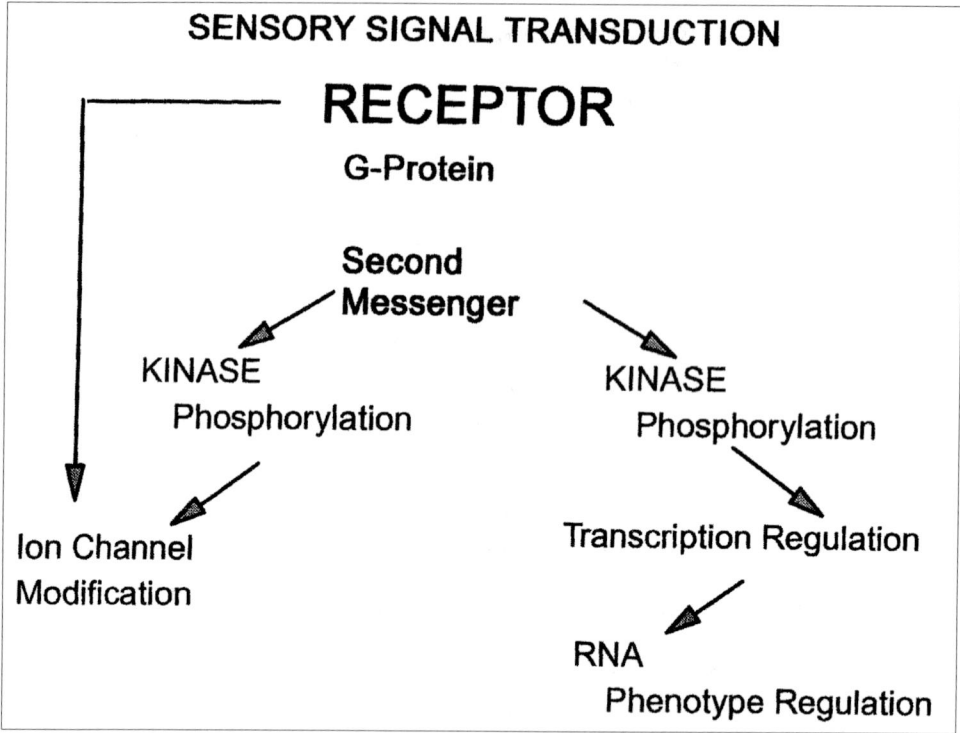

Figure 2. Chemical transduction by sensory neurons. Receptors are coupled directly with ion channels or indirectly *via* G-proteins and second messengers to change ion conductance or cell phenotype.

of nerve impulses *via* dorsal root fibers into the spinal cord where further amplification and modulation of somatosensory signals occurs.

Chemical receptors on afferent nerve terminals have been characterized pharmacologically using selective agonists and antagonists. Many receptors have also been identified, sequenced and cloned using molecular biological methods. As in other excitable membranes many receptors are coupled *via* G-proteins and second messenger systems to regulate intracellular ion concentration and to alter membrane ion permeability. For example protein kinases may be activated to induce changes in ion channel activity following the phosphorylation of ion channel proteins. These effects produce changes in cellular excitability. In addition activation of cellular transcription factors regulates cell phenotype resulting in changes in the activity of RNA polymerases and a consequent increase or decrease of the production of mRNA necessary for coding the synthesis of various peptides and proteins (Figure 2). Such changes provide the potential for long lasting alterations in cell excitability and biochemistry as well as inducing structural modification of cell cytoarchitecture and connectivity. Finally some receptors may be an integral part of the ion channel protein complex and ligand binding can alter membrane excitability by coupling directly with the ion channels.

Several types of ion channel are expressed in sensory neurons, as in other excitable cells [80] (Figure 3). There are two major types of sodium channel; as in other neurons one is sensitive to blockade by TTX while the other channels are TTX-insensitive. In the latter cells the activation and inactivation of membrane sodium conductance is slower. Potassium channels comprise the delayed rectifier channel, as in most neurons, which is responsible for rapid membrane repolarization after the action potential. Another fast, potassium channel opens rapidly and transiently during depolarization and is important for maintaining nerve excitability. Calcium-activated potassium conductance occurs in some types of sensory neurons, especially in the viscera. This conductance is responsible for the prolonged afterspike hyperpolarization. This is important for regulating excitability and for keeping cells quiescent for longer periods between action-potentials. Interestingly some inflammatory mediators block this conductance mechanism and thus allow cells to fire repetitively upon stimulation [113]. This mechanism has been suggested as a likely cellular explanation for the hypersensitivity and hyperalgesia during inflammation. However the prolonged spike after hyperpolarization is not prominent in somatic sensory neurons [86].

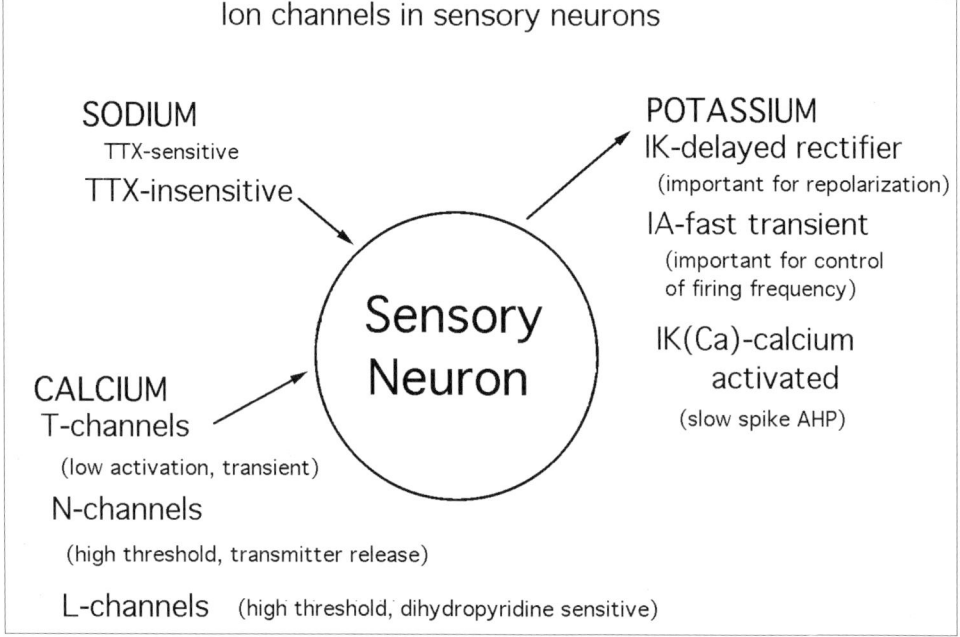

Figure 3. Ion channels in sensory neurons. For the most part sodium, potassium and calcium channels are similar to those in other neurons. Sensory neurons also possess TTX-resistant sodium channels. See text for further description of the properties of these ion channels.

In common with other neurons, there are three major types of voltage dependent calcium channels. T-channels have a low activation threshold and generate a transient current which makes a significant contribution to the excitability of sensory neurons.

N-channels have a higher activation threshold and are important in signal propagation for they control the release of neurochemicals from sensory neurons both in the periphery and also in the spinal cord during synaptic transmission. N-channels can be blocked with some degree of selectivity by ω-conotoxin. Finally L-channels have the highest activation threshold and remain open for longer periods. These channels can can be blocked by dihydropyridines and a number of chemical transmitters (opioids, GABA).

Products of tissue injury

Many substances produced upon tissue injury or during inflammation can effect sensory neurons. Amongst the best studied of these are bradykinin, serotonin, prostanoid products of arachidonic acid metabolism and more recently protons.

Bradykinin

Bradykinin is a nonapeptide formed by proteolytic (kallikrein enzymes) cleavage of circulating and tissue derived precursor proteins, the kininogens. Bradykinin is made *de novo* only during adverse conditions including local tissue anoxia, tissue injury and inflammation. In the vasculature the synthesis of bradykinin may be closely regulated by kallikrein enzymes activity but in tissues a number of proteolytic enzymes, activated upon tissue damage, can induce bradykinin synthesis. In addition bradykinin production can be induced in several different types of cells by the actions of other mediators, *e.g.* cytokines.

Bradykinin is one of the most potent endogenous algogenic substance and induces pain by stimulating nociceptors directly (skin, joint, muscle) but may also sensitize nociceptors to other stimuli, including mechanical stimulation [86]. There is a strong synergism between the actions of bradykinin and other algogenic substances, *e.g.* prostaglandins, 5-hydroxytryptamine. Bradykinin may also induce secondary effects *via* the release of prostaglandins and cytokines from a variety of cells and can degranulate mast cells to release histamine and other inflammatory mediators. Bradykinin may have other functions in tissue injury and repair since it promotes lymphocyte movement [66], possibly to sites of injury, and has been shown to exert mitogenic activity [43]. Postganglionic sympathetic neurons are also activated by bradykinin and this is important for mediating plasma extravasation during inflammation of the joint [44]. Sympathetic neurons may also be involved in bradykinin mediated mechanical hyperalgesia [102] though in the skin sympathectomy did not alter heat hyperalgesia induced by bradykinin [53, 71].

Bradykinin mediates its effects *via* two types of receptor, B1 and B2, which have been characterized pharmacologically [35]. Des-Arg^9-bradykinin, the major active metabolite of bradykinin, is the prefered ligand for the B1 receptor while another analogue, which does not occur naturally, Des-Arg^9-Leu^8-bradykinin, acts as a selective B1 receptor antagonist. The B1 receptor is constitutively expressed in certain tissues such as arteries, but in other tissues it is expressed less frequently and appears to be synthesised *de novo* under conditions of inflammation or infection. The physiological significance of this behaviour is not yet clear. However the majority of the acute effects of bradykinin are mediated *via* the B2 receptor and selective antagonists of B2 receptors show that bradykinin makes a major contribution to inflammatory pain and hyperalgesia [29]. However in conditions of persistent inflammation there is an expression of B1 receptors which make an additional contribution to the persistent hyperalgesia [29, 82].

Both molecular cloning and biochemical studies [13, 29] have shown that the B2 receptor is coupled to other effector systems *via* a G-protein. In sensory neurons, bradykinin acts mainly through the G protein-mediated activation of phospholipase C. This generates two intracellular second messengers, 1,4,5- inositol-trisphosphate (IP3) and diacylglycerol (DAG) following cleavage of membrane phospholipids [29, 86]. IP3 may stimulate the release of calcium from intracellular stores and produces a rise in the free calcium concentration within the cell but this may be of minor importance for changing cell excitability. The effect of DAG is to activate protein kinase C (PKC) which phosphorylates various cellular proteins including membrane receptors and ion channels. PKC plays a key role in the excitation of sensory fibers since staurosporine, a protein kinase C inhibitor, attenuated afferent fiber stimulation by bradykinin in the skin [31]. Further bradykinin-induced membrane depolarisation and the associated calcium entry could be mimicked by phorbol esters, which activate protein kinase C, and could be reduced or abolished by inhibition or down-regulation of protein kinase C [14]. Bradykinin has also been shown to inhibit voltage-gated calcium currents in sensory neurons : this effect being ascribed to activation of PKC [34]. This is hard to reconcile with the well documented ability of bradykinin to evoke calcium-dependent neuropeptide release from sensory neurons [41].

The release of intracellular calcium by IP3 seems to make little contribution to the activation of sensory neurons by bradykinin. However intracellular free calcium may regulate calcium-activated potassium channels, which normally show a low susceptibility to opening. Indeed other calcium-dependent effects of bradykinin in sensory neurons, such as neuropeptide release and generation of cGMP [15], require the presence of extracellular calcium which enters the cell through voltage-gated channels. Bradykinin also stimulates arachidonic acid production in sensory neurons through an indirect mechanism involving activation of phospholipase C and metabolism of DAG [86]. There is little evidence that bradykinin induces prostanoid production in mammalian sensory neurons though it directly activates phospholipase A2, to generate prostanoids, in avian sensory neurons and in many other types of cell. However bradykinin-induced excitation of sensory neurons is mediated in part through the actions of prostaglandins since cyclo-oxygenase inhibitors reduce, but do not abolish, the excitation of nociceptors by bradykinin [90]. This effect most likely involves the release of prostaglandins from other tissues.

The depolarization of sensory neurons by bradykinin [14, 68] is associated with an inward ionic current and an increase in membrane conductance, mainly to sodium ions. However in visceral sensory neurons increased excitability is associated with the inhibition of a long-lasting spike after-hyperpolarisation (slow-AHP). This is a calcium activated potassium conductance mechanism which is regulated by a cAMP dependent process. The slow-AHP following a single action potential produces a state of inexcitability thus limiting the number of action potentials that can be evoked [113]. Prostaglandins and bradykinin, through prostanoid formation, inhibit the slow-AHP by stimulating cAMP formation and allows the cell to fire repetitively following depolarisation. This mechanism can account for sensitization of sensory neurons. On the other hand, cGMP dependent mechanisms also regulate B2 receptors on sensory neurons. Thus bradykinin-induced IP3 production and activation of sensory neurons is reduced in the presence of cGMP possibly *via* desensitization of the receptor [15, 31, 68]. This mechanism is initiated *via* NO production since inhibitors of NOS attenuated bradykinin-induced desensitization in cultured sensory neurons [68].

5-Hydroxytryptamine (5-HT)

5-HT can be released from platelets and mast cells during tissue damage and acts on sensory neurons in several ways. It may directly excite sensory neurons which would explain the mild and transient pain produced by 5-HT following application to a human blister base [87]. This may involve an action of 5-HT_3 receptors since the sensation of pain and the 5HT-induced depolarization and sodium dependent inward current produced in small sensory neurons could be antagonised by 5HT_3 receptor blockers [87, 88]. Indeed molecular cloning experiments have shown that the 5-HT_3 binding site is part of a cation (Na^+) selective ion channel [62], which opens to depolarize and activate sensory neurons. 5-HT also activates sensory neurons *via* 5-HT_2 receptors which are linked through G-proteins to close potassium channels, which are normally open in the resting membrane. This results in membrane depolarization and neuronal firing [107]. 5-HT may also sensitize nociceptors by lowering their threshold to other stimuli (heat, pressure) [4, 89, 105]. This sensitization involves both 5-HT_1 and 5-HT_2 receptors but not 5HT_3 receptors [89, 105]. Conversely, in the human blister base, 5-HT- induced enhancement of the bradykinin-evoked pain was blocked by the 5-HT_3 antagonist ICS 205.930 [87]. Moreover this antagonist inhibited the hyperalgesia, but not the oedema, associated with experimental carageenan induced inflammation [33] suggesting that 5-HT_3 receptors are also involved in inflammatory hyperalgesia. Perhaps some of these antinociceptive actions occur within the spinal cord [42]. ICS 205.930 also blocks the 5-HT_4 receptor which is normally linked to adenylate cyclase system. It is therefore possible that several 5HT receptors mediate nociceptor sensitization and hyperalgesia through a common second messenger system rather than *via* 5HT_3-receptors coupled directly with ion channels. In support of this hyperalgesia was shown to be blocked by RpcAMPS, an inhibitor of cAMP dependent kinase, and augmented by a phospho-diesterase inhibitor [105]. Collectively these observations suggest that a cAMP mediated phosphorylation process is required for sensitization by 5-HT. Moreover the sensitization produced by 5-HT is likely to be a direct effect on sensory neurons. Thus sympathectomy and depletion of polymorphonuclear leukocytes had no effect on 5-HT mediated hyperalgesia [105] while indomethacin did not affect 5-HT-mediated sensitization [89, 105], suggesting that cyclo-oxygenase products are not involved.

Another explanation for 5-HT-induced sensitization in some sensory neurons is by a reduction of the slow-AHP that follows the action potential [16]. This increases neural excitability due to a cAMP-mediated reduction in K^+ permeability. The overall effect is to increase the likelihood that the neurone will respond to a weak stimulus with a train of action potentials rather than with a single spike.

Arachidonic acid metabolites (prostanoids)

These include the products of the cyclo-oxygenase and lipoxygenase enzyme pathways and have been reported to either excite nociceptors or, more usually, to sensitize them to other stimuli and thus contribute to hyperalgesia.

Prostanoids

Large amounts of prostaglandins are produced during inflammatory diseases such as rheumatoid arthritis or after experimental inflammation. NSAIDs prevent prostaglandin production by inhibiting cyclo-oxygenase activity, and thereby induce algesia and an anti-inflammatory action. A major effect of prostaglandins is to sensitize nociceptors to noxious stimuli [10, 72, 96]. However not all prostaglandins do this. Thus PGE_2 and PGI_2 commonly induce sensitization but PGD_2 does not [90]. Sensitization by prostaglandins involves cAMP production [36]. Indeed agents that elevate cAMP may also induce hyperalgesia [103]. The ionic mechanisms of sensitization have not yet been fully elucidated. In visceral neurons prostaglandins increase excitability *via* cyclic AMP-mediated inhibition of the slow-AHP.

It is uncommon for prostaglandins to activate sensory neurons directly and they do not evoke pain when injected intradermally into human skin [21]. But PGE_1 and prostacyclin (PGI_2) have been shown to increase the activity of nociceptors in rat articular nerves [10, 95] and PGE_2 stimulates the release of substance P sensory neurons in culture [78]. These findings certainly suggest that during inflammation prostanoids may contribute directly to the activation of afferent neurons. Indeed PGE_2 induced a direct depolarization produced, at least in part, by increasing membrane Na^+ conductance [84].

Lipoxygenase products

Leukotriene B_4 (a product of the 5-lipoxygenase pathway) or 8R,15S-diHETE (a product of the 15-lipoxygenase pathway) decrease the mechanical and thermal thresholds for nociception after intradermal injection [56, 65]. The action of LTB_4 is unaffected by block of cyclooxygenase activity and appears to be mediated indirectly *via* the release of 8R,15S-diHETE from polymorphonuclear leukocytes [56]. Indeed 8R,15S-diHETE also produces hyperalgesia directly by decreasing the mechanical and thermal thresholds of C-fibers [64]. The hyperalgesic effect of 8R,15S-di HETE and LTB_4, can be inhibited by the isomer 8S,15S-diHETE [56] indicating that some prostanoid fragments depress nociceptor sensitivity.

LTD4 also sensitizes sensory neurons [85] by a number of mechanisms involving the release of eicosanoids as well as the production of DAG and inositol phosphates in macrophages and basophils [20].

Protons and capsaicin

Protons activate myelinated afferent neurons as well as those with unmyelinated fibers. Activation of the latter groups of fibers accounts for the sharp stinging pain produced by local injections of acidic solutions and may contribute to the sensation of aching and discomfort following tissue acidosis after muscle exercise. Indeed the localized production of protons may provide an important stimulus for the continuous regulation of the sensitivity and excitability of sensory nerve terminals. Protons may have additional effects during pathological condition since the pH of the extracellular environment is known to fall in several conditions such as hypoxia / anoxia as well as in inflammation [18]. Proton-induced excitation of sensory neurons does not rapidly adapt whereas the actions of some inflammatory mediators undergo a rapid tachyphylaxis. Moreover solutions of low pH enhance the effects of a number of other inflammatory mediators [51].

Two types of proton-induced depolarization have been studied in sensory neurons. One type, seen commonly in several types of sensory neuron, is associated with a rapid, transient increase in membrane cation permeability and is evoked by pH changes in the normal physiological range. The second type of depolarization is associated with a more prolonged increase in membrane permeability and evoked by a greater lowering of extracellular pH, similar to that which gives rise to the sustained nerve activation. This type of depolarization shows a much slower rate of inactivation [9] and is likely to make a significant contribution to nociceptive responses. Moreover it is also likely to be the basis for the prolonged sensory neuron activation seen with low pH solutions and for the enhanced responsiveness of mechanosensitive afferent fibers [99]. It is likely that protons activate nociceptors by acting on the external membrane surface but activation by CO_2 application was abolished by carbonic anhydrase inhibition suggesting that activation by the intracellular generation of protons is also possible [99].

Several characteristics of the prolonged increase in membrane permeability produced by protons are shared by capsaicin, but not by other sensory neuron activators such as GABA or ATP [9]. Capsaicin, an exogenous chemical, is a major pungent principle in

Capsicum peppers. It is distinguished by its highly specific action on polymodal nociceptors and heat sensitive sensory neurons [28]. Thus like protons, capsaicin activates nociceptors to elicit a sensation of burning pain but later provokes a secondary hyperalgesia in the surrounding tissue due to a sensitization of central nociceptive mechanisms [54]. Afferent fiber activation also results in autonomic effects either through reflex actions on the viscera, *via* the release of neuropeptides and other transmitters, or *via* the release of substances from leaky microvessels following the induction of plasma protein extravasation [61]. Capsaicin interacts with a specific membrane receptor indicated by earlier structure-activity studies and more recently by the competitive antagonist, capsazepine [6, 26].

The presence of an ion channel in sensory neurons, permeable to both monovalent and divalent cations and which is uniquely sensitive to capsaicin-receptor activation, suggests that this channel may be operated by an endogenous ligand. So far no endogenous capsaicin-like molecule has been identified, but the sustained proton evoked membrane permeability change shows a striking similarity to that evoked by capsaicin [5]. Furthermore responsiveness to both agents is controlled by nerve growth factor (NGF) [8]. Although protons appear to activate the capsaicin operated ion channel, the binding site for protons and capsaicin differ as capsazepine has no effect on proton-induced activation [7, 30]. On the other hand, proton-induced neuropeptide release from visceral sensory neurons (heart, trachea) is inhibited by capsazepine [58, 94] suggesting that the activation mechanism of these cells may be different from somatic sensory neurons. Finally a number of second messengers can be generated by capsaicin in sensory neurons (arachidonic acid, DAG) although this is thought to be secondary to increasing calcium permeability and a rise in intracellular free calcium [114].

Sensory neurogenic factors

The release of neuropeptides from the peripheral endings of sensory nerves has been well characterised. An important function here is related to efferent or trophic activities (reviewed by Holzer [50]). However a more extensive function in the regulation of immune cells activity has also been proposed [112].

A number of sensory neuropeptides have an important role in neurogenic inflammation and the accompanying hyperalgesia. During inflammation sprouting of peripheral fibers occurs with an increase in their content of neuropeptide. There is some evidence that NGF is an important stimulus for increasing the synthesis of specific sensory neuropeptides [27] as NGF is also increased in inflammatory conditions (*see* later). During inflammation many fibers also show a coexistence of SP and CGRP and these fibers can often be seen in close proximity to immune cells, particularly macrophages and mast cells [112]. Substance P, NKA and CGRP also induce hyperalgesia upon repeated injection [76]. It is not clear whether this results from indirect actions *via* sympathetic nerve fibers or the vasculature. However the release of substance P can stimulate NO synthesis from vascular endothelium, thereby causing vasodilation. In addition SP-induced contraction of endothelial cells induces plasma extravasation, *via* a specific receptor action [3]. This allows substances such as bradykinin, ATP, 5HT, histamine and blood cells such macrophages and monocytes access to sites of tissue injury and to afferent nerve terminals. Substance P may also degranulate mast cell allowing the release of other inflammatory mediators, particularly histamine and proteolytic enzymes which catalyse the production of bradykinin. Interestingly CGRP does not itself produce plasma extravasation but is a powerfull arteriolar vasodilator and thus acts synergistically with substance P by allowing an increased blood flow into venules [11, 39]. Other sensory peptides such as galanin and somatostatin may lessen neurogenic inflammation since they reduce substance P release from sensory fibers [40]. These interactions provide important clues to alternative ways of treating inflammatory diseases for it has been suggested that substance P plays a critic role in the etiology of rheumatoid arthritis [56] in which pain relief can be obtained by injections of somatostatin into the joint [66].

Substance P also contributes to inflammation by recruiting inflammatory cells. There are several aspects to this : stimulation of chemotaxis [62], enhancement of lymphocyte proliferation [81], stimulation of macrophages and monocytes [12, 109]. Indeed lymph organs are innervated by capsaicin sensitive afferent fibers containing substance P and CGRP [83, 111].

Nitric oxide (NO)

Several important mediators of inflammatory hyperalgesia, including substance P and bradykinin stimulate vascular endothelial cells to release the vasodilator, nitric oxide. NO is a readily diffusable but unstable molecule which is considered to be important in intercellular communication in peripheral tissue and in the nervous system, including nociceptive pathways. Nitric oxide is formed from l-arginine following the activation of nitric oxide synthase (NOS) by calcium and other co-factors. NO then alters cellular processes mainly *via* the activation of guanylate cyclase and the production of cGMP [73].

Many types of sensory neurons are able to make NO, but increased cGMP has been seen only in satellite cells in the DRG following stimulation with an NO donor such as nitroprusside [75]. Indeed at present there is little evidence for direct activation of sensory neurons by NO [68]; but NO can indirectly affect their excitability. Thus the tachyphylaxis to bradykinin seen in cultured sensory neurons can be mimicked by NO donors and prevented by NOS inhibitors [68]. However NO donors have been postulated to activate cerebral sensory fibers directly causing the release of CGRP which then produces vasodilatation *via* guanylate cyclase stimulation [110]. These mechanisms may contribute to migraine and other types of head pain. In addition, systemic administration of L-arginine analogues which are inhibitors of NOS produced antinociceptive activity in neuropathic [71] and chemically-induced pain [46, 74]. In these latter situations it is likely that the effects were mediated centrally by the inhibition of NO-induced activation of NMDA receptors [70]. Paradoxically a number of NOS-inhibitors prevented the peripheral antinociceptive action of acetylcholine and morphine [32, 37].

Presently, it is unclear how NO is involved in peripheral nociception and to what extent it is involved in the actions of bradykinin or substance P in peripheral hyperalgesia and glutamate in central hyperalgesic mechanisms. During inflammation a calcium-independent form of NOS can be induced in macrophages [73] and in microglia while in peripheral nerve injury inducible NOS is seen in many sensory neurons [108]. Further studies are required however to see how the NO that is generated by the inducible form of NOS affects nociception.

Sympathetic neurons

Substance P and other neurokinins produce slow depolarization of postganglionic sympathetic neurons following the stimulation of visceral afferent fibers or distension of hollow organs. These effects are involved in the integration and regulation of visceral reflexes but can also be evoked following noxious stimulation of the viscera. In somatic regions similar interactions may be possible and produce local alterations in sympathetic fiber activity. This may alter vascular caliber, induce changes in local blood flow, and indirectly affect plasma extravasation. On the other hand direct interactions of sympathetic nerves or sympathetic transmitters with afferent fibers have not been easy to demonstrate [55] except after peripheral nerve damage or inflammation. However recent studies show that sympathetic nerve stimulation and noradrenaline directly excited some C-fiber afferents after a partially injury to a sensory nerve trunk [94]. Indeed during inflammation, afferent fibers can be sensitized by the release of prostanoids from sympathetic fibers [102]. Sympathetic fibers are also important for plasma extravasation since sympathectomy reduces plasma extravasation induced by noxious stimulation [17, 27]. However both sympathetic transmitters noradrenaline and neuropeptide Y reduced plasma extravasation in the knee joint [44] probably due to an inhibition of neuropeptide release from sensory fibers. Indeed both noradrenaline and NPY have been shown to inhibit calcium permeability and the consequently calcium dependent transmitter release in sensory neurons [34].

Immune cell products

Cytokines

A variety of cytokines (interleukins, interferons, tumor necrosis factor-α) are released by phagocytotic and antigen presenting cells of the immune system. These peptides are important pro-inflammatory agents which influence sensory neurons indirectly *via* products released from other cell types. IL-1β, IL-6 and IL-8 induce a mechanical hyperalgesia [22, 23, 38] which develops over about one hour but the basis for this differs. Thus the hyperalgesia produced by IL-8 but not IL-1β is blocked by β-adrenoceptor and dopamine (D_1) antagonists, and the sympathetic neurone blocking drug, guanethidine suggesting that the effects of IL-8 involve sympathetic nerves [23]. Furthermore, α-melanocyte stimulating hormone and tri-peptides related to Lys-D-Pro-Thr are able to block the effects of IL-1β and IL-6 but not IL-8 induced hyperalgesia [23, 38]. One possibility is that IL-1β and IL-6, but not IL-8, evoke the release of prostaglandins from cells such as mononuclear blood cells and fibroblasts and that the prostaglandins in turn act on the sensory nerves [22, 23, 38].

Tumor necrosis factor (TNF-α) also induces mechanical hyperalgesia which can be attenuated but not abolished by antisera to IL-1, IL-6 and IL-8 [22]. Furthermore the effect of TNF-α was attenuated by Lys-D-Pro-Thr, indomethacin and a β-adrenergic receptor antagonist. Significantly, carrageenin and LPS induced inflammatory hyperalgesia was reduced by TNF-α antiserum suggesting that this cytokine was an important mediator of inflammatory hyperalgesia and that TNF-α production initiated a cascade of other cytokine release.

Opioids

A variety of studies have indicated that exogenous as well as endogenous opioids can act on peripheral nociceptors to produce an antinociceptive effect. This phenomenon is particularly striking when hyperalgesia has been induced by the production of a local inflammation [36, 51, 101]. Indeed inflammation induces an increase in opioid receptors in peripheral cutaneous nerve fibers and opioid peptides are synthesized by immune cells stimulated during inflammation [48, 101]. In addition behavioural studies show that opioids produce analgesia *via* specific interactions with peripheral sensory neurons that have become sensitized following inflammation or exposure to certain inflammatory mediators such as prostanoids [36, 92]. The analgesic effect of opioids may be attributed in part to a decrease in sympathetic fiber activity [104] since postganglionic sympathetic nerve fibers are involved in inflammatory hyperalgesia. Recent studies further indicate that opioids depress excitability in peripheral sensory neurons following a peripheral nerve injury [2]. At the sensory nerve membrane the effects of opioids appear to be exerted in part *via* a receptor-coupled activation of a G-protein and inhibition of adenylate cyclase. The inhibition of neural activity is likely to involve a reduction of membrane calcium conductance and/or increased potassium ion conductance [19, 97].

Vascular factors

Several substances already described in other sections are derived from the vasculature (blood and endothelium) following injury to blood vessels or after the extravasation of blood-born cells, proteins and neuroactive chemicals during inflammation. Amongst these factors are products of mast cell degranulation or platelet activation, *e.g.* histamine, serotonin, ATP ; products derived from monocytes and macrophages (nitric oxide, cytokines) ; plasma proteins such as kininogens (kinin precursors) or small molecular weight factors such as bradykinin, sympathomimetics and NO.

Neurotrophic factors (neurotrophins)

Nerve growth factor (NGF) has been the most extensively characterized of the neurotrophic factors produced by a range of cell types (*e.g.*, fibroblasts, Schwann cells) and peripheral target tissues [57]. NGF and other neurotrophic factors act on a specific membrane receptor. In sensory neurons this is mainly trk-A, that belongs to the tyrosine kinase (trk) family of receptors. Following activation the NGF-receptor complex is transported to the cell body where gene transcription is altered by activation of specific transcription factors such as Oct-2 [115]. NGF is essential for the survival of sensory and sympathetic neurons in the early stages of development, but is no longer required for survival of adult neurons. In addition NGF promotes the differentiation of developing neurons and treatment of neonatal animals with anti-NGF prevents the differentiation of Aδ fibers into high threshold mechanoreceptors [57]. In adults however NGF regulates gene expression and the encoding of a number of important cellular proteins. Thus the presence of NGF produces an increased of mRNA and corresponding synthesis, axoplasmic transport and neuronal content of substance P and CGRP [27]. Furthermore NGF regulates a number of other sensory neuron proteins such as the capsaicin receptor [114], the proton activated ion channel and the TTX resistant Na^+ channel. In each case, NGF promotes the expression while removal of NGF produces a reduction or complete loss of the receptor or channel activity. NGF may be one of a number of factors which promotes axonal sprouting at the periphery thereby increasing the receptive field of sensory neurons [25]. If a similar phenomenon occurred at the central terminals of nociceptive neurons it would provide an explanation for an increased strength of synaptic interaction between sensory and dorsal horn neurons observed during NGF induced hyperalgesia.

Besides its normal physiological role in maintaining sensory neuronal phenotype NGF is important in the pathophysiology of inflammatory pain. Thus NGF levels are elevated in blister fluid, in pleurisy, in keratinocytes after skin injury with UV irradiation and in the synovial fluid from patients with rheumatoid arthritis [1]. NGF may therefore induce the increased chemosensitvity, exaggerated responsiveness and synaptic efficacy seen during inflammatory hyperalgesia. This would be consistent with studies showing that injection of NGF produces increased sensitivity to noxious stimuli while animals exposed to anti-NGF antibodies have a reduced response to painful and inflammatory stimuli [57].

There is an important interplay between nerves, invading inflammatory cells as well as resident tissues cells at sites of tissue damage in which NGF also plays a critical role. Thus NGF promotes the differentiation of eosinophils, basophils and mast cells. It also stimulates IgM secretion from b-lymphocytes and the release of histamine as well as the lipid mediators (LTC_4) from human basophils. On the other hand the synthesis of NGF is stimulated by cytokines such as IL- 1β and TNF-α which are produced during inflammation and the production of these and other cytokines is, in turn, upregulated by substance P released from the sensory nerves [86]. Thus, NGF initates a cascade of events, triggering interactions between neuropeptides, cytokines and immune cells in chronic inflammation.

In addition to the long term effects of NGF on sensory neurons which are mediated by changes in gene expression, shorter term hyperalgesic effects have also been described. For example an amino terminal octapeptide, cleaved from NGF by an endogenous endopeptidase, has been thought responsible for a rapidly occurring mechanical hyperalgesia following NGF. The basis for this hyperalgesia is unclear, although an interaction between sensory and sympathetic nerves appeared likely [103]. More recently NGF has been shown to produce a rapid thermal hyperalgesia due to the release of bradykinin or 5HT following mast cell degranulation [91]. The importance of these effects is not clear at present since they were produced following the administration of large amounts of NGF, likely to be far in excess of the concentrations found in inflammed tissues.

Conclusions

It is difficult to over-emphasize the importance of the chemical environment for the activity of sensory neurons. These neurons appear to be uniquely equipped with an array of receptors coupled to biochemical processes which have also been found in other sensory systems. This would allow cells to respond to changes of the chemical environment occurring during normal physiological processes. There is also provision for flexibility including long-term changes in sensitivity and activity. These are provided by changes in gene expression; usually determined by trophic and growth factors which are secreted from target tissues or other supporting cell. However there is an added dimension to the activity of fine peripheral fibers exhibited during adverse conditions such as inflammation and tissue injury in which afferent and efferent capability is increased. This is manifested in two ways; the triggering of adaptive processes to increase the sensitivity for detection and amplification of potentially adverse signals and the adjustment of cellular neurochemistry to boost the signalling capability and interactions with surrounding tissues. These processes can thus be viewed as both reactive (to exogenous stimuli) and interactive since there is a dynamic chemical exchange between secretions produced by the "afferent" neuron and those chemical signals that surrounding (or circulating) tissues generate.

To date we have a rather simplistic image of the environment of the sensory nerve terminal during inflammation in which it may be bathed by a "soup " of chemical mediators from whose ingredients it can "taste" at any given moment. Clearly it would be helpfull to know the concentrations of various factors generated during inflammation. It may also be the case that the presentation of chemicals to the nerve terminal is highly organised. Indeed interactions between different kinds of tissues (immune cells, sympathetic nerve varicosities) and sensory nerve terminals are likely to be diverse but highly regulated. For instance chemo-attractive factors, specific activation and deactivation of cellular adhesion molecules as well as the time dependent migration of cells might occur. Signalling by certain cell types and specific chemicals might also occur at specific loci (hot spots) on the nerve terminal which may themselves be undergoing structural modifications, *e.g.* sprouting or repair. Indeed areas of membrance specialization occur outside the Schwann cell envelope of fine nerve terminals [49]. These features may allow sensory nerve terminals to integrate signals since it is conceivable that many interactions would be occurring simultaneously at different sites on the same terminal or at one of the branches. In addition chemosensitive afferents are likely to be heterogeneity both in terms of their function (efferent/afferent) and biochemistry sensitivity. Presently we are hampered by methodological limitations to address some of these issues. It is clear however that the multitude of chemical entities undergo molecular interactions *via* an equally large number of receptors but which are coupled with a limited repertoir of other cellular regulatory intermediates that have also been found in many other types of cell.

References

1. Aloe L, Tuveri MA, Carcassi U, Levi-Montalcini R. Nerve growth factor in the synovial fluid of patients with chronic arthritis. *Arthritis Rheum* 1992 ; 35 : 351-5.
2. Andreev N, Urban K, Dray A. Opioids suppress activity of polymodal nociceptors in rat paw skin induced by ultraviolet irradiation. *Neuroscience* 1994 ; 58 : 793-8.
3. Andrews PV, Helm RD, Thomas KL. NK1 receptor mediation of neurogenic plasma extravasation in the rat skin. *Br J Pharmacol* 1989 ; 97 : 1232-8.
4. Beck PW, Handwerker HO. Bradykinin and serotonin effects on various types of cutaneous nerve fibers. *Pflugers Arch* 1974 ; 347 : 209-22.
5. Bevan S, Forbes CA, Winter J. Protons and capsaicin activate the same ion channels in rat isolated dorsal root ganglion neurons. *J Physiol* 1993 ; 459 : 401.
6. Bevan S, Hothi S, Hughes G, James IF, Rang HP, Shah K, Walpole CSJ, Yeats JC. Capsazepine : a competitive antagonist of the sensory neurone excitant capsaicin. *Br J Pharmacol* 1992 ; 197 : 544-52.
7. Bevan S, Rang HP, Shah K. Capsazepine does not block the proton induced activation of rat sensory neurons. *Br J Pharmacol* 1992 ; 107 : 235.
8. Bevan S, Szolcsanyi J. Sensory neuron-specific actions of capsaicin : mechanisms and applications. *TIPS* 1990 ; 11 : 330-3.
9. Bevan S, Yeats J. Protons activate a cation conductance in a subpopulation of rat dorsal root ganglion neurons. *J Physiol* 1991 ; 433 : 145-61.
10. Birrell GJ, McQueen DS, Iggo A, Coleman RA, Grubb BD. PGI_2 induced activation and sensitization of articular mechanonociceptors. *Neurosci Lett* 1991 ; 124 : 5-8.

11. Brain SD, Williams TJ. Inflammatory oedema induced by synergism between calcitonin gene related peptide and mediators of increased vascular permeability. *Br J Pharmacol* 1985 ; 86 : 855-60.
12. Brunelleschi S, Vanni L, Ledda F, Giotti A, Maggi CA, Fantozzi R. Tachykinins activate guinea-pig alveolar macrophages : involvement of NK-2 and NK-l receptors. *Br J Pharmacol* 1990 ; 100 : 417-20.
13. Burch RM, Kyle DJ. Recent developments in the understanding of bradykinin receptors. *Life Sci* 1992 ; 50 : 829-38.
14. Burgess GM, Mullaney J, McNeil M, Dunn P, Rang HP. Second messengers involved in the action of bradykinin on cultured sensory neurons. *J Neurosci* 1989 ; 9 : 3314-25.
15. Burgess GM, Mullaney I, McNeill M, Coote PR, Minhas A, Wood JN. Activation of guanylate cyclase by bradykinin in rat sensory neurones is mediated by calcium influx : possible role of the increase in cyclic GMP. *Neurochem* 1989 ; 53 : 1212-8.
16. Christian EP, Taylor GE, Weinreich D. Serotonin increases excitability of rabbit C-fiber neurons by two distinct mechanisms. *J Appl Physiol* 1989 ; 67 : 584-91.
17. Coderre TJ, Basbaum AI, Levin JD. Neural control of vascular permeability; interaction between primary afferents, mast cells, and sympathetic efferents. *J Neurophysiol* 1989 ; 62 : 48-58.
18. Corbe SM, Poole-Wilson PA. The time of onset and severity of acidosis in myocardial ischaemia. *J Mol Cell Cardiol* 1980 ; 12 : 745-60.
19. Crain SM, Shen KF. Opioids can evoke direct receptor-mediated excitatory effects on sensory neurons. *TIPS* 1990 ; 11 : 77-81.
20. Crook ST, Mattern M, Sarau HM, Winkler JD, Balcarek J, Wong A, Bennett FC. The signal transduction system of the leukotriene D_4 receptor. *TIPS* 1989 ; 10 : 103-7.
21. Crunkhorn P, Willis AL. Cutaneous reaction to intradermal prostaglandins. *Br J Pharmacol* 1971 ; 41 : 49-56.
22. Cunha FQ, Poole S, Lorenzetti BB, Ferreira SH. The pivotal role of tumor necrosis factor α in the development of inflammatory hyperalgesia. *Br J Pharmacol* 1992 ; 107 : 660-4.
23. Cunha FQ, Lorenzetti BB, Poole S, Ferreira SH. Interleukin-8 as a mediator of sympathetic pain. *Br JPharmacol* 1991 ; 104 : 765-7.
24. Davies A. Cell death and the trophic requirements of developing sensory neurons. In : Scott SA ed. *Sensory neurons : diversity, development and plasticity*. New York : Oxford University Press, 1991 : 194-214.
25. Diamond J, Holmes M, Coughlin M. Endogenous NGF and nerve impulses regulate the collateral sprouting of sensory axons in the skin of the adult rat. *J Neurosci* 1992 ; 12 : 1454-66.
26. Dickenson AH, Dray A. Selective antagonism of capsaicin by capsazepine : evidence for a spinal receptor site in capsaicin-induced antinociception. *Br J Pharmacol* 1991 ; 104 : 1045- 9.
27. Donnerer J, Schuligoi R, Stein C. Increased content and transport of substance P and calcitonin gene-related peptide in sensory nerves innervating inflamed tissue : evidence for a regulatory function of nerve growth factor *in vivo*. *Neuroscience* 1992 ; 49 : 693-8.
28. Dray A. Neuropharmacological mechanisms of capsaicin and related substances. *Biochem Pharmacol* 1992 ; 44 : 611-5.
29. Dray A, Perkins M. Bradykinin and inflammatory pain. *TINS* 1993 ; 16 : 99-104.
30. Dray A, Patel I, Naeem S, Rueff A, Urban L. Studies with capsazepine on peripheral nociceptor activation by capsaicin and low pH : evidence for a dual effect of capsaicin. *Br J Pharmacol* 1992 ; 107 : 236
31. Dray A, Patel IA, Perkins MN, Rueff A. Bradykinin-induced activation of nociceptors: receptor and mechanistic studies on the neonatal rat spinal cord-tail preparation *in vitro*. *Br J Pharmacol* 1992 ; 107 : 1129-34.
32. Duarte IDG, Lorenzetti BB, Ferreira SH. Peripheral analgesia and activation of the nitric oxide-cyclic GMP pathway. *Eur J Pharmacol* 1990 ; 186 : 289-93.

33. Eschalier A, Kayser V, Guilbaud G. Influence of specific 5-HT_3 antagonists on carageenan-induced hyperalgesia in the rat. *Pain* 1989 ; 36 : 249-55.
34. Ewald DA, Matthies JG, Perney TM, Walker MW, Miller RJ. The effect of down regulation of protein kinase C on the inhibition of dorsal root ganglion neuron Ca^{2+} currents by neuropeptide Y. *J Neurosci* 1988 ; 8 : 2447-51.
35. Farmer SG, Burch RM. Biochemical and molecular pharmacology of kinin receptors. *Annu Rev Pharmacol* 1992 ; 32 : 511-36.
36. Ferreira SH, Nakamura M. Prostaglandin hyperalgesia : the peripheral analgesic activity of morphine, enkephalin and opioid-antagonists. *Prostaglandins* 1979 ; 18 : 191-200.
37. Ferreira SH, Duarte IDG, Lorenzetti BB. The molecular mechanism of action of morphine analgesia : stimulation of the cGMP system via nitric oxide. *Eur J Pharmacol* 1991 ; 201 : 121-2.
38. Ferreira SH, Lorenzetti BB, Bristow AF, Poole S. Interleukin 1β as a potent hyperalgesic agent antagonized by a tripeptide analogue. *Nature* 1988 ; 334 : 698-700.
39. Gamse R, Saria A. Potentiation of tachykinin-induced plasma protein extravasation by calcitonin gene-related peptide. *Eur J Pharmacol* 1985 ; 114 : 61-6.
40. Gazelius B, Brodin E, Olgart L, Panopoulos P. Evidence that substance P is a mediator of antidromic vasodilatation using somatostatin as a release inhibitor. *Acta Phys Scand* 1981 ; 113 : 155-9.
41. Geppetti P, Tramontana M, Santicolli P, Del Bianco E, Giulani S, Maggi CA. Bradykinin-induced release of CGRP from capsaicin-sensitive nerves in guinea-pig atria : mechanism of action and calcium requirements. *Neuroscience* 1990 ; 38 : 687-92.
42. Glaum SR, Proudfit HK, Anderson EG. 5-HT_3 receptors modulate spinal nociceptive reflexes. *Brain Res* 1990 ; 510 : 12-6.
43. Goldstein RH, Wall M. Activation of protein formation and cell division by bradykinin and des-Arg^9-bradykinin. *J Biol Chem* 1984 ; 259 : 9263-8.
44. Green PG, Luo J, Heller P, Levine JD. Modulation of bradykinin-induced plasma extravasation in the rat knee joint by sympathetic co-transmitters. *Neuroscience* 1993 ; 52 : 451-8.
45. Habler HJ, JanigW, Kolzenburg M. Activation of unmyelinated afferent fibers by mechanical stimuli and inflammation of the urinary bladder in the cat. *J Physiol* 1990 ; 425 : 545-62.
46. Haley JA *et al*. Electrophysiological approaches to the study of bradykinin and nitric oxide in inflammatory pain. *Agents Actions* 1992 ; Suppl. 38 : 358-65.
47. Handwerker HO, Kilo S, Reeh PW. Unresponsive afferent nerve fibers in the sural nerve of the rat. *J Physiol* 1991 ; 435 : 229-42.
48. Hassan AHS, Ableiter A, Stein C, Herz A. Inflammation of the rat paw enhances axonal transport of opioid receptors in the sciatic nerve and increases their density in the inflamed tissue. *Neuroscience* 1993 ; 55 : 185-95.
49. Hepplemann B, Messlinger K, Neiss WF, Schmidt RF. Ultrastructural three-dimensional reconstruction of Group III and Group IV sensory nerve endings ("Free nerve endings") in the knee joint capsaule of the cat : evidence for multiple receptive sites. *J Comp Neurol* 1990 ; 292 : 103-16.
50. Holzer P. Local effector functions of capsaicin-sensitive sensory nerve endings : involvement of tachykinins, calcitonin gene-related peptide, and other neuropeptides. *Neuroscience* 1988 ; 24 : 739-68.
51. Joris J, Costello A, Dubner R, Hargreaves KM. Opiates suppress carrageenan-induced edema and hyperthermia at doses that inhibit hyperalgesia. *Pain* 1990 ; 43 : 95-103.
52. Kessler W, Kirchoff C, Reeh PW, Handwerker HO. Excitation of cutaneous afferent nerve endings *in vitro* by a combination of inflammatory mediators and conditiong effect of substance P. *Exp Brain Res* 1992 ; 91 : 467-76.

53. Kolzenburg M, Kress M, Reeh PW. The nociceptor sensitization by bradykinin does not depend on sympathetic neurons. *Neuroscience* 1992 ; 46 : 465-73.
54. LaMotte RH, Lundberg LER, Torebjork HE. Pain, hyperalgesia and activity in nociceptive C units in humans after intradermal injection of capsaicin. *J Physiol* 1992 ; 448 : 749-64.
55. Lang E, Nowak A, Reeh P, Handwerker HO. Chemosensitivity of fine afferents from rat skin *in vitro. J Neurophysiol* 1990 ; 63 : 887-901.
56. Levine JD, Lam D, Taiwo YO, Donatoni P, Goetzl EJ. Hyperalgesic properties of 15-lipoxygenase products of arachidonic acid. *Proc Nat Acad Sci USA* 1986 ; 83 : 5331-4.
57. Lewin GR, Mendell LM. Nerve growth factor and nociception. *TINS* 1993 ; 16 : 353-8.
58. Lou YP, Lundberg JM. Inhibition of low pH evoked activation of airway sensory nerves by capsazepine, a novel capsaicin-receptor antagonist. *Biochem Biophys Res Comm* 1992 ; 189 : 537-44.
59. Maggi CA. Capsaicin and primary afferent neurons : from basic science to human therapy ? *J Auton Nerv Syst* 1991 ; 33 : 1-14.
60. Maggi CA, Meli A. The sensory-efferent function of capsaicin-sensitive neurons. *Gen Pharrnacol* 1988 ; 19 : 1-43.
61. Maggi CA, Patacchini R, Rovero P, Giachetti A. Tachykinin receptors and tachykinin receptor antagonists . *J Auton Pharmacol* 1992 ; 13 : 23-93.
62. Marasco WA, Showell HL, Becker EL. Substance P binds to formyl peptide chemotaxis receptor on the rabbit neutrophil. *Biochem Biophys Res Commun* 1981 ; 99 : 1065-72.
63. Maricq AV, Peterson AS, Brake AJ, Meyers RM, Julius D. Primary structure and functional expression of the $5HT_3$ receptor, a serotonin-gated ion channel. *Science* 1991 ; 254 : 432-7.
64. Martin HA. Leukotriene B_4 induced decrease in mechanical and thermal thresholds of C-fiber mechanociceptors in rat hairy skin. *Brain Res* 1990 ; 509 : 273-9.
65. Martin HA, Basbaum AI, Kwiat GC, Goetzl EJ, Levine JD. Leukotriene and prostaglandin sensitization of cutaneous high threshold C- and A-delta mechanoreceptors in the hairy skin of rat hindlimbs. *Neuroscience* 1987 ; 22 : 651-9.
66. Matucci C, Marabini S. Somatostatin treatment for pain in rheumatoid arthritis : a double blind versus placebo study in knee involvement. *Med Sci Res* 1988 ; 16 : 223-34.
67. McFadden RG, Vickers KE. Bradykinin augments the *in vitro* migration of nonsensitized lymphocytes. *Clin Invest Med* 1989 ; 12 : 247-53.
68. McGehee DS, Goy MF, Oxford GS. Involvement of the nitric oxidecyclic GMP pathway in the desensitization of bradykinin responses of cultured rat sensory neurons. *Neuron* 1992 ; 9 : 315-24.
69. McMahon SB. Mechanisms of sympathetic pain. *Br Med Bull* 1991 ; 47 : 584-600.
70. Meller ST, Gebhart GF. Nitric oxide (NO) and nociceptive processing in the spinal cord. *Pain* 1993 ; 52 : 127-36.
71. Meyer RA, Davis KD, Raja SN, Campbell JN. Sympathectomy does not abolish bradykinin induced cutaneous hyperalgesia in man. *Pain* 1992 ; 51 : 323-7.
72. Mizumura K, Sato J, Kumazawa T. Effects of prostaglandins and other putative chemical intermediaries on the activity of canine testicular polymodal receptors studied *in vitro. Pflugers Arch* 1987 ; 408 : 565-72.
73. Moncada S, Palmer RM, Higgs EA. Nitric Oxide : physiology, pathophysiology, and pharmacology. *Pharmacol Rev* 1991 ; 43 : 109-42.
74. Moore PK, Oluyomi AO, Babbedge P, Wallace P, Hart SL. L-N^G-nitro arginine methyl ester exhibits antinociceptive activity in the mouse. *Br J Pharmacol* 1991 ; 102 : 198-202.
75. Morris R, Southam E, Braid DJ, Garthwaite J. Nitric oxide may act as a messenger between dorsal root ganglion neurones and their satellite cells. *Neurosci Lett* 1992 ; 137 : 29-32.
76. Nakamura-Craig M, Gill BK. Effect of neurokinin A, substance P and calcitonin gene related peptide in peripheral hyperalgesia in the rat paw. *Neurosci Lett* 1991 ; 124 : 49-51.

77. Neugebauer V, Schaible HG, Schmidt RF. Sensitization of articular afferents for mechanical stimuli by bradykinin. *Pflugers Arch* 1989 ; 415 : 330-5.
78. Nicol GD, Klingberg DK, Vasko MR. Prostaglandin E_2 increases calcium conductance and stimulates release of substance P in avian sensory neurons. *J Neurosci* 1992 ; 12 : 1917-27.
79. Nilsson G, Alving K, Ahlstedt S, Hokfelt T, Lundberg JM. Peptidergic innervation of rat lymphoid tissue and lung : relation of mast cells and sensitivity to capsaicin ane immunization. *Cell Tissue Res* 1990 ; 262 : 125-33.
80. Nowycky M. Voltage gated ion channels in dorsal root ganglion neurons. In : Scott SA ed. *Sensory neurons : diversity, development and plasticity.* New York : Oxford University Press, 1992.
81. Payan DG, Levine JD, Goetzl EJ. Modulation of immunity and hypersensitivity by sensory neuropeptides. *J Immunol* 1984 ; 132 : 1601-4.
82. Perkins MN, Campbell E, Dray A. Anti-nociceptive activity of the B_1 and B_2 receptor antagonists desArg^{9}Leu^{8}Bk and HOE 140, in two models of persistent hyperalgesia in the rat. *Pain* 1993 ; 53 : 191-7.
83. Popper P, Mantyh CR, Vigna SR, Maggios JE, Mantyh PW. The localization of sensory nerve fibers and receptor binding sites for sensory neuropeptides in canine mesenteric lymph nodes. *Peptides* 1988 ; 9 : 257-67.
84. Puttick RM. Excitatory action of prostaglandin E_2 on rat neonatal cultured dorsal root ganglion cells. *Br J Pharmacol* 1992 ; 105 : 133.
85. Rackham A, Ford-Hutchinson AW. Inflammation and pain sensitivity : effects of leukotrienes D_4, B_4 and prostaglandin E_1 in the rat paw. *Prostaglandins* 1983 ; 25 : 193-203.
86. Rang HP, Bevan S, Dray A. Chemical activation of nociceptive peripheral neurons. *Br Med Bull* 1991 ; 47 : 534-8.
87. Richardson BP, Engel G, Donatsch P, Stadler PA. Identification of serotonin M-receptor subtypes and their specific blockade by a new class of drugs. *Nature* 1985 ; 316 : 126-31.
88. Robertson B, Bevan S. Properties of 5-hydroxytrypatamine$_3$ receptorgated currents in adult dorsal root ganglion neurones. *Br J Pharmacol* 1991 ; 102 : 272-6.
89. Rueff A, Dray A. 5-Hydroxytryptamine-induced sensitization and activation of peripheral fibers in the neonatal rat are mediated via different 5-hydroxytryptamine-receptors. *Neuroscience* 1992 ; 50 : 899-905.
90. Rueff A, Dray A. Sensitization of peripheral afferent fibers in the *in vitro* neonatal rat spinal cord-tail by bradykinin and prostaglandins. *Neuroscience* 1993 ; 54 : 527-35.
91. Rueff A, Lewin GR, Mendell LM. Peripheral and central mechanisms of NGF-induced hyperalgesia. *Soc Neurosci* 1993 ; 643-2 : 1563 (Abstract).
92. Russell N, Jamieson A, Callen T, Rance M. Peripheral opioid effects upon neurogenic plasma extravasation and inflammation. *Br J Pharmacol* 1985 ; 86 : 788.
93. Santicioli P, Del Bianco E, Giachetti AM, Maggi CA. Capsazepine inhibits low pH-and capsaicin-induced release of calcitonin gene-related peptide (CGRP) from rat soleus muscle. *Br J Pharmacol* 1992 ; 107 : 464
94. Sato J, Perl ER. Adrenergic excitation of cutaneous pain receptors induced by peripheral nerve injury. *Science* 1991 ; 251 : 1608-10.
95. Schaible HG, Schmidt RF. Excitation and sensitization of fine articular afferents from cat's knee joint by prostaglandin E_2 *J Physiol* 1988 ; 403 : 91-104.
96. Schaible HG, Schmidt RF. Time course of mechanosensitivity changes in articular afferents during a developing experimental arthritis. *J Neurophysiol* 1988 ; 60 : 2180-95.
97. Shen KF, Crain SM. Dynorphin prolongs the action potential of mouse sensory ganglion neurons by decreasing a potassium conductance whereas another specific kappa opioid does so by increasing a calcium conductance. *Neuropharmacol* 1990 ; 29 : 343-9.

98. Shepherd GM. Sensory transduction : entering the mainstream of membrane signaling. *Cell* 1991 ; 67 : 845-51.
99. Steen KH, Reeh PW, Anton F, Handwerker HO. Protons selectively induce lasting excitation and sensitization to mechanical stimuli of nociceptors in rat skin, *in vivo. J Neurosci* 1992 ; 12 : 86-95.
100. Stein C. Peripheral analgesic actions of opioids. *Pain Sympt Manag* 1991 ; 6 : 119-24.
101. Stein C, Hassan AHS, Przewlocki R, Gramsch C, Peter K, Herz A. Opioids from immunocytes react with receptors on sensory nerves to inhibit nociception in inflammation. *Proc Natl Acad Sci USA* 1990 ; 87 : 5935-9.
102. Taiwo YO, Levine JD. Characterization of the arachidonic acid metabolite mediating bradykinin and norepinephrine hyperalgesia. *Brain Res* 1988 ; 492 : 397-9.
103. Taiwo YO, Levine JD. Further confirmation of the role of adenyl cyclase and of cAMP-dependent protein kinase in primary afferent hyperalgesia. *Neuroscience* 1991 ; 44 : 131-5.
104. Taiwo YO, Levine JD. κ- and δ-opioids block sympathetically dependent hyperalgesia. *J Neurosci* 1991 ; 11 : 928-32.
105. Taiwo YO, Heller PH, Levine JD. Mediation of serotonin hyperalgesia by the cAMP second messenger system. *Neuroscience* 1992 ; 48 : 479-83.
106. Taiwo YO, Levine JD, Burch RM, Woo JE, Mobley WC. Hyperalgesia induced in the rat by the amino-terminal octapeptide of nerve growth factor. *Proc Natl Acad Sci USA* 1991 ; 88 : 5144-8.
107. Todorovic S, Anderson EG. 5-HT_2 and 5-HT_3 receptors mediate two distinct depolarizing responses in rat dorsal root ganglion neurons. *Brain Res* 1990 ; 511 : 71-9.
108. Verge VMK, Xu Z, Xu XJ, Wiesenfelt-Hallin Z, Hokfelt T. Marked increase in nitric oxide synthase mRNA in rat dorsal root ganglia after peripheral axotomy : in situ hybridization and functional studies. *Proc Natl Acad Sci USA* 1992 ; 89 : 11617-21.
109. Wagner F, Fink T, Hart R, Dancygier H. Substance P enhance interferon γ production of human peripheral blood mononuclear cells. *Regul Pept* 1987 ; 19 : 355-64.
110. Wei P, Moskowitz MA, Boccalini P, Kontos HA. Calcitonin gene-related peptide mediates nitroglycerin and sodium nitroprusside-induced vasodilatation in feline cerebral arterioles. *Circulation Res* 1992 ; 70 : 1313-9.
111. Weihe E, Muller S, Fink T, Zentel HJ. Tachykinins, CGRP and neuropeptide Y in nerves of the mammalian thymus : interactions with mast cells in autonomic and sensory neuroimmunomodulation ? *Neurosci Lett* 1989 ; 100 : 77-82.
112. Weihe E, Nohr D, Muller SD, Buchler M, Friess H, Zentel HJ. The tachykinin neuroimmune connection in inflammatory pain. *Ann NY Acad Sci* 1991 ; 632 : 283-95.
113. Weinreich D, Wonderlin WF. Inhibition of calcium-dependent spike after-hyperpolarization increases excitability of rabbit visceral sensory neurons. *J Physiol* 1987 ; 394 : 415-27.
114. Winter J, Forbes CA, Sternberg J, Lindsay JM. Nerve growth factor (NGF) regulates adult rat culture dorsal root ganglion neuron responsive to the excitatoxin capsaicin. *Neuron* 1988 ; 1 : 973-81.
115. Wood JN, Coote PR, Minhas A, Mullaney I, McNeill M, Burgess GM. Capsaicin-induced ion influxes increase cGMP but not cAMP levels in rat sensory neurones in culture. *J Neurochem* 1989 ; 53 : 1203-11.
116. Wood JN, Lillycrop KA, Dent KL, Ninkina NN, Beech MM, Willoughby JJ, Winter J, Latcham DS. Regulation of expression of the neuronal POU protein Oct-2 by nerve growth factor. *J Biol Chem* 1992 ; 267 : 17787-91.

6

Capsaicin sensitivity of primary sensory neurones and its regulation

G. JANCSÓ, A. AMBRUS

Department of Physiology, Albert Szent-Gyorgyi Medical University, Szeged, Hungary.

The potential of capsaicin as a highly selective sensory neurotoxin has been exploited in exploring the structural and neurochemical traits of a population of primary afferent neurones whose functional significance is now being increasingly recognized. In spite of extensive investigations, the factors which might be involved in the regulation/modulation of neuronal capsaicin sensitivity in vivo are largely unknown. Previous studies have shown that the perineural application of capsaicin results in a selective blockade of the function of C-fiber polymodal nociceptor afferents associated with an inhibition of axonal transport processes and a depletion of specific macromolecules in small primary sensory neurones.

The present paper describes ganglionic and transganglionic changes which commence after perineural capsaicin treatment assessed with the aid of the capsaicin gap technique, and demonstrates the potential of this approach in the detection of cellular processes involved in the regulation/modulation of neuronal capsaicin sensitivity.

Experiments were performed on adult male Wistar rats weighing 200-250 g at the beginning of the study. Initial surgery involving the application of capsaicin or its vehicle onto the right and left sciatic nerves was performed under anaesthesia. Animals were given a single subcutaneous injection of capsaicin 1-120 days later and killed 2-8 hours afterwards. The 5th lumbar dorsal root ganglia and segments $L_2 L_6$ of the spinal cord were removed and processed for light microscopic histological examination.

In lumbar sensory ganglia relating to the control (vehicle-treated) sciatic nerve, quantitative morphological and morphometric analyses revealed substantial numbers of degenerating small neurones at all survival times examined. These nerve cells comprised 14-21% of the total neuronal population in these ganglia. Similar results were obtained in the ganglia 1 day after the ipsilateral sciatic nerve had been treated with capsaicin. In sharp contrast, ganglia relating to the capsaicin-treated nerve contained very low numbers of degenerating neurones at survival times of 4 days or more. These amounted to only 2-5 % of the total neuronal population. A significant decrease in the total neuronal numbers of ganglia relating to the capsaicin-treated sciatic nerve could be detected after long (90 days), but not after short (1-8 days) postoperative survival periods.

In the spinal cord, heavy axon terminal degeneration was demonstrated in the entire medio-lateral aspect of the marginal zone and the substantia gelatinosa ipsilateral to the vehicle-treated nerve at all postoperative times. Ipsilateral to the capsaicin-treated sciatic nerve, the distribution of degeneration argyrophilia was similar 1-8 days postoperatively. However, from the 15th postoperative day on, unstained gaps were detected within the otherwise continuous argyrophilic band of the superficial layers of the dorsal horn. These "capsaicin gaps", which became more prominent after longer survival periods, correspond to the spinal projection regions of the sciatic nerve.

The present findings indicate that perineural treatment with capsaicin resulted in a rapid decrease in the capsaicin sensitivity of sensory ganglion cells. It is suggested that an altered expression of capsaicin binding sites, due to an impairment of intraneuronal transport mechanisms and/or changes in cellular metabolism, leads to changes in neuronal capsaicin sensitivity. In turn, maintenance of axonal transport processes may be critical with respect to the regulation of neuronal capsaicin sensitivity. The results also imply that different systems may operate in the regulation of the perikaryal and axon terminal sensitivity to capsaicin. Further investigations in this line may reveal important clues for an understanding of the molecular basis of neuronal capsaicin sensitivity and its regulation, and may provide new information on the significance of these mechanisms in the response of the nerve cell to injury.

Capsaicin is a highly potent neurotoxin which has proved to be critical in exploration of the structural and functional characteristics of primary sensory neurones [17, 30, 31]. Capsaicin-sensitive ganglion cells form a separate division of the sensory system and are involved in nociceptive, reflex and local regulatory functions of many tissues and organs [16, 26, 35]. Study of the consequences of elimination and/or functional blockade of this particular population of sensory neurones, through utilization of the selective neurotoxic effect of capsaicin, has become the strategy most commonly employed to explore their functional significance [5, 12, 16, 39]. Sensitivity to capsaicin seems to be a common trait of mammalian sensory ganglion cells [24, 39, 40]. However, in spite of extensive investigations, the factors which might be involved in the modulation/regulation of neuronal capsaicin sensitivity *in vivo* remain largely unknown.

Perineural treatment with capsaicin is one of the approaches most frequently used to produce a blockade of capsaicin-sensitive nociceptive afferent fibers. This method has the advantage that its effects are confined to primary sensory neurones whose peripheral branches run in the treated nerve [18, 20]. The actions of capsaicin applied directly onto a peripheral nerve involve a substantial reduction in the nociceptive responses evoked by chemical irritants and heat, and a complete abolition of the neurogenic inflammatory response. These changes have proved to be dose-dependent and apparently permanent [9, 18, 24, 25]. Electrophysiological studies extended these observations and indicated that the perineural application of capsaicin may be regarded as a specific chemodenervation technique which produces a permanent and selective loss and/or blockade of C-fiber polymodal nociceptor afferents [6, 41, 45]. Additionally, the marked alterations observed in the functional properties of spinal and medullary dorsal horn neurones provide evidence of significant central changes following perineural capsaicin treatment [10, 36].

These functional alterations are accompanied by marked changes in the chemistry of the primary sensory neurones. Histochemical and biochemical investigations have revealed a marked depletion of peptides and other sensory neurone-specific macromolecules from the central terminals and the perikarya of small sensory ganglion neurones [13, 15, 27]. Although these findings indicated profound changes in the chemistry of the primary sensory neurones, they yielded little information on the nature of these changes. In particular, it is unclear whether these changes are associated with an irreversible structural impairment of primary afferent terminals or merely reflect a depletion of these peptides and proteins from these neurones.

A salient feature of the structural changes accompanying peripheral nerve damage involving all classes of afferent fibers is a delayed degeneration of the central terminals of myelinated primary afferents [2, 4, 28]. Efforts to demonstrate similar transganglionic degenerative changes in unmyelinated C-fiber primary afferents remained unsuccessful [2, 28]. In an attempt to reveal possible morphological alterations in C-fiber primary sensory neurones in response to perineural capsaicin treatment, we have recently developed a new experimental approach, termed the capsaicin gap technique, which permits the recognition of previously undetected structural changes in C-fiber dorsal root ganglion neurones after peripheral nerve injury [23, 28, 29].

The present report deals with the ganglionic and transganglionic changes which commence after perineural capsaicin treatment, assessed with the aid of the capsaicin gap technique, and demonstrates the potential of this approach in the detection of cellular processes involved in the regulation/modulation of neuronal capsaicin sensitivity.

Materials and methods

The "capsaicin gap" technique

This technique relies firstly on the fact that peripheral nerves are represented in a strict somatotopic manner in the spinal dorsal horn [38, 42, 44], and secondly, on the selective neurodegenerative action of capsaicin. Systemic administration of capsaicin to adult rats results in a selective, rapid degeneration of a subpopulation of primary sensory neurones with unmyelinated axons whose degenerating central terminals can be detected with silver impregnation techniques in the superficial laminae of the spinal dorsal horn [22, 24]. This phenomenon provides a reliable method of examination of the topographical distribution of capsaicin-sensitive C-fiber primary afferent terminals within the spinal dorsal horn [29]. The principle of the capsaicin gap technique is illustrated in Figure 1. It was assumed that ipsilateral to the control nerve all the capsaicin-sensitive primary afferent terminals undergo degeneration after a systemic injection of capsaicin. We surmised that if prior treatment of a peripheral nerve with capsaicin resulted in an irreversible destruction of primary afferent terminals, including those which undergo degeneration after a systemic administration of capsaicin, then the spinal projection regions of that particular nerve would be free of degeneration following a subsequent systemic injection of capsaicin. Accordingly, somatotopically related regions served by the treated nerve would appear as prominent unstained gaps within the heavy argyrophilic band in the superficial dorsal horn formed by degenerating axonal endings confined to the marginal zone and the substantia gelatinosa.

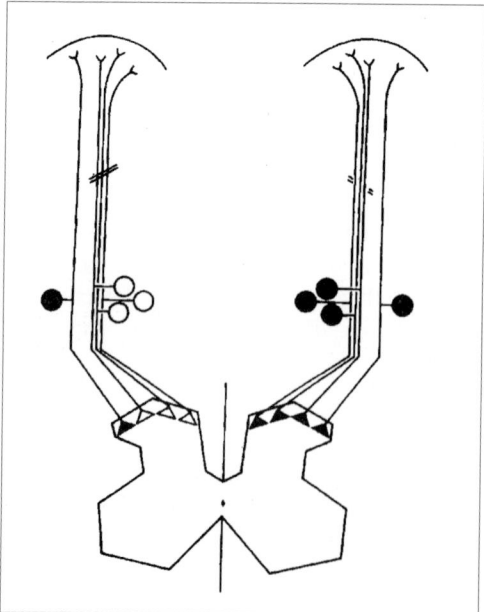

Figure 1. This scheme illustrates the principle of the capsaicin gap technique. It shows the capsaicin-sensitive small dorsal root ganglion neurones and the topographical arrangement of their central projections in the superficial spinal dorsal horn. Open and filled symbols represent intact and degenerating ganglion cells or axon terminals, respectively. The sites of treatment with capsaicin and its vehicle are indicated by continuous and interrupted parallel bars, respectively. For further explanation, see the text.

To test this hypothesis, experiments were performed on adult male rats weighing 200-250 g at the beginning of the study. Both sciatic nerves were exposed in the thigh under anaesthesia and one nerve was treated with capsaicin (50 μl of a 1 % solution) while the other nerve was treated with its vehicle. Sixty to ninety days later, the animals were anaesthetized again and given a systemic injection of capsaicin (100 mg/kg, subcutaneously) 7-8 hours prior to sacrifice. The rats were perfused transcardially with 10% formalin, and the fifth lumbar dorsal root ganglia, up to 85 per cent of the neuronal population of which consists of cell bodies giving rise to afferent fibers running within the sciatic nerve [3, 47], and segments L_2-L_6 of the spinal cord were removed for histological examination. Serial sections of 4 μm in thickness were cut from each ganglion and stained with Methylene Blue. Normal and degenerating neurones which exhibited a clear-cut nucleolus were counted separately in every section taken at a regular interval of 80 μm throughout the ganglion. Increased basophilia of the cytoplasm and of the pyknotic nucleus, and heavy vacuolization of the perikaryon, were used as the criteria for defining degenerating neurones. The number of nucleoli was converted to the number of ganglion cells according to formula 4 of Königsmark [34] and the actual number of neurones in the ganglion was calculated. In the spinal cord, axon terminal degeneration was demonstrated with silver impregnation techniques [8, 11].

Results and discussion

Transganglionic degenerative changes in C-fiber primary afferents

The distribution pattern of degeneration argyrophilia demonstrated with silver impregnation techniques was studied in transverse sections cut from the spinal cord. Ipsilateral to the vehicle-treated nerve, degenerating axon terminals formed a continuous argyrophilic band extending throughout the entire medio-lateral aspect of the marginal zone and the substantia gelatinosa (Figure 2A). However, ipsilateral to the capsaicin-treated nerve, prominent unstained gaps were seen within this strongly argyrophilic band of the superficial dorsal horn (Figure 2B). These gaps correspond to the known projection regions of the sciatic nerve [7, 38, 42].

In earlier studies we have shown that in adult animals, including rats, many neurones in sensory ganglia undergo a rapid degeneration process following a systemic injection of capsaicin [22, 24, 29]. These degenerating neurons can be reliably identified in semithin sections under the light microscope : they display increased nuclear and cytoplasmic basophilia and severe cytoplasmic vacuolization.

Two quantitative procedures were utilized to detect long-term ganglionic changes 60-90 days after perineural treatment with capsaicin. First, the total numbers of nerve cells were determined in the ganglia relating to the capsaicin or vehicle-treated nerves. Second, the proportion of degenerating neurones was estimated in these ganglia 2-3 hours after a systemic injection of capsaicin. In addition, size-frequency distribution histograms of sensory neurones were generated by measuring their sizes by means of a light microscope equipped with a camera lucida and a digitizing tablet connected to a computerized system.

In ganglia relating to the vehicle-treated sciatic nerves, a substantial proportion of the neurones (comprising up to 21 per cent of the total ganglion cell population) exhibited degenerative alterations following a systemic injection of capsaicin. Size-frequency distribution histograms showed that the degenerating ganglion cells belong exclusively to the population of small neurones (Figure 3A). In contrast, in ganglia relating to the capsaicin-treated nerves, the small cells which displayed degenerative changes comprised only 2-4 per cent of all neurones (Figure 3B, Table I). Examination of the size-frequency distribution histograms indicated an overall reduction in the proportion of small neurones of ganglia relating to the capsaicin-treated nerves. In accord with this latter finding, the quantitative data revealed a substantial decrease in the number of neurones in these ganglia (Table I). It is to be emphasized that capsaicin treatment resulted in a selective loss of small neurones, unlike other types of peripheral nerve lesions, which cause an indiscriminate loss of ganglion cells of all sizes [2, 28].

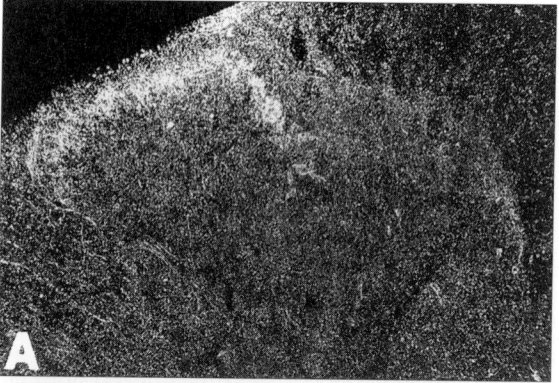

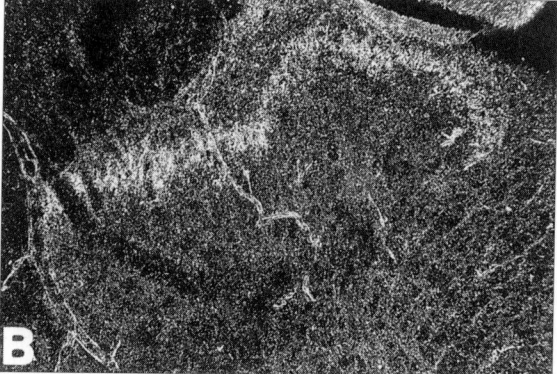

Figure 2. Dark-field light microscopic photomicrographs showing the effects of perineural capsaicin treatment on the distribution of degeneration argyrophilia within the spinal dorsal horn. The sciatic nerve on one side was treated with capsaicin, and that on the other side was treated with its vehicle, and 90 days later the animal was given a single subcutaneous injection of capsaicin 3 hours prior to being killed. Ipsilateral to the vehicle-treated nerve (B), degenerating axon terminals appearing as bright irregular particles form a continuous band and are confined to the marginal zone and the substantia gelatinosa. Ipsilateral to the capsaicin-treated nerve (A), the medial section of the marginal zone and of the substantia gelatinosa is devoid of degenerating axonal endings. Gallyas' technique, x70.

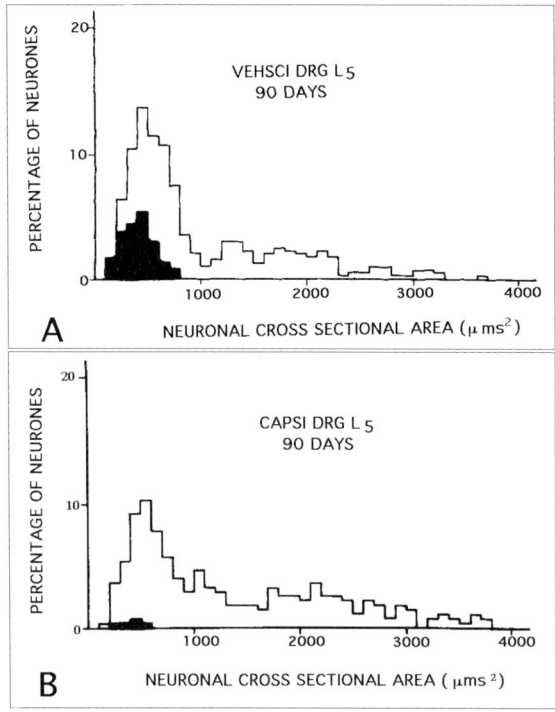

Figure 3. Size-frequency distribution histograms of fifth lumbar dorsal root ganglion neurones. The sciatic nerve on one side was treated with capsaicin, and that on the other side was treated with its vehicle, and 90 days later the animal was given a single subcutaneous injection of capsaicin 3 hours prior to being killed. Histograms were obtained from the ganglion ipsilateral to the vehicle- (A) and capsaicin-treated (B) nerves, respectively. The clear histograms represent the total neuronal population in the ganglion, whereas the overimposed filled histograms represent only the degenerating neurones. The numbers of cells measured were 393 and 311 for the histograms in A and B, respectively. It should be noted that degenerating neurones belong exclusively in the small-sized cell population. The histograms demonstrate that perineural treatment with capsaicin resulted in a diminution in the proportion of small neurones and a striking reduction in the percentage of degenerating ganglion cells.

Table I. Calculated numbers of neurones in the fifth lumbar dorsal root ganglia 90 days after perineural treatment of the sciatic nerve in the rat.

	Vehicle**			Capsaicin***			C/V ratio****	
	Number of neurones		Percentage	Number of neurones		Percentage	Total	DEG
	Total	DEG	DEG	Total	DEG	DEG		
1	8522	1789	21.0	7076	424	6.0	0.83	0.24
2	6687	1290	19.3	5290	101	1.9	0.79	0.07
3	9077	1279	14.1	6400	288	4.5	0.71	0.23
4	12468	1633	13.1	8164	440	5.3	0.65	0.27
5	7003	912	13.0	6011	277	4.6	0.86	0.30
6	6422	1109	17.2	5277	89	1.6	0.82	0.08
mean	8363	1335	16.29	6369*	270*	4.01		
± S.E.M.	±927	±133	±1.38	±454	±61	±0.73		
Change*****(%)				-24	-80			

* : Significantly different (p<0.05) from vehicle-treated control.
The sciatic nerve on one side was treated with capsaicin, and that on the other side was treated with its vehicle. Ninety days later, the rats were given a single systemic injection of capsaicin and killed 3 h afterwards.
** : Neuronal counts in ganglia ipsilateral to vehicle-treated nerves.
*** : Neuronal counts in ganglia ipsilateral to capsaicin-treated nerves.
**** : Ratio of number of neurones relating to capsaicin- and vehicle-treated nerve, respectively.
***** : Percentage change in mean number of ganglion cells as compared with vehicle-treated control side.
DEG = degenerating.

These findings indicated that perineural capsaicin treatment induces profound transganglionic changes in the spinal dorsal horn in the adult rat. The most probable explanation of the results is that perineural application of capsaicin resulted in an irreversible destruction of at least that population of C-fiber primary afferent terminals which undergo degeneration after a systemic injection of capsaicin. Substantial reductions in both the absolute number of dorsal root ganglion neurones and the proportion of degenerating neurones ipsilateral to a capsaicin-treated nerve support this assumption and provide evidence that transganglionic degeneration of C-fiber primary afferent terminals may be causally related to ganglionic cell loss. The few degenerating nerve cells seen in the ganglia relating to a capsaicin-treated nerve most likely represent neurones whose peripheral processes run in other peripheral nerves.

Possible mechanisms of the regulation of neuronal capsaicin sensitivity *in vivo*

Investigations into the progression of structural changes observed after perineural capsaicin treatment furnished information not only on the time course of these alterations, but, more importantly, provided new insight into the possible mechanisms of the regulation of neuronal capsaicin sensitivity *in vivo*.

To study the temporal characteristics of the morphological alterations which commence after perineural capsaicin treatment, animals were given a single subcutaneous injection of capsaicin 1, 4, 14 or 30 days after surgery and were sacrificed 3-8 hours later. The respective sensory ganglia and segments of the spinal cord were examined as described above.

One day after surgery, it was found that the size distribution, the total number of neurones and the proportion of degenerating nerve cells were comparable in ganglia ipsilateral to the capsaicin or vehicle-treated nerves (Figure 4A B, Table II).

The results obtained on animals which underwent surgery 4 or 8 days before systemic capsaicin treatment and sacrifice were rather different. As illustrated in Figure 5, in ganglia relating to the vehicle-treated nerve, degenerating neurones were frequent, whereas such neurones were scarcely seen in ganglia relating to the capsaicin-treated nerve. These observations were supported by the quantitative data which demonstrated that, in ganglia ipsilateral to the vehicle- and capsaicin-treated nerves, the proportion of small degenerating neurones was 14-18% and 2-5%, respectively. The quantitative results in Table III also show that the ratio of the neuronal numbers for the left and right fifth lumbar dorsal root ganglia displayed little variation. Similarly, there was little if any difference in the size-frequency distribution of neurones on the two sides (Figure 6). These findings therefore indicate that the perineural application of capsaicin results in a rapid and profound reduction in the proportion of degenerating nerve cells, which is not associated with a significant change in the total numbers of neurones in the affected ganglia.

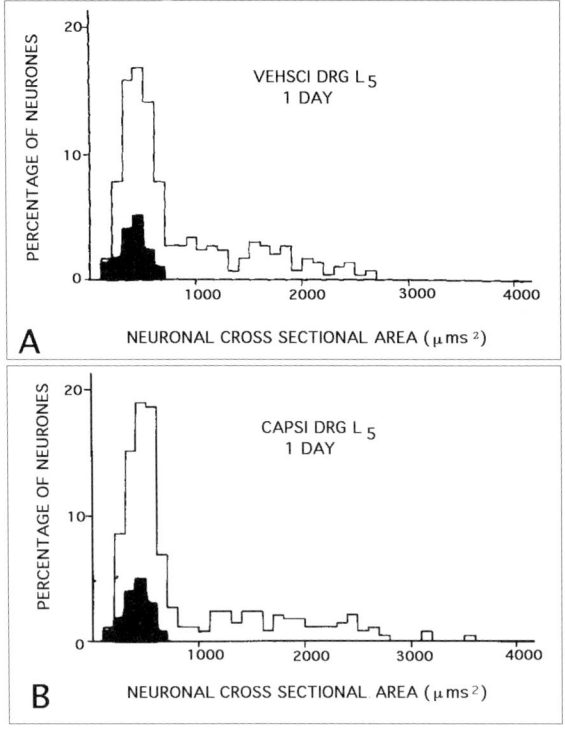

Figure 4. Size-frequency distribution histograms of fifth lumbar dorsal root ganglion neurones. The sciatic nerve on one side was treated with capsaicin, and that on the other side was treated with its vehicle, and 1 day later the animal was given a single subcutaneous injection of capsaicin 3 hours prior to being killed. Histograms were obtained from the ganglion ipsilateral to the vehicle- (A) and capsaicin-treated (B) nerves, respectively. The clear histograms represent the total neuronal population in the ganglion, whereas the overimposed filled histograms represent only the degenerating neurones. The numbers of cells measured were 298 and 305 for the histograms in A and B, respectively. The histograms demonstrate that perineural treatment with capsaicin had no effect on the proportions of the different neuronal populations 1 day after treatment.

Table II Calculated numbers of neurones in the fifth lumbar dorsal root ganglia 1 day after perineural treatment of the sciatic nerve.

	Vehicle*			Capsaicin**			C/V ratio***	
	Number of neurones		Percentage	Number of neurones		Percentage	Total	DEG
	Total	DEG	DEG	Total	DEG	DEG		
1	7575	1156	15.26	8754	1473	16.8	1.15	1.27
2	6917	1020	14.75	6758	1042	15.4	0.98	1.02
3	7756	1330	17.15	9933	1480	14.9	1.28	1.11
4	7597	1087	14.30	6713	1067	15.9	0.88	0.98
5	6112	1088	17.80	5556	766	13.7	0.91	0.70
mean	7191	1136	15.85	6542	1165	15.36		
± S.E.M.	±305	±53	±0.68	±1617	±137	±0.50		
Change****(%)					+9.1	+2.5		

The sciatic nerve on one side was treated with capsaicin, and that other side was treated with its vehicle. One day later, the rats were given a single systemic injection of capsaicin and killed 3 h afterwards.
* : Neuronal counts in ganglia ipsilateral to vehicle-treated nerves.
** : Neuronal counts in ganglia ipsilateral to capsaicin-treated nerves.
*** : Ratio of number of neurones relating to capsaicin- and vehicle-treated nerve, respectively.
**** : Percentage change in mean number of ganglion cells as compared with vehicle-treated control side.
DEG = degenerating.

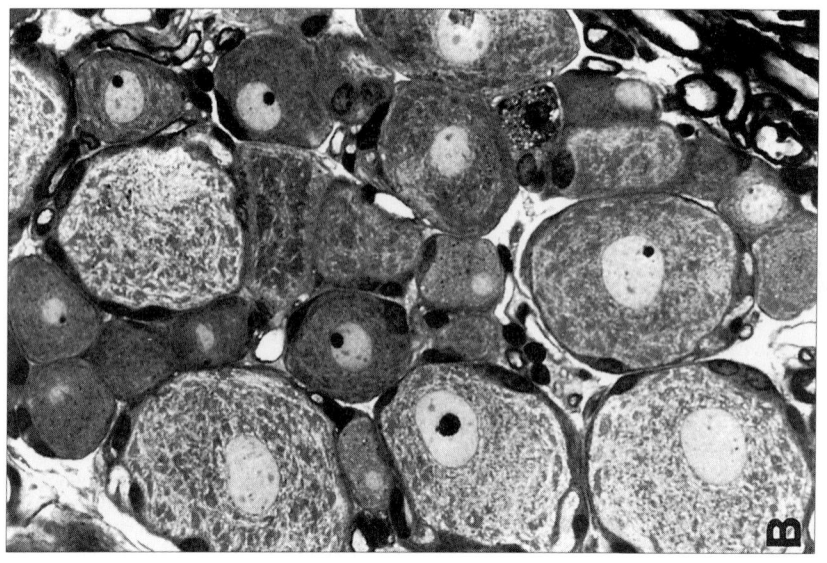

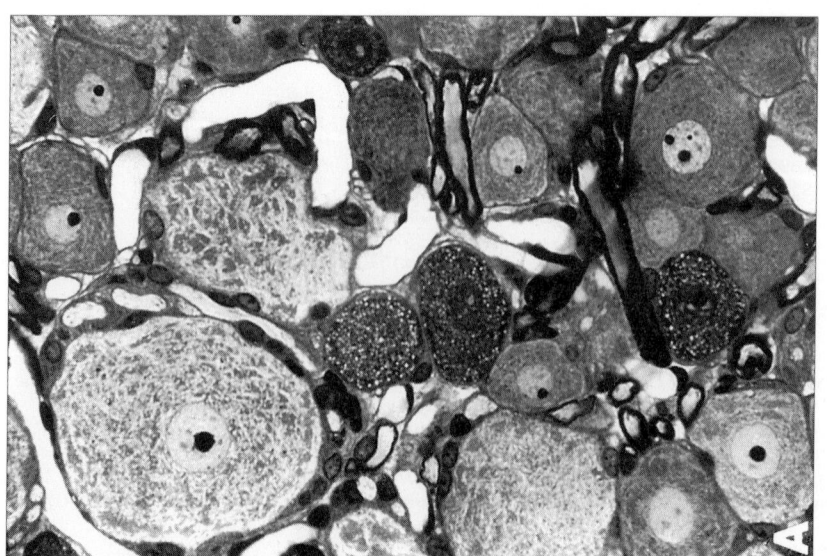

Figure 5. Light microscopic photographs showing details of the fifth lumbar dorsal root ganglia. The sciatic nerve on one side was treated with capsaicin, and that on the other side was treated with its vehicle, and 4 days later the rat was given a systemic injection of capsaicin (100 mg/kg) 3 hours prior to sacrifice. It should be noted that ipsilateral to the capsaicin-treated nerve (A) numerous small neurones display an increased nuclear and cytoplasmic basophilia and severe vacuolization of the perikaryon. Large cells are not affected. Ipsilateral to the vehicletreated nerve, degenerating neurones are scarce. Methylene blue-stained semithin sections. x580.

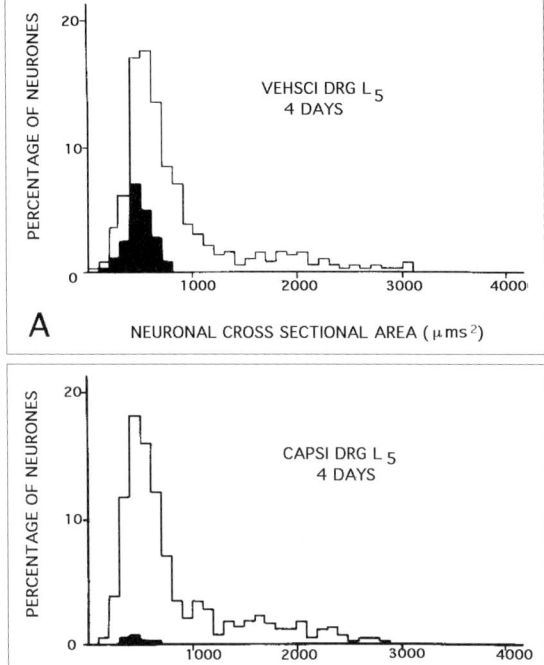

Figure 6. Size-frequency distribution histograms of fifth lumbar dorsal root ganglion neurones. The sciatic nerve on one side was treated with capsaicin, and that on the other side was treated with its vehicle, and 4 days later the animal was given a single subcutaneous injection of capsaicin 3 hours prior to being killed. Histograms were obtained from the ganglion ipsilateral to the vehicle- (A) and capsaicin-treated (B) nerves, respectively. The clear histograms represent the total neuronal population in the ganglion, whereas the overimposed filled histograms represent only the degenerating neurones. The numbers of cells measured were 390 and 440 for the histograms in A and B, respectively. The histograms demonstrate that perineural treatment with capsaicin had no effect on the overall distribution of the total neuronal population, but resulted in a striking reduction in the proportion of degenerating neurones ipsilateral to the capsaicin-treated nerve.

Table III. Calculated number of neurones in the fifth lumbar dorsal root ganglia 4 days after perineural treatment of the sciatic nerve in the rat.

	Vehicle*			Capsaicin**			C/V ratio***	
	Number of neurones		Percentage	Number of neurones		Percentage	Total	DEG
	Total	DEG	DEG	Total	DEG	DEG		
1	8632	1396	16.1	9796	370	3.7	1.13	0.26
2	6951	1169	16.8	8084	206	2.6	1.16	0.17
3	5702	1016	17.8	6041	148	2.5	1.05	0.14
4	8833	1332	15.1	8071	190	2.3	0.91	0.14
5	8378	1544	18.4	7765	232	2.99	0.92	0.15
mean	7699	1291	16.8	7951	229	2.8	1.03	0.17
± S.E.M.	±598	±91	±0.58	±596	±37	±0.24		
Change**** (%)				+3.2	-83			

The sciatic nerves were treated with either capsaicin or its vehicle. Four days later the rats were given a single system injection of capsaicin and killed 3 h afterwards.
* : Neuronal counts in ganglia ipsilateral to the vehicle-treated nerves.
** : Neuronal counts in ganglia ipsilateral to the capsaicin-treated nerves.
*** : Ratio of the number of neurones related to the capsaicin- and vehicle-treated nerve, respectively.
**** : Percentage change in the mean number of ganglion cells as compared with the vehicle-treated control side.
DEG = degenerating.

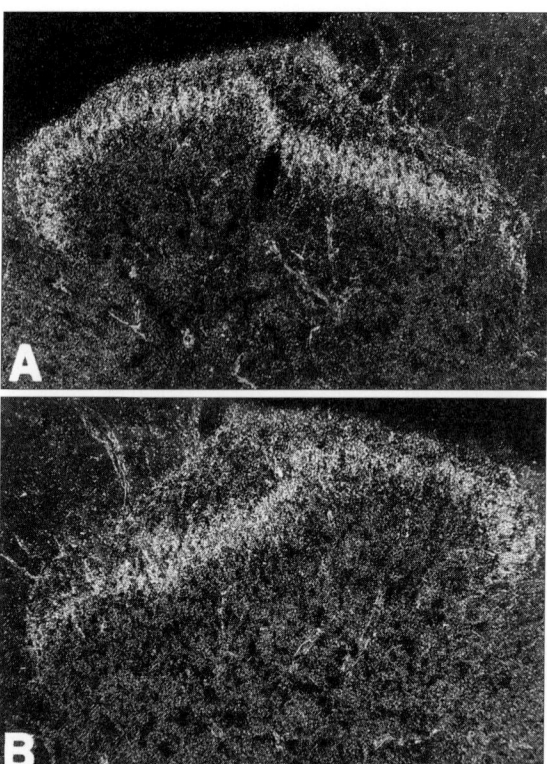

Figure 7. Dark-field light microscopic photomicrographs showing the effect of perineural capsaicin treatment on the distribution of degeneration argyrophilia within the spinal dorsal horn. The sciatic nerve on one side was treated with capsaicin, and that on the other side was treated with its vehicle, and 4 days later the animal was given a single subcutaneous injection of capsaicin 3 hours prior to being killed. There is no apparent difference in the distribution of degeneration argyrophilia between the sides relating to the capsaicin-treated (A) and the vehicle-treated sciatic nerve, respectively. Gallyas' technique, x70.

To reveal the time course of transganglionic changes, degeneration argyrophilia was examined in the spinal dorsal horn at different times after perineural treatment. Study of the topographical distribution and extent of axon terminal degeneration in the spinal dorsal horn revealed a seemingly identical pattern on both sides 1, 4 or 8 days after perineural treatment of the sciatic nerves with capsaicin or its vehicle, respectively (Figure 7). A considerable reduction in the degeneration argyrophilia in the dorsal horn relating to the capsaicin-treated nerve was noted only after a post-treatment interval of 14 days or more (Figure 8).

The present findings indicate a substantial, rapid decrease in the capsaicin sensitivity of sensory ganglion cells whose peripheral branches have been exposed previously to capsaicin. Prior perineural treatment with capsaicin apparently protects the affected sensory ganglion cells from the neurotoxic effect of systemically injected capsaicin. This may be related to an altered expression of putative capsaicin receptors on these sensory ganglion cells. Resiniferatoxin binding sites demonstrated in membrane preparations of sensory ganglia have been suggested to represent such receptors [43].

It is not possible to explain the mechanism of this phenomenon on the basis of the present experiments. It can be argued, however, that the inhibition of intraneuronal transport processes in C-fiber afferent fibers demonstrated in previous morphological

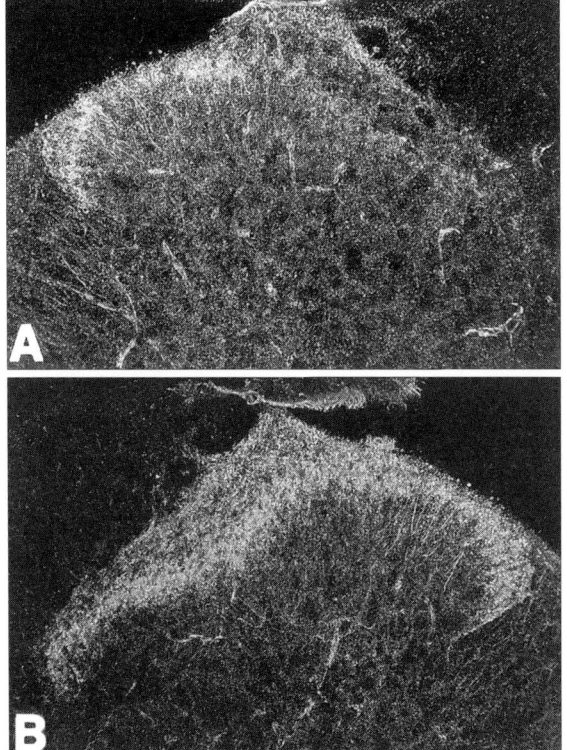

Figure 8. Dark-field light microscopic photomicrographs showing the effect of perineural capsaicin treatment on the distribution of degeneration argyrophilia within the spinal dorsal horn. The sciatic nerve on one side was treated with capsaicin, and that on the other side was treated with its vehicle, and 14 days later the animal was given a single subcutaneous injection of capsaicin 3 hours prior to being killed. It should be noted that there is a marked reduction in degeneration argyrophilia in the marginal zone and the substantia gelatinosa ipsilateral to the capsaicin-treated nerve (A), whereas degenerating axon terminals form a continuous band in the superficial dorsal horn ipsilateral to the vehicle-treated nerve (B). Gallyas' technique, x70.

and biochemical studies [13, 21, 24, 25] may contribute significantly to this change in perikaryal capsaicin sensitivity. It may be suggested that, under normal conditions, a peripherally derived substance which reaches the perikaryon through retrograde intra-axonal transport plays a crucial role in the regulation of neuronal capsaicin sensitivity. Therefore, inhibition of axonal transport processes may result in a depletion of this substance that is essential for the synthesis of specific molecules which may interact with capsaicin. Nerve growth factor, which is known to be taken up by sensory nerve endings and transported to the parent cell body [32], appears to be a likely candidate regulating the expression of such molecules. This assumption is supported by recent findings that nerve growth factor deprivation markedly decreases the sensitivity of cultured dorsal root ganglion neurones to capsaicin [1, 46]. Additionally, a decreased level of peripherally injected nerve growth factor has been measured in guinea pig sensory ganglia after systemic capsaicin treatment, which was accounted for by an inhibition of retrograde axonal transport processes [37].

Alternatively, it can be suggested that the perineural application of capsaicin results in an altered cellular metabolism, leading, for example, to an increased synthesis and/or accumulation of substances which might interfere with the deleterious effects of capsaicin. Peripheral nerve lesions, including perineural treatment with capsaicin, have been shown to induce the expression of "injury peptides" which may promote recovery of damaged neurones [28]. Blockade of axonal transport processes has also been demonstrated to result in the expression of such peptides [33]. Therefore, it cannot be excluded that perikaryal synthesis and/or the accumulation of certain protective substances due to an axonal transport inhibition by capsaicin may contribute to the altered sensitivity of sensory ganglion cells to capsaicin.

The results revealed a mismatch of ganglionic and spinal degenerative alterations evoked by a systemic injection of capsaicin in early survival periods after perineural capsaicin treatment. Thus, although the proportions of degenerating neurones differed markedly in ganglia relating to the capsaicin- and vehicle-treated nerves, degeneration argyrophilia in the spinal dorsal horn was pronounced and comparable on the two sides. Accordingly, a "capsaicin gap" could not be observed in the spinal dorsal horn at these early postoperative survival times. A possible explanation of this phenomenon may be that a "capsaicin gap" develops only after irreversible degeneration of the central terminals of the affected sensory ganglion cells. The destruction of the central terminals may ensue as a result of damage to and a consequent loss of the affected sensory ganglion cells induced by chemodenervation of the peripheral nerve by capsaicin.

By showing that degeneration of the central terminals may be unrelated to ganglion cell degeneration, these findings imply a differential regulation of the capsaicin sensitivity of the separate domains of the sensory neurones. This assumption is strongly supported by our previous findings that degeneration of primary afferent terminals might occur without ganglion cell death. In fact, degeneration of the central terminals of trigeminal and spinal capsaicin sensitive sensory ganglion cells without apparent structural, neurochemical and functional changes in their perikarya and peripheral endings has been demonstrated after an intracisternal injection of capsaicin [14, 19].

In conclusion, we suggest that the integrity of the peripheral branches of the primary sensory neurones and axonal transport processes are critical with respect to neuronal capsaicin sensitivity. We also assume that different systems may operate to maintain the expression of perikaryal and axon terminal sensitivity to capsaicin. Further studies are needed to explore whether the blockade of axonal transport processes by colchicine, for example, might influence neuronal capsaicin sensitivity, and in turn whether perineural capsaicin treatment might interfere with the effects of other toxic agents affecting sensory ganglion neurones. Finally, it remains to be seen whether cellular events underlying capsaicin sensitivity, or changes in this, are of any relevance to the normal functioning of primary sensory neurones. Investigations in this line may reveal not only important clues for an understanding of the molecular basis of neuronal capsaicin sensitivity and its regulation, but also provide new information on the significance of these mechanisms in the response of the nerve cell to injury.

Acknowledgements

This work was supported by grants from OTKA (2710) and ETT (PT-65/1990). We wish to thank Mrs. Krisztina Mohacsi for skilful technical assistance and Dr. D. Durham for linguistic revision of the text.

References

1. Aguay LG, Whit G. Effects of nerve growth factor on TTX and capsaicin sensitivity in adult rat sensory neurons. *Brain Res* 1992 ; 570 : 61-7.
2. Aldskogius H, Arviddson J, Grant G. The reaction of primary sensory neurons to peripheral nerve injury with particular emphasis on transganglionic changes. *Brain Res Rev* 1985 ; 10 : 27-46.
3. Aldskogius H, Wiesenfeld-Hallin Z, Kristensson K. Selective neuronal destruction by ricinus communis agglutinin I and its use for the quantitative determination of sciatic nerve dorsal root ganglion cell numbers. *Brain Res* 1988 ; 461: 215-20.
4. Arvidsson J, Ygge J. A quantitative study of the effects of neonatal capsaicin treatment and of subsequent peripheral nerve transection in adult rat. *Brain Res* 1986 ; 397 : 130-6.
5. Buck STH, Burks TF. The neuropharmacology of capsaicin : review of some recent observations. *Pharmacol Rev* 1986 ; 38 : 179-226.
6. Chung JM, Lee KH, Hori Y, Willis WD. Effects of capsaicin applied to a peripheral nerve on the responses of primate spinothalamic tract cells. *Brain Res* 1985 ; 329 : 27-38.
7. Devor M, Claman D. Mapping and plasticity of acid phosphatase afferents in the rat dorsal horn. *Brain Res* 1980 ; 190 : 17-28.
8. Eager RP. Selective staining of degenerating axons in the central nervous system by a simplified silver method : spinal cord projections to external cuneate and inferior olivary nuclei in the cat. *Brain Res* 1970 ; 22 : 137-41.
9. Fitzgerald M, Woolf CJ. The time course and specificity of the changes in the behavioural and dorsal horn responses to noxious stimuli following peripheral nerve capsaicin treatment in the rat. *Neuroscience* 1982 ; 7 : 2051-6.
10. Fitzgerald M. Alterations in the ipsi- and contralateral afferent inputs of dorsal horn cells produced by capsaicin treatment of one sciatic nerve in the rat. *Brain Res* 1982 ; 248 : 92-107.
11. Gallyas F, Wolff JR, Bottcher H, Zaborszky L. A reliable and sensitive method to localize terminal degeneration and lysosomes in the central nervous system. *Stain Technol* 1980 ; 55 : 299-306.
12. Gamse R, Holzer P, Lembeck F. Decrease of substance P in primary afferent neurones and impairment of neurogenic plasma extravasation by capsaicin. *Br J Pharmacol* 1980 ; 68 : 207-13.
13. Gamse R, Petsche U, Lembeck F, Jancsó G. Capsaicin applied to peripheral nerve inhibits axoplasmic transport of substance P and somatostatin. *Brain Res* 1982 ; 239 : 447-62.
14. Gamse R, Jancsó G, Kiraly E. Intracisternal capsaicin : a novel approach for studying nociceptive sensory neurons. In : Chahl LA, Szolcsanyi J, Lembeck F, eds. *Neurogenic inflammation and antidromic vasodilatation*. Budapest : Akadémiai Kiado, 1984 : 93-110.
15. Gibson SJ, McGregor G, Bloom SR, Polak JM, Wall PD. Local application of capsaicin to one sciatic nerve of the adult rat induces a marked depletion in the peptide content of the lumbar dorsal horn. *Neuroscience* 1982 ; 7 : 3153-62.
16. Holzer P. Capsaicin : cellular targets, mechanisms of action, and selectivity for thin sensory neurons. *Pharmacol Rev* 1991 ; 43 : 143-201.

17. Jancsó G, Kiraly E, Jancsó-Gabor A. Pharmacologically induced selective degeneration of chemosensitive primary sensory neurones. *Nature* 1977 ; 270 : 741-3.
18. Jancsó G, Kiraly E, Jancsó-Gabor A. Direct evidence for an axonal site of action of capsaicin. *Naunyn-Schmiedeberg's Arch Pharmacol* 1980 ; 313 : 91-4.
19. Jancsó G. Intracisternal capsaicin : selective degeneration of chemosensitive primary sensory afferents in the adult rat. *Neurosci Lett* 1981 ; 27 : 41-5.
20. Jancsó G, Such G. Effects of capsaicin applied perineurally to the vagus nerve on cardiovascular and respiratory functions in the cat. *J Physiol Lond* 1983 ; 341 : 359-70.
21. Jancsó G, Ferencsik M, Such G, Kiraly E, Nagy A, Bujdosó M. Morphological effects of capsaicin and its analogues in newborn and adult mammals. In : Hakanson R, Sundler F, eds. *Tachykinin antagonists.* Amsterdam, New York, Oxford : Elsevier, 1985 : 35-44.
22. Jancsó G, Kiraly E, Joó F, Such G, Nagy A. Selective degeneration by capsaicin of a subpopulation of primary sensory neurons in the adult rat. *Neurosci Lett* 1985 ; 59 : 209-14.
23. Jancsó G, Lawson SN. Perineural capsaicin treatment of the sciatic nerve in adult rat causes transganglionic changes in the spinal cord dorsal horn. *J Physiol Lond* 1987 ; 394 : 109.
24. Jancsó G, Kiraly E, Such G, Joó F, Nagy A. Neurotoxic effect of capsaicin in mammals. *Acta Physiol Hung* 1987 ; 69 : 295-313.
25. Jancsó G, Such G, Rodel C. A new approach to selective regional analgesia. In : Sicuteri F, Vecchiet L, Fanciullacci M, eds. *Trends in cluster headache.* Amsterdam, New York, Oxford : Elsevier Science Publishers BV, 1987 : 59-68.
26. Jancsó G. B-afferents : a system of capsaicin-sensitive primary sensory neurons ? *Behav Brain Sci* 1990 ; 13 : 306-7.
27. Jancsó G, Lawson SN. Ganglionic changes associated with transganglionic degeneration of capsaicin-sensitive primary sensory afferents : a quantitative morphometric and immunohistochemical study. *Regul Pept* 1988 ; 22 : 97-7.
28. Jancsó G. Pathobiological reactions of C-fiber primary sensory neurones to peripheral nerve injury. *Exp Physiol* 1992 ; 77 : 405-31.
29. Jancsó G, Lawson SN. Transganglionic degeneration of capsaicin-sensitive C-fiber afferent terminals. *Neuroscience* 1990 ; 39 : 501-11.
30. Jancsó N. Role of the nerve terminals in the mechanism of inflammatory reactions. *Bull Millard Fillmore Hosp (Buffalo NY)* 1960 ; 7 : 53-77.
31. Jancsó N. Desensitization with capsaicin as a tool for studying the function of pain receptors. In : Lim RKS, ed. *Pharmacology of pain.* Oxford : Pergamon Press, 1968 : 33-55.
32. Johnson EM, Rich KM, Yip HK. The role of NGF in sensory neurons *in vivo. TINS* 1986 ; 9 : 33-7.
33. Kashiba H, Senba E, Kawai Y, Ueda Y, Tohyama M. Axonal blockade induces the expression of vasoactive intestinal polypeptide and galanin in rat dorsal root ganglion neurons. *Brain Res* 1992 ; 577 : 19-28.
34. Konigsmark BW. Methods for the counting of neurons. In : Nauta WJH, Ebbesson SOE, eds. *Contemporary research methods in neuroanatomy.* Springer, Berlin 1970 : 315-40.
35. Maggi CA, Meli A. The sensory-efferent function of capsaicin-sensitive sensory neurons. *Gen Pharmacol* 1988 ; 19 : 1-43.
36. McMahon SB, Wall PD, Granum SL, Webster KE. The effects of capsaicin applied to peripheral nerves on responses of a group of lamina I cells in adult rats. *J Comp Neurol* 1984 ; 227 : 393-400.
37. Miller MS, Buck SH, Lipes IG, Yamamura HI, Burks TF. Regulation of substance P by nerve growth factor : disruption by capsaicin. *Brain Res* 1982 ; 250 : 193-6.
38. Molander C, Grant G. Laminar distribution and somatotopic organization of primary afferent fibers from hindlimb nerves in the dorsal horn. A study by transganglionic transport of horseradish peroxidase in the rat. *Neuroscience* 1986 ; 19 : 297-312.

39. Nagy JI. Capsaicin : a chemical probe for sensory neuron mechanism. In : Iversen LL, Iversen SD, Snyder SH, eds. *Handbook of psychopharmacology,* Vol. 15. New York : Plenum Press, 1982 : 185-235.
40. Pierau FK, Szolcsanyi J, Sann H. The effect of capsaicin on afferent nerves and temperature regulation of mammals and bird. *J Therm Biol* 1986 ; 11 : 95-100.
41. Pini A, Baranowski R, Lynn B. Long-term reduction in the number of C-fiber nociceptors following capsaicin treatment of a cutaneous nerve in adult rats. *Eur J Neurosci* 1990 ; 2 : 89-97.
42. Swett JE, Woolf CJ. The somatotopic organization of primary afferent terminals in the superficial laminae of the rat spinal cord. *J Comp Neurol* 1985 ; 231 : 66-77.
43. Szallasi A, Blumberg PM. Resiniferatoxin and its analogs provide novel insights into the pharmacology of the vanilloid (capsaicin) receptor. *Life Sci* 1990 ; 47 : 1399-408.
44. Szentagothai J, Kiss T. Projection of dermatomes on the substantia gelatinosa. *Arch Neurol Psychiatry* 1949 ; 62 : 734-44.
45. Welk E, Petsche U, Fleischer E, Handwerker HO. Altered excitability of afferent C-fibers of the rat distal to a nerve site exposed to capsaicin. *Neurosci Lett* 1983 ; 38 : 245-50.
46. Winter J, Forbes CA, Sternberg J, Lindsay RM. Nerve growth factor (NGF) regulates adult rat cultured dorsal root ganglion neuron responses to the excitotoxin capsaicin. *Neuron* 1988 ; 1 : 973-81.
47. Yip HK, Rich KM, Lampe PA, Johnson EM Jr. The effects of nerve growth factor and its antiserum on the postnatal development and survival after injury of sensory neurons in the rat dorsal root ganglia. *J Neurosci* 1984 ; 4 : 2986-92.

7

A new site of coupling between sympathetic neurones and afferent neurones following peripheral nerve lesions

W. JÄNIG*, M. DEVOR**, E.M. MCLACHLAN***, M. MICHAELIS*

* *Physiologisches Institut, Christian-Albrechts-Universität, Kiel, Germany.*
** *Department of Cell and Animal Biology, Institute of Life Sciences, Hebrew University, Jerusalem, Israël.*
*** *Prince of Wales Medical Research Institute, Randwick, Australia.*

Conceptual and clinical background

Basically the sympathetic nervous system is associated with pain in two ways :
- First, it shows well-orchestrated generalized as well as specific localized reactions to noxious, tissue-damaging events. The generalized reactions are organized in the hypothalamus and suprahypothalamic brain structures and described phenomenologically as the "defence reaction" ; they enable the organism to cope with dangerous situations. There are also specific reactions which are organized within the spinal cord and in the periphery, *i.e.* somatosympathetic, viscero-sympathetic and viscero-visceral reflexes (*see* [21]). Both levels of reaction are presumably protective under normal biological conditions and associated with activation of both the adreno-cortical system of the hypothalamo-hypophyseal axis and the somato-motor system.
- Second, tissue damage in the extremities with and without any obvious nerve lesion is sometimes followed by diffuse burning pain and hyperalgesia which can be best relieved by blockade of the (efferent) sympathetic activity to the affected extremity. Spontaneous pain and hyperalgesia may be associated with changes of blood flow and sweating, changes of active and passive movements including an increase in physiological tremor, and trophic changes in skin and subcutaneous tissues. These changes are thought to be, directly or indirectly, associated with the sympathetic

nervous system. Like the pain, these changes may be alleviated by blockade of sympathetic activity although this sometimes needs to be repeated several times to be successful [5, 6]. Pain syndromes of this type are called "reflex sympathetic dystrophy" (RSD) and "sympathetically maintained pain" (SMP), terms which were initially introduced by Evans [16] and Roberts [47], respectively. It is important to remember that the term "reflex sympathetic dystrophy" is purely descriptive and does not imply primary mechanisms (*see* [24]).

It is the second of these aspects which has puzzled clinicians very much since the turn of the century and has led to considerable confusion speculation as far as the underlying mechanisms are concerned. Several observations strongly argue that the sympathetic nervous system is involved in the generation of pain and the other associated changes in patients with RSD and SMP [3, 4, 12, 22, 23, 30, 51].

1) Pain is relieved following sympathetic block (by local anaesthetics applied to paravertebral ganglia [6], by regional application of guanethidine [20], or by phentolamine injected intravenously [2, 9, 45]). It is not relevant in the present context that the sympathetic block is sometimes only temporarily successful and in some cases does not lead to permanent relief of pain.

2) Pain can be rekindled or enhanced by an alpha-adrenoceptor agonist applied to the affected extremity (*e.g.* iontophoretically through the skin in patients with superficial burning pain and hyperalgesia), as has been observed by Wallin *et al.* [59] and Davis *et al.* [11].

3) Guanethidine injected intravenously into the affected extremity initially elicits pain which is presumably generated by noradrenaline released from postganglionic terminals [4].

4) Continuous electrical stimulation of decentralised thoracic sympathetic ganglia in conscious causalgic patients who underwent surgery reproducibly elicited the tingling and burning pain after latencies of 4-20 seconds [57]. White and Sweet [61] confirmed this observation.

These observations made on patients with pain after peripheral trauma are strongly in support of the notion that efferent sympathetic nervous activity is actively involved in the generation of pain. The problem focusses on the question "How is the sympathetic nervous system coupled in the periphery to primary afferent neurones so as to produce the peripheral components of pain in these patients" ? (*see* Figure 1). This coupling has to be postulated in order to explain the beneficial effects of sympathetic block in some pathophysiological conditions. The type of coupling must be such that primary afferent neurones are excited and that the activity enters the nociceptive pathways in the central nervous system, otherwise it is almost impossible to explain the relatively prompt effects of sympathetic block or of "sympathetic" stimulation in the patients.

Confusion does not only exist about the underlying mechanisms but also about the clinical diagnosis of patients who develop pain after trauma with nerve injury. Basic research can be applied to models developed on the basis of testable hypotheses.

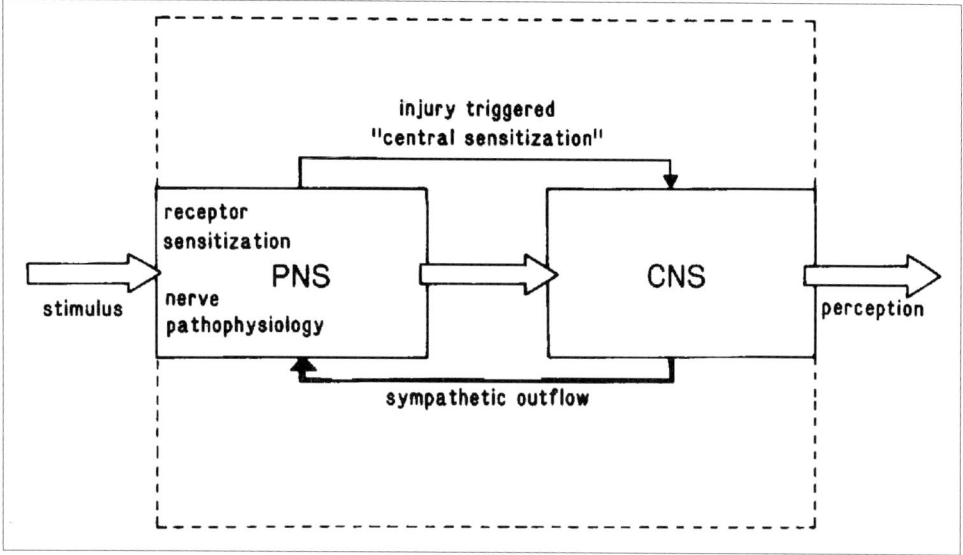

Figure 1. Schematic diagram showing the components of our understanding of mechanisms of pain in which the sympathetic nervous system may be involved. Note that sensitization of peripheral nociceptors and ectopic impulse generation may be maintained by a positive feedback loop *via* the sympathetic system. This may be combined with sensitization of neurons of the central nociceptive system. (Modified from [12].)

Whether a model (and therefore also the therapeutic strategy which follows from that model) might apply to a particular group of patients depends on the clinical diagnosis. Thus consensus about clinical diagnosis is critical (*see* [24]).

Several ways of coupling sympathetic and afferent neurones have been proposed and tested in the last few years (Figure 2). These include :
- direct chemical coupling between the noradenergic terminal and the afferent terminal, leading to excitation or sensitization of the afferent fibers ;
- indirect coupling, most proposed mechanisms being still rather hypothetical ;
- coupling in the traumatized nerve, which is possible but has yet to be experimentally supported ;
- ephaptic coupling between sympathetic and afferent fibers which seems unlikely to occur at all.

Details about these types of coupling are discussed by Jänig and Koltzenburg [25, 27] and Jänig and McLachlan [29].

Here we report a novel type of chemical coupling between sympathetic postganglionic neurones and afferent neurones which develops after a peripheral nerve lesion in rats and which occurs in the dorsal root ganglion proximal to the nerve lesion (d in Figure 2) [14, 40]. Whether or not this new type of coupling can occur in patients needs to be tested.

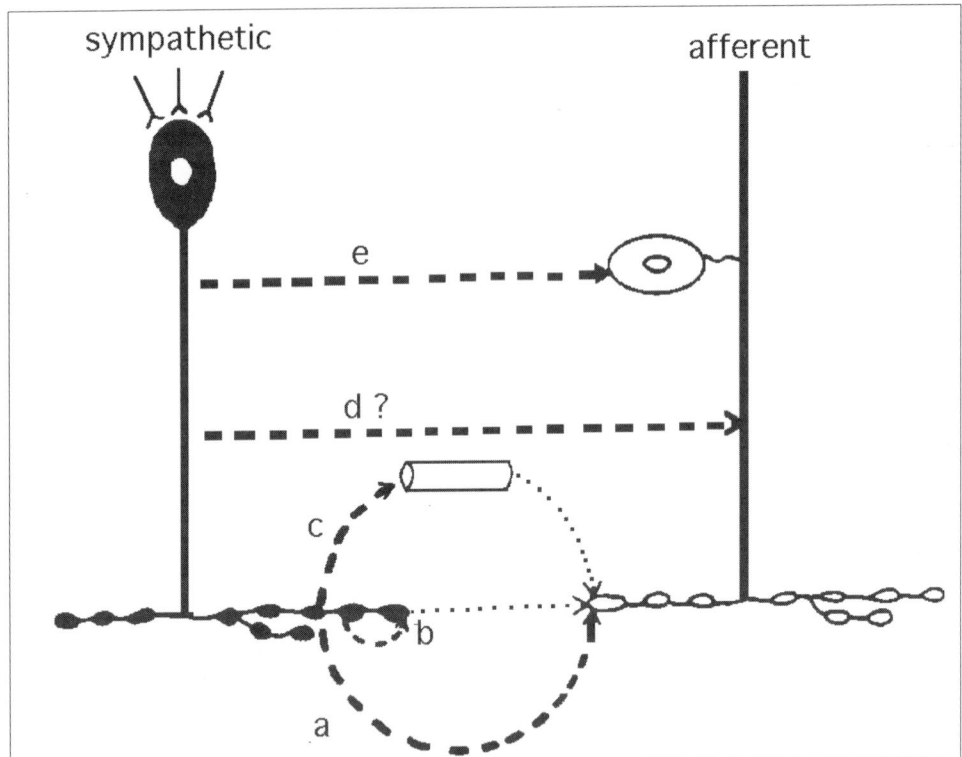

Figure 2. Possible ways of coupling between sympathetic postganglionic neurons and afferent neurons under pathological conditions. a : Noradrenergic (and non-noradrenergic ?) chemical coupling in the periphery. This may occur after nerve lesions. b : Indirect chemical coupling. Noradrenaline acts prejunctionally at the varicosities via alpha$_2$-adrenoceptors and triggers release of other substances (*e.g.* prostaglandins). This may be relevant during states of chronic inflammation [37]. c : Indirect coupling via the vascular bed (changes in neurovascular transmission, development of hyperreactivity of the vascular bed). This may occur after various forms of trauma with or without nerve lesion [26, 32]. d : Interaction along the nerve. This may occur after nerve lesions during regeneration and sprouting in the nerve (hypothetical). e : Noradrenergic coupling in the dorsal root ganglion. This may occur after a remote nerve lesion. Summary scheme composed from [25, 27].

Electrophysiology

Somata in dorsal root ganglia are (with a few exceptions in the rat [58]) almost silent in normal conditions *in vivo* and are not activated when neigbouring cells are excited. A few may discharge when all neigbouring somata are activated synchronously [15]. However, after a complete or partial nerve lesion (*e.g.* of the sciatic nerve in the rat), many more DRG somata exhibit ectopic discharges and cross-excitation (Figure 4 left) [15, 34, 54, 58]. Can the afferent neurones also be driven *via* their somata from the sympathetic nervous system ? Under normal conditions most sympathetic endings in the DRG innervate local blood vessels. Rare reports have suggested that a few end in relation to neuronal somata (*see* below). The question we asked was : "Is it possible to activate primary afferent neurons *via* their cell bodies by electrical stimulation of the sympathetic outflow ?"

Methods

In anaesthetized Wistar-derived Sabra strain rats we tested under standardized experimental conditions whether afferent neurones can be activated by stimulation of sympathetic neurones 4 to 22 days after axotomy (ligating and cutting the sciatic nerve). The experimental setup is shown in Figure 3 and the details of the methods used are described in Devor *et al.* [14]. In brief, activity of afferent neurons was recorded from their peripherally cut axons which were isolated from the sciatic nerve rostral to the neuroma (R1 in Figure 3) and identified by electrical stimulation of dorsal roots L4 and L5 (S1 in Figure 3) which contain the central branches of the afferent neurones projecting in the sciatic nerve. Preganglionic sympathetic axons in ventral roots between T12 and L2 were stimulated electrically. These segments contain the preganglionic sympathetic neurons that form synapse with postganglionic neurones projecting through the grey rami to the spinal nerves L4 and L5 [1]. Afferent axons in the sciatic nerve were stimulated distal to the recording site (S2 in Figure 1). Successful activation of the sympathetic outflow was monitored by recording the mass volley from

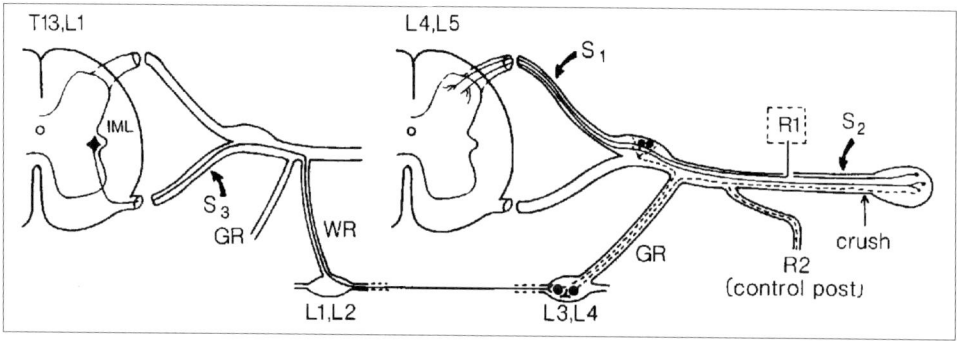

Figure 3. Diagram of the experimental set-up showing the arrangement of the stimulating (S) and recording (R) electrodes. Cell bodies of most afferent neurons that project into the sciatic nerve are situated in DRGs L4 and L5. Cells bodies of most postganglionic sympathetic neurons that project into the sciatic nerve are situated in paravertebral ganglia L3 and L4. The corresponding preganglionic neurons are situated mostly in spinal segments T13 to L2 [1]. R1, electrode for recording afferent activity in microfilaments teased from the sciatic nerve about 30 mm proximal to the neuroma. R2, electrode for monitoring the postganglionic volley (elicited by S3 stimulation) from a branch of the posterior or anterior biceps muscle nerve (*see* Figure 2). S1, stimulating electrode(s) on DRs L4 and L5, used for identification of afferent axons. S2, electrode, placed about 8 mm proximal to neuroma, used for stimulating neighboring afferent axons. S3, electrode on VRs T13 and L1, or L1 and L2, used for stimulating preganglionic sympathetic axons. Crush, site at which the sciatic nerve was crushed in some experiments. GR, grey ramus. WR, white ramus.(From [14] with permission.)

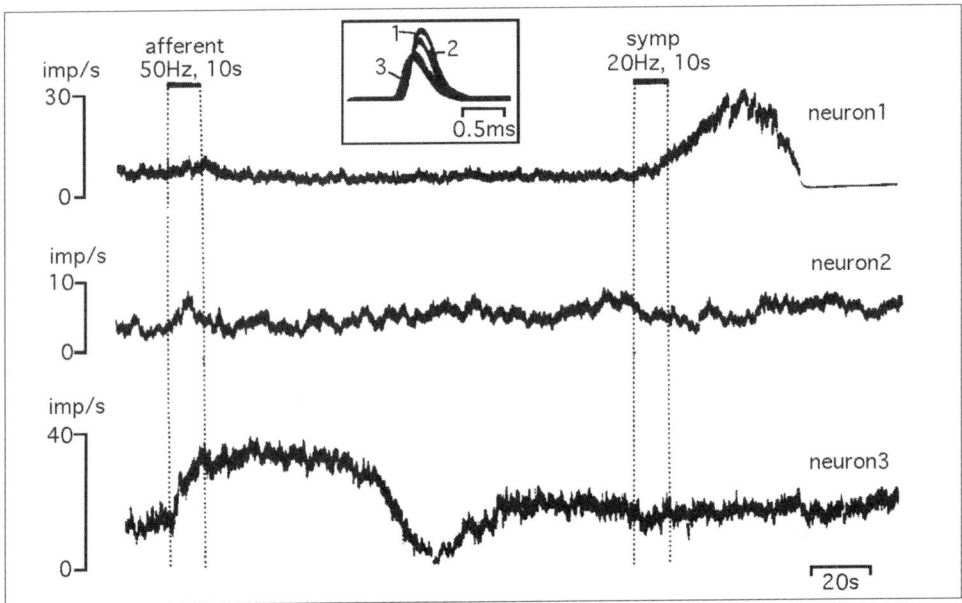

Figure 4. Responses of afferent neurons with myelinated axons to electrical stimulation of neighboring sciatic nerve afferents (afferent, left side, S2 electrode in Figure 1, 50 Hz stimulation for 10s, stimulus strength maximal for myelinated fibers), and to stimulation of sympathetic preganglionic efferents in VRs T13 and L1 (symp, right side, S3 electrode in Figure 1, 20 Hz stimulation for 10s, stimulus strength maximal for preganglionic axons). Activity was recorded simultaneously from the axons of three neurons each with spontaneous background activity. Neuron 1 exhibited weak cross-excitation to stimulation of neighboring afferents, and strong sympathetic excitation followed by aftersuppression. Neuron 2 showed afferent crossexcitation, and suppression to sympathetic stimulation. Neuron 3 exhibited strong afferent cross-excitation followed by aftersuppression, but was not affected by sympathetic stimulation. Inset shows the superimposed action potentials of neurons 1, 2 and 3. (From [14] with permission.)

a branch of the hamstring nerve (R2 in Figure 3) ; pairs of segmental adjacent ventral roots were chosen which generated maximal postganglionic volleys for each experimental animal (S3 in Figure 3).

Results

Responses to electrical stimulation of the preganglionic sympathetic axons with brief trains of 10s duration (S3 in Figure 3) were observed in 55% of the spontaneously active afferent units and in a few silent afferent units. With one exception, all afferent neurones had fast conducting axons (conduction velocity 7.8 - 60 m/s) and were therefore myelinated.

About 60% of the responding afferent units were activated by repetitive sympathetic stimulation (Figure 4 right, Figure 5 upper trace, Figure 6) whereas the rest were depressed (Figure 5 lower trace). The activation began 5-50s (mean + 8.9 s) after the

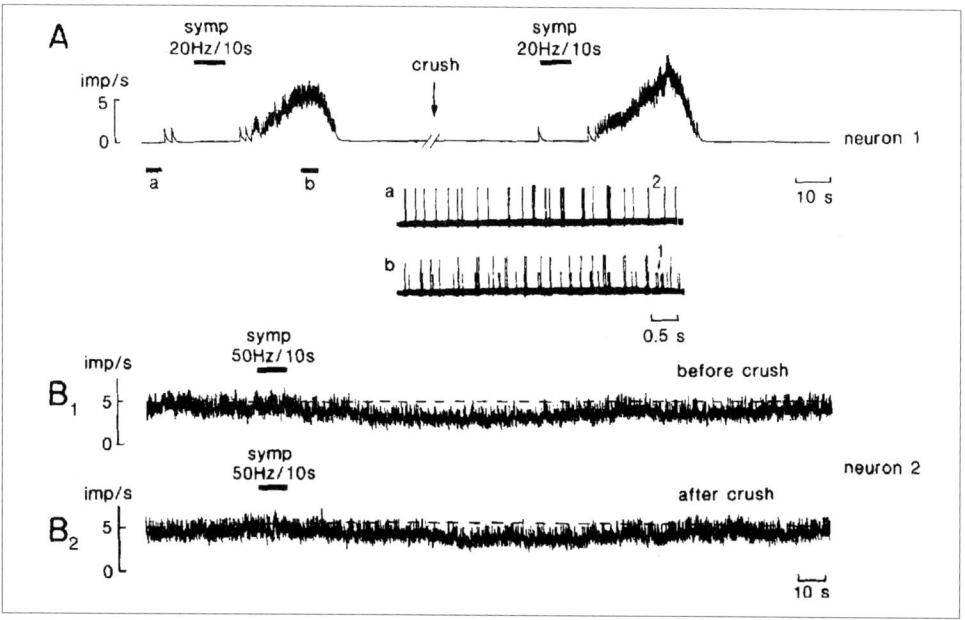

Figure 5. Excitation (A) and depression of activity (B1, B2) in two simultaneously recorded afferent neurons upon sympathetic stimulation (symp, S3 in Figure 1). The insets a and b show the activity in neuron 2 before and in neuron 1 and 2 after sympathetic stimulation (time periods of the insets marked by bars a,b). Crushing the sciatic nerve between the S2 electrode and the neuroma (Figure 1) did not block the responses (compare A left and right, B1 *versus* B2).(From [14] with permission.)

start of the stimulus train and continued to rise for about 10-20s until the responses reached their peaks. Afterwards the firing rate fell below resting levels in some neurones, the subsequent recovery taking several 10s (*see* neuron 1 in Figure 3). Four of the 26 neurons which were activated were initially silent (Figure 5A, Figure 6).

In 40% of the responding afferent units, spontaneous activity was depressed without an initial excitation by sympathetic stimulation (Figure 5B). Latency and duration of this depression was the same as or somewhat longer than that following excitation in the other responding units.

The responses increased in amplitude and duration with increasing frequency of stimulation from about 5 Hz and were maximal at 20 to 50 Hz. Single pulse stimulation of sympathetic axons never elicited a response. The response to sympathetic stimulation did not depend on sympathetic-afferent interaction within the neuroma at the lesion site of the sciatic nerve [13]. Crushing or cutting the sciatic nerve between the neuroma and the recording site (*see* "crush" in Figure 3) did not affect the responses to electrical stimulation of the sympathetic axons in 6 experiments (Figure 5).

The responses elicited in the afferent neurones by sympathetic stimulation were mimicked by adrenaline given *via* an intra-arterial catheter in the common carotid artery (0.5-2 μg ; Figure 6). Both the response to electrical sympathetic stimulation and that

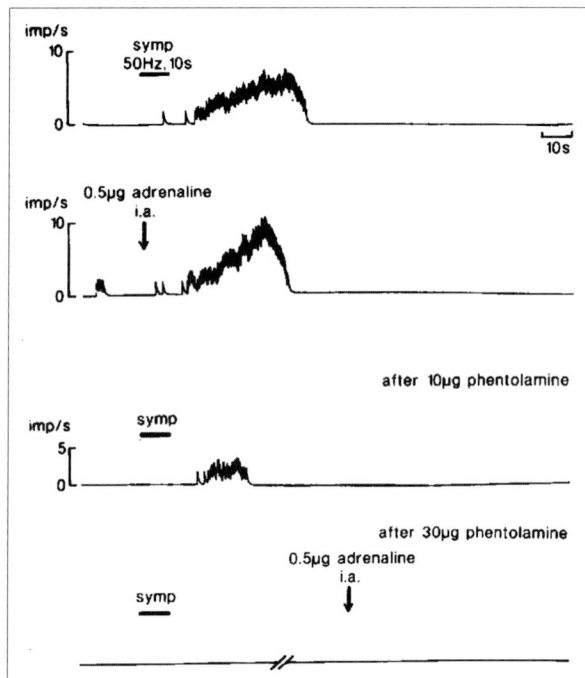

Figure 6. Responses of an afferent neuron to stimulation of sympathetic preganglionic axons (symp, S3 in Figure 1) and to systemic injection of 0.5 μ9 adrenaline, before (upper traces) and after (lower traces) i.a. injection of phentolamine (initially 10μ9, followed by an additional 20μ9). (From [14] with permission.)

to systemic application of adrenaline were substantially reduced or eliminated by the alpha-adrenoceptor antagonist phentolamine (1050Mg i.a. ; Figure 6), as was the depression of activity. Cross-afterdischarges which were elicited in afferent neurones by stimulation of other adjacent afferent neurones (Figure 4) were not affected by phentolamine.

Virtually no responses are initiated from the sympathetic supply and mediated at the cell body in the DRG in control preparations ; so far only one afferent neurone (with a fast conducting axon) has been observed to be excited in control preparations (Devor and Michaelis, unpublished observation).

Morphology

These neurophysiological results led immediately to the possibility that there was morphological coupling between sympathetic postganglionic axons and afferent neurones in the dorsal root ganglion. Postganglionic varicose noradrenergic axons in the dorsal root ganglion (DRG) are normally found around small diameter blood vessels and only very rarely amongst the afferent cell bodies [36]. Since Cajal [8], it has from time to time been reported in the literature that occasional DRG cells may be surrounded or contacted by axon profiles. However, the frequency and origin of these terminals remain unclear. We have put forward the hypothesis that peripheral nerve injury might lead to noradrenergic axons growing into dorsal root ganglia and forming connections with afferent neurones on or near their somata.

Methods

In anaesthetized Wistar rats, the left sciatic nerve was ligated and cut at mid-thigh level. After 2-70 days, the reanaesthetized animals were perfused with oxygenated saline and dorsal root ganglia (DRG) L3-L6, the paravertebral ganglia L3-L5, the spinal nerves L4 and L5 and the sciatic nerves on the lesioned side as well as on the contralateral side were removed. The tissues were rapidly frozen in moulds, and serial (20μm) cryostat sections processed using a modified version of the glyoxylic acid method [32]. Direct demonstration of catecholamine was preferred over immunohistochemistry for transmitter-synthesizing enzymes or neuropeptides because non-catecholaminergic neurones may express these substances after peripheral nerve lesions [41, 56]. Unoperated animals served as controls.

Results

After the experimental lesions of the sciatic nerve many fine catecholamine containing axons were present within the DRGs which contained somata with lesioned axons. The sprouts were fine and showed very faint catecholamine fluorescence in the first three weeks after the peripheral nerve injury. At later times, some somata were partially or completely surrounded by varicose catecholaminergic terminals. The number and frequency of these synaptic-like structures increased at least for 70 days after the nerve lesion (Figure 7). Quantitative analysis of the morphological data revealed the following characteristics (Figure 8 [40]) :
- noradrenergic axons sprouted preferentially in DRGs L4 and L5 which contain somata projecting in the lesioned sciatic nerve. Brightness and extent of the sprouts increased with time after the nerve lesion ;
- some sprouting also occurred within the corresponding contralateral DRGs L4 and 5, which contained only sensory cell bodies with intact axons. Sprouting contralaterally was more than in control ganglia from unoperated rats (# in Figure 8) and significantly less than in the ipsilateral DRGs with axotomized cell bodies (* in Figure 8) ;
- varicose catecholaminergic varicose terminals surrounded preferentially DRG cells with large diameters on the ipsilateral side ;
- many of the sensory cell bodies which were surrounded by noradrenergic nerve terminals appeared to be axotomized.

The sympathetic neurones that sprouted into the DRGs were unlikely to be those that previously projected into the lesioned nerve. The fine catecholaminergic axons visible in the normal sciatic nerve disappeared proximally within a few days after ligation and by 10-14 days virtually no noradrenergic axons were detectable in the lesioned nerve except in scar tissue adjacent to the neuroma ([19], McLachlan and Jänig unpublished).

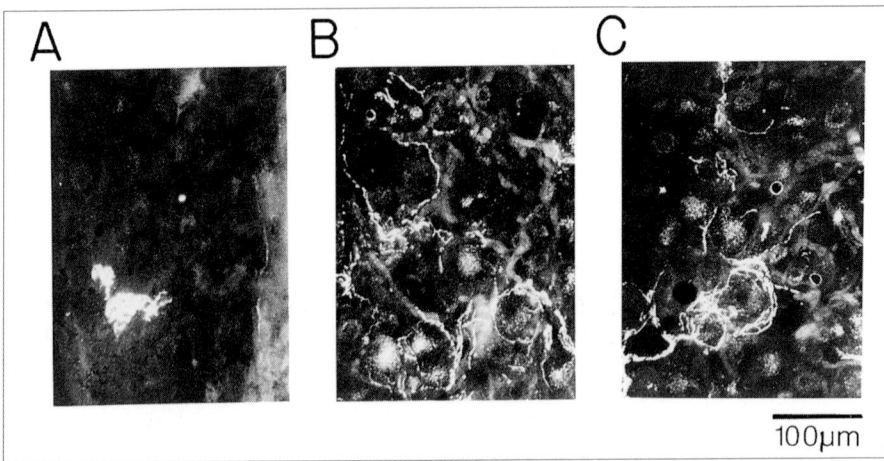

Figure 7. Catecholamine-fluorescent axons in a L5 dorsal root ganglion (DRG) of normal (control) rats (A) and 50 days after ligation of the left sciatic nerve (B,C). Almost all fluorescent axons are perivascular in the control DRG. In the lesioned DRG, many fluorescent axons run between the somatic profiles (B) ; some form varicose "rings" around sensory cell bodies.

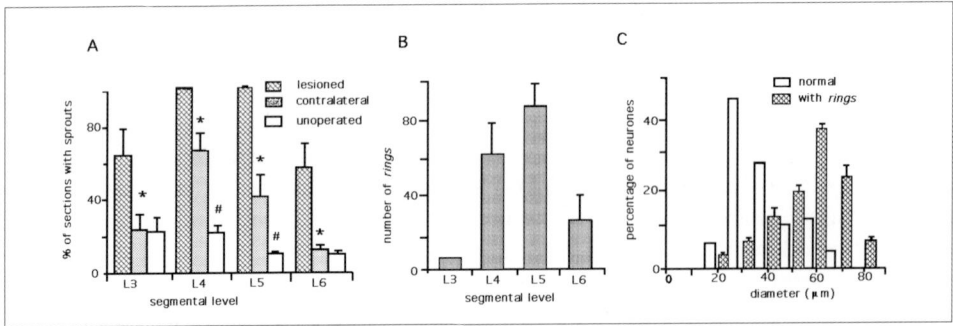

Figure 8. Quantitative analysis of experimental data regarding sprouting of noradrenergic axons in dorsal root ganglia (DRGs) following ligation of the sciatic nerve in rats. A : Frequency of sprouting in DRGs >30 days after ligating the sciatic nerve. The ordinate scale gives the percentage of sections containing fluorescent axon sprouts. Data are mean + 1 s.e.m, n=5-7 animals. B : Numbers of profiles surrounded by fluorescent axons in DRGs 50 days after ligating the sciatic nerve. Mean + 1 s.e.m. (n=4 animals for L4-L6, n=2 for L3). C : Diameter of profiles surrounded by fluorescent axons (hatched columns) in lesioned DRGs. Data from 4 animals 50 days after ligating the left sciatic nerve (mean + 1 s.e.m.). White columns show distribution of soma diameter in control DRG L5. (Modified from [40].)

This suggests that many ligated sympathetic axons degenerate retrogradely, lose their capacity to synthesize noradrenaline and/or die [28]. However, sprouts were seen to arise from perivascular plexuses in the DRGs. These perivascular axons were not injured directly by the sciatic nerve lesion.

Thus in these experiments the peripheral nerve lesion led to sprouting of noradrenergic neurones located proximal to the lesion site. The mechanism leading to noradrenergic sprouting in DRGs is unknown. It is unlikely to be triggered by a transneuronal signal within the paravertebral ganglia following lesioning of the postganglionic axons because sprouting occurred contralaterally. The sprouting observed in contralateral DRGs resembles that reported for sensory [35] and motor axons [48] after nerve lesions which has been explained by crossed intraspinal signals. On the lesioned side, some chemotactic signal generated within the DRG seems a likely trigger for sprouting, but it will be necessary to identify which of several possible mechanisms are responsible.

Interpretation of the neurophysiological and morphological results

Figure 9 summarizes the neurophysiological and morphological results and puts them into a broader context : under normal conditions, postganglionic neurons and afferent neurons are separate and form specific connections with distinct targets : most postganglionic neurons projecting to the periphery innervate blood vessels, sweat glands or erector pili muscles ; those projecting to the DRG innervate small blood vessels within them. Afferent neurons project to different laminae of the dorsal horn according to their function (Figure 9A). Following sciatic nerve ligation, noradrenergic perivascular axons sprout into the DRG and form basket-like structures around large

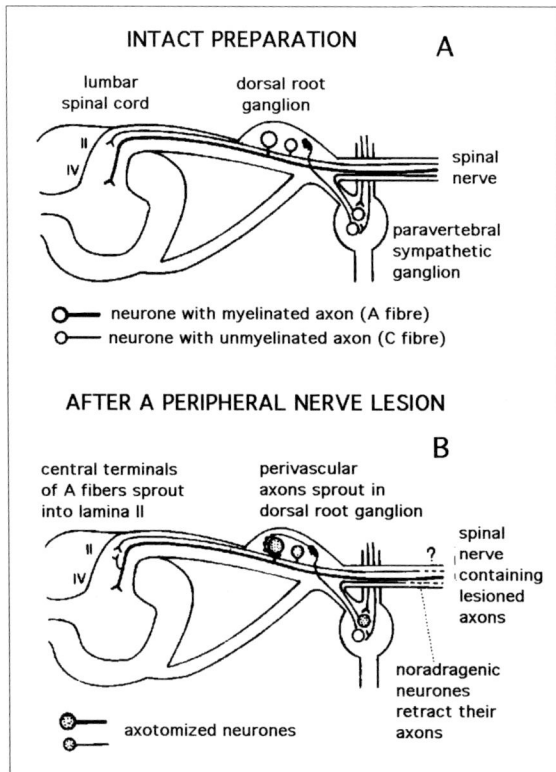

Figure 9. Relation between afferent neurons, sympathetic postganglionic neurons and their projections in the lumbar outflow. A : Myelinated and unmyelinated afferent neurons and postganglionic neurons form separate projections to the periphery and to the spinal cord and do not interact in normal conditions. B : After ligating and cutting the sciatic nerve, noradrenergic perivascular axons sprout into the dorsal root ganglia and form basketlike structure around large diameter axotomized sensory neurons. Repetitive sympathetic stimulation can generate bursting activity in such neurons. Central axons of sensory neurons with myelinated axons may sprout in their spinal projections into lamina II to gain access to the central nociceptive system (see [50, 62]).

diameter axotomized sensory cell bodies. Stimulation of the sympathetic outflow can activate these afferent neurons (Figure 9B). The aberrant pathological connections might account for spontaneous pain and allodynia in those patients who have evidence for pain which is dependent on sympathetic activity after peripheral nerve lesions.

The same type of nerve lesion has been shown to induce sprouting of large diameter DRG neurons into lamina II of the dorsal horn. These sprouts may fill vacated synaptic sites on the lamina II neurons [50, 62]. Thus, mechanisms exist by which mechano-sensitive large-diameter afferents may have access to the nociceptive system and activity in these afferents may be induced or enhanced by sympathetic activity.

What mechanisms underlie the sympathetic responses in DRG neurones ?

We now have experimental evidence of a new site for direct chemical coupling between sympathetic postganglionic terminals and primary afferent neurones after peripheral nerve injury. The neurones with which the coupling is made have predominantly large diameter axons, and so are likely to have been low threshold mechanoreceptor neurones, but activity in these neurones (as well as in nociceptor neurones) can give rise to pain sensations.

The effects of sympathetic activation are mediated *via* alpha-adrenoceptors. The alpha sub-type receptor has not yet been tested. There is almost no evidence of noradrenaline sensitivity in uninjured DRG neurones or their terminals in anaesthetized animals. This applies whether noradrenaline is "applied" by stimulation of sympathetic nerves or by introduction of relatively high concentrations (up to 5 microg/kg) into the circulation. In the experiment performed by Devor *et al.* [14], only one primary afferent neuron with large diameter has been found which was activated by sympathetic stimulation in control animals. This does not exclude the possibility that other DRG cells *in situ* can be affected by noradrenaline, but that these effects are subthreshold. When noradrenaline is applied at relatively high concentrations directly to the soma membrane, then some effects can be measured. Li *et al.* [38] and Wang *et al.* [60] have shown in preparations of toad dorsal root ganglia that noradrenaline can induce either depolarization or hyperpolarization of DRG somata. Depolarization was mediated by $alpha_1$-adrenoceptors and involved in a decrease of membrane conductance. Hyperpolarization was mediated by $alpha_2$-adrenoceptors and involved increase of membrane conductance, presumably a potassium conductance.

Exogenous noradrenaline has been shown to exert two distinct responses in mammalian central neurones. Increased excitability is due primarily to a decrease in the resting conductance of potassium ions ; noradrenaline at concentrations of 1-100 microM leads to depolarization of the membrane associated with an increase in input resistance. This response is mediated by either beta- or $alpha_1$ adrenoceptors in different cells, the latter involving a change in phosphoinositide turnover [42]. This conductance change would be consistent with the alpha-mediated excitatory responses described here. In other neurones, hyperpolarization arising from an increase in potassium conductance follows activation of $alpha_2$-adrenoceptors ; many of these neurones have a slow IPSP sensitive to $alpha_2$-adrenoceptor blockade [42]. This conductance change would be consistent with the alpha-mediated inhibitory responses described here. Thus the most simple way to explain sympathetically induced excitation and inhibition in DRG cells would be by decreases and increases of potassium conductance respectively (Figure 10). In many cases, the response of DRG neurones to lumbar sympathetic stimulation after a nerve lesion was excitation followed by inhibition ; if the mechanisms described above exist in axotomized DRG cells, both receptor types may be present. It is notable that there are other central neurones in which the pharmacology of the alpha receptor subtype is not at all clear ; blockade by specific antagonists and activation by specific agonists do not give consistent results. This may also be the case for the sympathetically-mediated responses in injured DRG neurones which have usually only been shown to be sensitive to phentolamine.

On the other hand, peripheral sensitivity to noradrenaline after a partial nerve lesion appears to be mediated *via* $alpha_2$-adrenoceptors [49]. If this is the case, a different cellular mechanism must be activated. A train of a few stimuli activating the postganglionic sympathetic terminals generates a slow $alpha_2$ mediated decrease in potassium conductance lasting about a minute in several vascular smooth muscles (tail artery : [10] ; vein : [55] ; spleen : [31]). The same intracellular pathway linking $alpha_2$-adrenoceptors to potassium channels might well be expressed in DRG cells after nerve lesions.

The intracellular mechanisms which operate in the DRG somata which show excitation and/or inhibition of activity to stimulation of the sympathetic outflow and to adrenaline remain to be clarified. It seems likely that they will be similar to those which have been shown for other neurones [42]. In future, intervention at adrenoceptor sites may be therapeutically successful. Whether interventions directed at the intracellular mechanisms can ever be used for therapy of sympathetically dependent pain is doubtful (Figure 10).

How do adrenoceptors appear in afferent neurones ?

There are a number of possible cellular mechanisms by which alpha-adrenoceptors might change so as to increase the noradrenaline sensitivity of large diameter DRG cells whichever type of alpha adrenoceptor is involved :
- novel appearance of alpha-adrenoceptor mRNA ;
- novel translation and/or transcription of mRNA leading to expression (synthesis) of alpha-adrenoceptors ;
- upregulation of the number of existing adrenoceptors ; the results reported above suggest they are present in some dissociated adult DRG cells ;

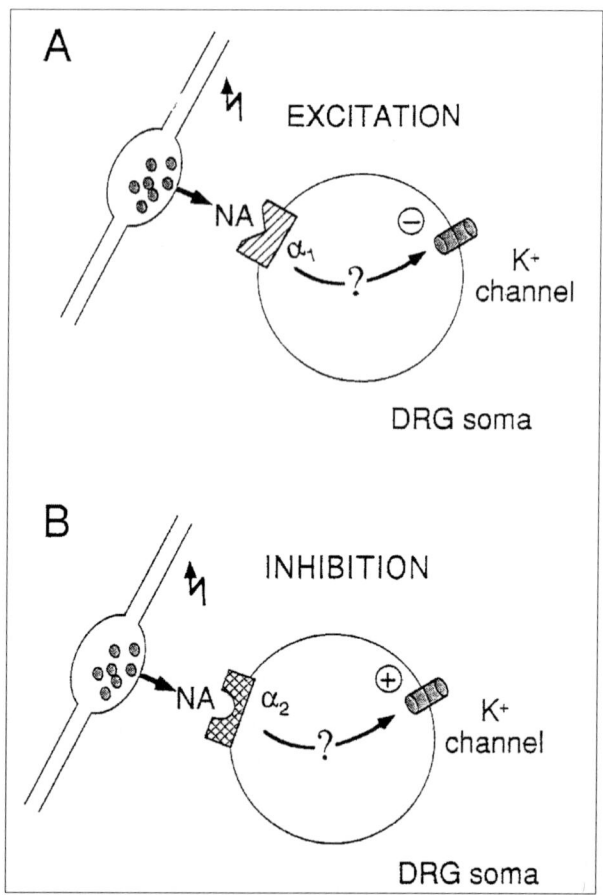

Figure 10. Putative adrenoceptors and intracellular pathways in DRG somata for mediating excitatory and inhibitory effects of noradrenaline (NA) released from the sympathetic varicosities close to the cell bodies during activation.
- inhibition, + activation.

- uncovering of "hidden" adrenoceptors, *i.e.* responses appear too quickly to be dependent on *de novo* protein synthesis.

It seems unlikely that the appearance of noradrenaline sensitivity can be explained by "upregulation" of adrenoceptors produced simply as a consequence of prolonged (nociceptor) neurone activity as suggested by Campbell *et al.* [9]. First, adrenosensitivity is not restricted to neurones which demonstrate ongoing activity [14]. Secondly, what prevents the appearance of this sensitivity in normal nociceptor neurones, *i.e* when there is no nerve injury ?

Further, the rekindling of pain following application of noradrenaline to the skin of some patients who had been successfully treated for spontaneous pain and hyperalgesia by sympathetic block or sympathectomy [11, 52, 59] indicates that the adrenoceptors persist on the terminals at a time when they were unlikely to be discharging (Figure 12).

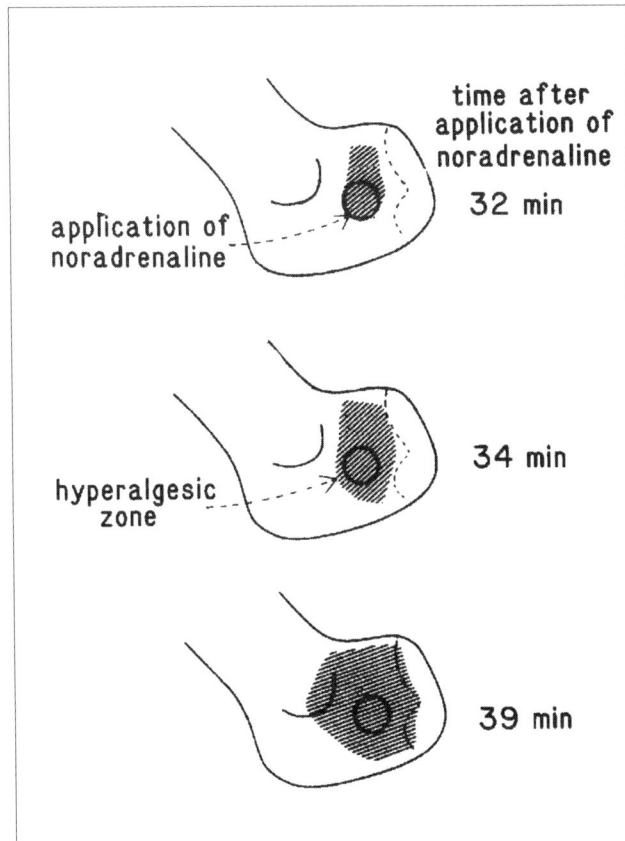

Figure 11. Patient 11 days after surgical sympathectomy of the lumbar sympathetic trunk. Spontaneous pain and mechanical hyperalgesia in the foot (toes amputated) disappeared. Iontophoretic application of noradrenaline (NA) to the previously hyperalgesic area (0.2 mg/ml to a 2 cm² area indicated by the solid circle). The skin became pale immediately after the application of NA; the skin temperature dropped by 3-4 degree Celsius. The temperature increased again after 5-7 min and the pallor persisted longer. About 30 min after NA application hyperalgesia to light touch (allodynia) developed, the intensity of hyperalgesia and the size of the hyperalgesic zone (hatched area) increased. When the hyperalgesia was maximal, the patient also felt some spontaneous pain. Pain and hyperalgesia had the same character as before the sympathectomy. Similar results were obtained from three other patients.(From [59] with permission.)

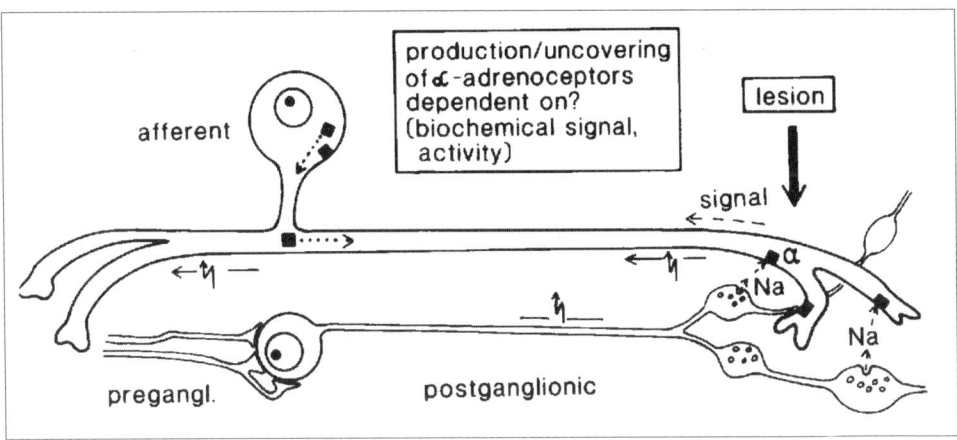

Figure 12. Upregulation or uncovering in adrenoceptors by afferent neurons after nerve lesion. Is this process related to activity in the afferent neurons, to the presence/absence of postganglionic noradrenergic neurons, to activity in the postganglionic neurons or even to sprouting of postganglionic and afferent neurons ? *See* text.

Perl ([44], *see* Perl, this volume) has proposed that the expression or upregulation of adrenoceptors in primary afferent neurones is related to the reduced number of axons in the target tissue, analogous to the development of the so-called "denervation supersensitivity" which is observed in effector tissues following their denervation [17]. If it were the loss of sympathetic axons that triggered the expression of alpha-adrenoceptors, then one would expect that afferent neurons become sensitive to catecholamine after sympathectomy. This has not directly been tested, but pain may develop in about 10% to 20% of the patients after surgical sympathectomy ("postsympathectomy neuralgia" [7, 43, 46, 53], "postsympathectomy neuralgia" [39]). Pain appears about 10 days after sympathectomy, lasts for a few weeks or months before disappearing. It would be interesting to know whether this pain can be relieved by an alpha-adrenoceptor antagonist.

In the rabbit ear [49], the main nerve was partially lesioned and excitation and sensitization to heat stimuli were produced in non-lesioned primary afferent polymodal nociceptors by sympathetic stimulation and by noradrenaline. What probably happens in this preparation is that partial denervation leads to collateral sprouting of the non-lesioned axons in the target tissue [18]. This might be in some way related to development of the catecholamine sensitivity of polymodal afferents. Sprouting of noradrenergic axons might lead to juxtaposition of noradrenergic terminals with axon terminals bearing alpha-adrenoceptors.

Acknowledgements

Supported by the Deutsche Forschungsgemeinschaft (WJ, MM), the German Israeli Foundation (WJ, MD) and the National Health & Medical Research Council of Australia (EM McL.)

References

1. Anderson CR, McLachlan EM, Srb-Christie O. Distribution of sympathetic preganglionic neurons and monoaminergic nerve terminals in the spinal cord of the rat. *J Comp Neurol* 1989 ; 283 : 269-84.
2. Arnér S. Intravenous phentolamine test : diagnostic and prognostic use in reflex sympathetic dystrophy. *Pain* 1991 ; 46 : 17-22.
3. Blumberg H, Jänig W. Changes of reflexes in vasoconstrictor neurons supplying the cat hindlimb following chronic nerve lesions : a model for studying mechanisms of reflex sympathetic dystrophy ? *J Auton Nerv Syst* 1983 ; 7 : 399-411.
4. Blumberg H, Jänig W. Clinical manifestations of reflex sympathetic dystrophy and sympathetically maintained pain. In : Wall PD, Melzack R, eds. *Textbook of pain*. Churchill Livingstone, 1993.
5. Bonica JJ. Causalgia and other reflex sympathetic dystrophies. In : Bonica JJ, Liebeskind JC, Albe-Fessard DG, eds. *Advances in pain research and therapy*. New York : Raven Press, 1979 ; 3 : 141-66.

6. Bonica JJ. Causalgia and other reflex sympathetic dystrophies. In : Bonica JJ, ed. *The Management of pain.* 2nd ed. Philadelphia, London : Lea & Febinger, 1990 : 220-43.
7. Brown GE, Adson AW. Physiologic effects of thoracic and of lumbar sympathetic ganglionectomy or section of the trunk. *Arch Neurol Psychiatry* 1929 ; 22 : 322-257.
8. Campbell JN, Meyer RA, Raja SN. Is nociceptor activation by alpha$_1$ adrenoreceptors the culprit in sympathetically maintained pain ? *Am Pain Soc J* 1992 ; 1 : 3-11.
9. Cajal, Ramon S. *Histologie du système nerveux de l'homme et des vertébrés.* Paris : Maloine, 1909-1911.
10. Cassell JF, McLachlan EM, Sittiracha T. The effect of temperature on neuromuscular transmission in the main caudal artery of the rat. *J Physiol* 1988 ; 397 : 31-44.
11. Davis KD, Treede RD, Raja SN, Meyer RA, Campbell JN. Topical application of clonidine relieves hyperalgesia in patients with sympathetically maintained pain. *Pain* 1991 ; 47 : 309-17.
12. Devor M, Basbaum AI, Bennett GJ, Blumberg H, Campbell JN, Dembowsky KP, Guibaud G, Jänig W, Koltzenburg M, Levine JD, Otten UH, Portenoy RK. Mechanisms of neuropathic pain following peripheral injury. In : Basbaum AI, Besson JM, eds. *Towards a new pharmacotherapy of pain.* Dahlem Workshop Reports. Chichester : John Wiley & Sons, 1991 : 417-40.
13. Devor M, Jänig W. Activation of myelinated afferents ending in a neuroma by stimulation of the sympathetic supply in the rat. *Neurosci Lett* 1981 ; 24 : 43-7.
14. Devor M, Jänig W, Michaelis M. Modulation of activity in dorsal root ganglion (DRG) neurons by sympathetic activation in nerve-injured rats. *J Neurophysiol* 1994 ; 71 : 38-47.
15. Devor M, Wall PD. Cross-excitation in dorsal root ganglia of nerve-injured and intact rats. *J Neurophysiol* 1990 ; 64 : 1733-46.
16. Evans JA. Reflex sympathetic dystrophy. *Surg Clin North Am* 1946 ; 26 : 780-90.
17. Fleming WW, Westfall DP. Adaptive supersensitivity. In : Trendelenburg W, Weiner N, eds. *Handbook of experimental pharmacology,* Vol 90/I Catecholamines I. Berlin, Heidelberg, New York : Springer Verlag, 1988 : 509-59.
18. Gloster A, Diamond J. Sympathetic nerves in adult rats regenerate normally and restore pilomotor function during an anti-NGF treatment that prevents their collateral sprouting. *J Comp Neurol* 1992 ; 326 : 362-74.
19. Goldstein RS, Raber P, Govrin-Lippmann R, Devor M. Contrasting time course of catecholamine accumulation and of spontaneous discharge in experimental neuromas in the rat. *Neurosci Lett* 1988 ; 94 : 58-63.
20. Hannington-Kiff JG. *Pain relief.* Philadelphia : Lippincott, 1974.
21. Jänig W. Systemic and specific autonomic reactions in pain : efferent, afferent and endocrine components. *Eur J Anaesth* 1985 ; 2 : 319-46.
22. Jänig W. Causalgia and reflex sympathetic dystrophy : in which way is the sympathetic nervous system involved ? *Trends Neurosci* 1985 ; 8 : 471-7.
23. Jänig W. The sympathetic nervous system in pain : physiology and pathophysiology. In : Stanton-Hicks M, ed. *Pain and the sympathetic nervous system.* Boston : Kluwer Academic Publishers, 1990 : 17-89.
24. Jänig W, Blumberg H, Boas RA, Campbell JA. The reflex sympathetic dystrophy syndrome : consensus statement and general recommendations for diagnosis and clinical reseach. In : Bond MR, Charlton JE, Woolf CJ, eds. *Pain research and clinical management* (Proceedings of the VIth World Congress on Pain) Amsterdam : Elsevier Science Publishers, 1991 : 372-5.
25. Jänig W, Koltzenburg M. What is the interaction between the sympathetic terminal and the primary afferent fiber ? In : Basbaum AI, Besson JM, eds. *Towards a new pharmacotherapy of pain,* Dahlem Workshop Reports. Chichester : John Wiley & Sons, 1991 : 331-52.
26. Jänig W, Koltzenburg M. Sympathetic reflex activity and neuroeffector transmission change after chronic nerve lesions. In : Bond MR, Charlton JE, Woolf CJ, eds. *Pain research and clinical*

management : Proceedings of the VIth World Congress on Pain, Vol 4. Amsterdam : Elsevier Science Publishers, 1991 : 365-71.
27. Jänig W, Koltzenburg M. Possible ways of sympathetic afferent interactions. In : Jänig W, Schmidt RF, eds. *Reflex sympathetic dystrophy. Pathophysiological mechanisms and clinical implications.* Weinheim : VCH Verlagsgesellschaft, 1992 : 213-45.
28. Jänig W, McLachlan E. On the fate of sympathetic and sensory neurons projecting into a neuroma of the superficial perineal nerve in the cat. *J Comp Neurol* 1984 ; 225 : 302-11.
29. Jänig W, McLachlan EM. The role of modifications in noradrenergic peripheral pathway after nerve lesions in the generation of pain. In : Fields HL, Liebeskind, eds. *Pharmacological approaches to the treatment of pain : new concepts and critical issues.* Vol 1. Seattle : IASP Press, 1994 : 101-28.
30. Jänig W, Schmidt FR. *Reflex sympathetic dystrophy. Pathophysiological mechanisms and clinical implications.* Weinhelm : VCH Verlagsgesellschaft, 1992.
31. Jobling P. Electrophysiological events during neuroeffector transmission in the spleen of guinea pig and rat. *J Physiol* 1994 : in press.
32. Jobling P, McLachlan EM. An electrophysiological study of responses evoked in isolated segments of rat tail artery during growth and maturation. *J Physiol* 1992 ; 454 : 83-105.
33. Jobling P, McLachlan EM, Jänig W, Anderson CR. Electrophysiological responses in the rat tail artery during reinnervation following lesions of the sympathetic supply. *J Physiol* 1992 ; 454 : 107-28.
34. Kajander KC, Wakisaka S, Bennett GJ. Spontaneous discharge originates in the dorsal root ganglion at the onset of a painful peripheral neuropathy in the rat. *Neurosci Lett* 1992 ; 138 : 225-8.
35. Kolston J, Lisney SJ, Mulholland MN, Passant CD. Transneuronal effects triggered by saphenous nerve injury on one side of a rat are restricted to neurones of the contralateral, homologous nerve. *Neurosci Lett* 1991 ; 130 : 187-9.
36. Kummer W, Gibbins IL, Stefan P, Kapoor V. Catecholamines and catecholamine-synthesizing enzymes in guinea-pig sensory ganglia. *Cell Tissue Res* 1990 ; 261 : 595-606.
37. Levine JD, Taiwo YO, Collins SD, Tam JK. Noradrenaline hyperalgesia is mediated through interaction with sympathetic postganglionic neurone terminals rather than activation of primary afferent nociceptors. *Nature* 1986 ; 323 : 158-60.
38. Li ZW, Wang AJ, Leng M, Yan XP. Actions of noradrenaline on alpha-adrenergic receptors of toad dorsal root ganglion neurones. *Acta Physiol Sin* 1988 ; 40 : 240-9.
39. Litwin MS. Postsympathectomy neuralgia. *Arch Surg* 1962 ; 84 : 591-5.
40. McLachlan EM, Jänig W, Devor M, Michaelis M. Peripheral nerve injury triggers noradrenergic sprouting within dorsal root ganglia. *Nature* 1993 ; 363 : 543-5.
41. Morris JL, Gibbins IL. Co-transmission and neuromodulation. In : Burnstock G, Hoyle CHV eds. *Autonomic neuroeffector mechanisms.* Chur Switzerland : Harwood Academic Publishers, 1992 : 33-119.
42. Nicoll RA, Malenka RC, Kauer JA. Functional comparison of neurotransmitter receptor subtypes in mammalian central nervous system. *Physiol Rev* 1990 ; 70 : 513-65.
43. Nystrom TG. Lumbar sympathectomy : late results in chronic obliterative arterial diseases of the legs. *Arch Chir Scand* Suppl 1949 ; 142 : 1-127.
44. Perl ER. Alterations in the responsiveness of cutaneous nociceptors : sensitization by noxious stimuli and the induction of adrenergic responsiveness by nerve injury. In : Willis WD, ed. *Hyperalgesia and allodynia.* New York : Raven Press, 1992 : 59-79.
45. Raja SN, Treede RD, Davis KD, Campbell JN. Systemic alpha-adrenergic blockade with phentolamine : a diagnostic test for sympathetically maintained pain. *Anesthesiology* 1991 ; 74 : 691-8.

46. Raskin NH, Levinson SA, Hoffman PM, Pickett JBE, Fields HL. Postsympathectomy neuralgia. Amelioration with diphenylhydantoin and carbamazepine. *Am J Surg* 1974 ; 128 : 75-8.
47. Roberts WJ. A hypothesis on the physiological basis for causalgia and related pains. *Pain* 1986 ; 24 : 297-311.
48. Rotshenker S. Multiple modes and sites for the induction of axonal growth. *Trends Neurosci* 1988 ; 11 : 363-6.
49. Sato J, Perl ER. Adrenergic excitation of cutaneous pain receptors induced by peripheral nerve injury. *Science* 1991 ; 251 : 1608-10.
50. Shortland P, Woolf CJ. Chronic peripheral nerve section results in a rearrangement of the central axonal arborizations of axotomized A beta primary afferent neurons in the rat spinal cord. *J Comp Neurol* 1993 ; 330 : 65-82.
52. Stanton-Hicks M. *Pain and the sympathetic nervous system.* Boston : Kluwer Academic Publishers, 1990.
53. Torebjork E. Clinical and neurophysiological observations relating to psychophysiological mechanisms in reflex sympathetic dystrophy. In : Stanton Hicks M, Jänig W, Boas RA, eds. *Reflex sympathetic dystrophy.* Boston : Kluwer Academic Publishers, 1990 : 71-80.
54. Tracy GD, Cockett FB. Pain in the lower limb after sympathectomy. *Lancet* 1957 ; 1 : 12-4.
55. Utzschneider D, Kocsis J, Devor M. Mutual excitation among dorsal root ganglion neurons in the rat. *Neurosci Lett* 1992 ; 146 : 53-6.
56. Van Helden DF. Electrophysiology of neuromuscular transmission in guinea-pig mesenteric veins. *J Physiol* 1988 ; 401 : 469-88.
57. Wakisaka S, Kajander KC, Bennett GJ. Effect of peripheral nerve injuries and tissue inflammation on the levels of neuropeptide Y-like immunoreactivity in rat primary afferent neurons. *Brain Res* 1992 ; 598 : 349-52.
58. Walker AE, Nulsen F. Electrical stimulation of the upper thoracic portion of the sympathetic chain in man. *Arch Neurol Psychiatry* 1948 ; 59 : 559-60.
59. Wall PD, Devor M. Sensory afferent impulses originate from dorsal root ganglia as well as from the periphery in normal and nerve injured rats. *Pain* 1983 ; 17 : 321-39.
60. Wallin G, Torebjork HE, Hallin RG. Preliminary observations on the pathophysiology of hyperalgesia in the causalgic pain syndrome. In : Zottermann Y, ed. *Sensory functions of the skin in primates.* Oxford : Pergamon, 1976 : 489-99.
61. Wang AJ, Li ZW, Hu MX, Wang SD, Leng M. Ionic mechanism of noradrenaline-induced membrane potential changes of neurones in dorsal root ganglion. *Acta Physiol Sin* 1989 ; 41 : 145-52.
62. White JC, Sweet WH. *Pain and the neurosurgeon.* Springfield, Illinois : Charles C. Thomas, 1969.
63. Woolf CJ, Shortland P, Coggeshall RE. Peripheral nerve iniury triggers central sprouting of myelinated afferents. *Nature* 1992 ; 355 : 75-8.

8

Capsaicin and pharmacology of nociceptors

J. SZOLCSÁNYI, R.PÓRSZÁSZ, G. PETHÖ

Department of Pharmacology, University Medical School of Pécs, Pécs, Hungary.

The selective site of action of capsaicin and their analogues on a subset of primary sensory neurons comprising the polymodal nociceptors opened new perspectives in afferent pharmacology and pain therapy. The chapter is an overview of some recent achievements, emphasizing possible explanations for unsettled issues in this field. The concept that sensory neurons with well defined types of exteroceptors belong to the capsaicin-sensitive (CS) afferentation is supported by single unit recordings from peripheral nerves. Generator region of CS subset of receptors seems to be chemoceptive in general and supplied by capsaicin/resiniferatoxin-operated nonselective cation channels suitable for activation by protons. CS receptors have bidirectional function. They serve for both afferent impulse initiation and mediator release for efferent neuroregulatory tissue responses. These transduction and effector functions can be analysed both in vivo *and* in vitro *with the aid of ruthenium red, a blocking agent of the CS cation channel, and by using resiniferatoxin a highly potent toxin acting on the capsaicin recognition site. Four stages in the action of capsaicin are suggested : (1) excitation ; (2) sensory neuron blockade ; (3) degenerative neurotoxic stage ; (4) irreversible cell destruction. Degeneration or axonal blockade alone does not explain the antinociceptive effects of capsaicin. Secondary changes after neonatal capsaicin treatment in the rat and mice confound the role of CS sensory neurons when testings are made in the adult age. The action of capsaicin on sensory neuropeptides is discussed from this point of view.*

Sensory effects of capsaicin have five hundred years of written history. Christopher Columbus in his letter to the Spanish Royal Majesties dated on 1493 described for the first time the very hot sensation induced by chilli peppers commonly used by the inhabitants of the New World [41, 77]. The considerable selective site of action of the pungent ingredient of red and green peppers on sensory fibers had been recognized already in the first research paper published on this topic in the last century [26]. The unexpected observation that capsaicin in high doses produces chemical analgesia without affecting nociception to mechanical stimuli raised the possibility to use it as a pharmacological tool in nociception and neurogenic inflammation [27-29]. First evidence for a selective action on C-polymodal nociceptors [68] with small B-type sensory neurons of the trigeminal and dorsal root ganglia [35, 78] formed the basis to define the target neurons for this drug. Capsaicin induced release and depletion of substance P from the primary afferent neurons and their processes [18, 33, 87, 94]. Thus, biochemical results also supported this remarkable selective new type of drug action and has added force to the neuropeptide research. Furthermore, with the aid of this compound drug development for analgesics acting on nociceptive primary afferent neurons has been initiated [7, 10, 50, 51, 76, 78, 80, 92].

The aim of this chapter is to summarize some recent achievements in this field and to reevaluate some earlier findings in order to help further research in pharmacology of nociceptors, particularly in respect of appropriate usage of capsaicin type agents.

Sensory receptors which are sensitive to capsaicin

Receptor types which are sensitive and insensitive to the stimulatory effect of capsaicin has been described in mammals using the single unit technique.

Cutaneous receptors

C-polymodal nociceptors were excited in all studies tested by close arterial injection in the rabbit [69, 73] and rat [82], by topical application onto the skin of the rat [36], cat [17], monkey [5] and humans [39] or by intradermal injection in the rabbit [73], rat [55] and monkey [5]. In the skin of monkey «heat nociceptors», mechanoheat insensitive «chemonociceptors» and warmth receptors were also excited by intradermal injection [5]. Other types of C-afferents as the high threshold mechanoreceptors (HTM), low threshold mechanoreceptors (LTM) or cold receptors were not activated in these studies.

A-delta polymodal nociceptors described as «mechanoheat sensitive nociceptors» showed also high chemical excitability to capsaicin in the rat [82] and monkey [5]. Other types of cutaneous A-afferents including the A-delta HTM (mechanonociceptors) and cold receptors as well as mechanoreceptors with A-beta fibers were insensitive to the action of capsaicin. More detailed discussion of these single unit data as well as description of the subclasses of capsaicin-sensitive interoceptors have been reviewed elsewhere [75, 77].

Corneal receptors

Topical application of capsaicin to the cat's cornea excited all polymodal nociceptors tested, but not the HTM or cold receptors. Intracorneal terminal part of the fiber of these receptors conducted in the C-fiber range, but their more proximal portion had myelinated axons conducting in the A-delta range [6].

Concept of capsaicin-sensitive afferents

Single unit data on exteroceptors suggest a selective site of action for capsaicin which is confined to well defined subsets of sensors and is not related to the conduction velocity of their axon *per se*. Therefore the concept of a pharmacological classification for afferents as «capsaicin-sensitive» and insensitive populations has been introduced to label primary afferent neurons under conditions when characterization was not performed by single unit recordings [70, 71, 76, 77]. No distinctive morphological or immunocytochemical marker for this neural population has been described yet [24, 25]. Nevertheless the selectivity of the drug and the concept for classification of afferents on this ground has gained strong support by functional, histochemical and biochemical data. Designation of a subgroup of afferents as capsaicin-sensitive is now in common usage [7, 23-25, 42, 47, 50].

Pharmacological differentiation among neurotransmission processes in the autonomic and motoric part of the peripheral neurons system by alkaloids as nicotine, atropin, curare etc. had been the starting point for fruitful development in the past. Molecular background of these observations, *i.e.* identification of the pharmacological recognition sites for these drugs, became a reality only many decades later. Structure activity relationships [79, 80] and marked species differences [28, 81] formed the basis to suggest a similar pharmacological receptive site for capsaicin on nociceptors [70, 79]. Recent binding studies and patch clamp recordings from isolated neurons of the dorsal root ganglia *in vitro* are in agreement with this suggestion and have provided a detailed insight into the ionic basis of the action of capsaicin type agents [7, 92].

Mechanism of capsaicin induced depolarization

Nanomolar concentrations of capsaicin open a nonselective cation channel on a subpopulation of primary afferent neurons. Anions such as Cl- do not contribute directly to the cell depolarization [7, 54, 93]. Thus, in physiological conditions, both calcium and sodium ions will flow into the cell while potassium will flow out. No second messenger systems are necessary for the capsaicin induced depolarization. This new type of cation channel can be activated by protons at the soma [8] and at the nociceptors in rat skin, *in vitro* [66].

Ruthenium red, (RR) an inorganic dye, blocks the capsaicin-operated cation channel [3], and capsazepine, a structural analogue of capsaicin, (Figure 1) blocks the capsaicin receptive site in a competitive manner [9, 15].

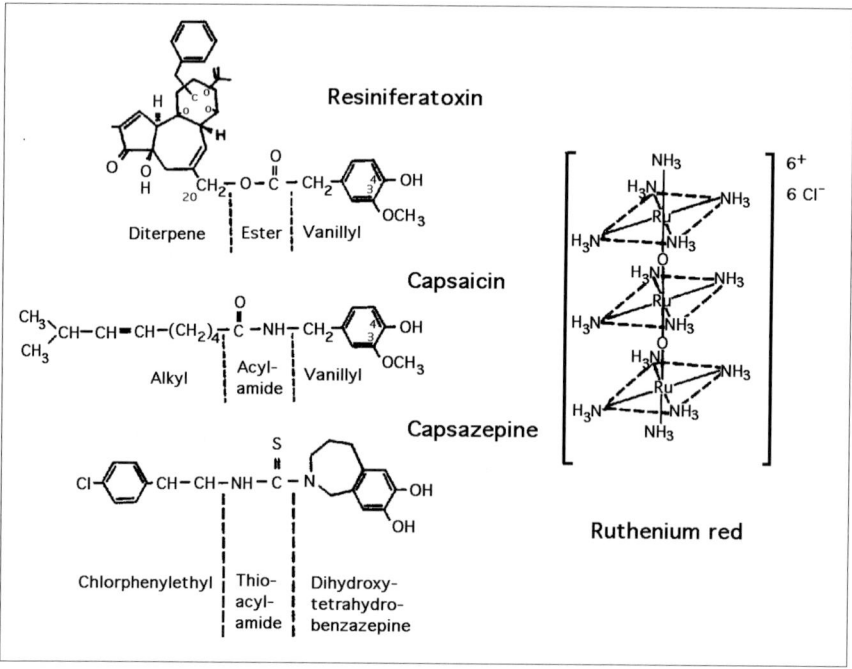

Figure 1. Chemical structure of resiniferatoxin, capsaicin, capsazepine and ruthenium red.

Resiniferatoxin (RTX), a natural product of plant origin, has an identical substituted ring as capsaicin but contains bulky more rigid diterpene apolar moity instead of an alkyl chain (Figure 1). This toxin is several hundred folds more potent than capsaicin, to open the capsaicin-operated cation channel [7, 48, 67, 83]. Depolarization of isolated sensory neurons by RTX has a much slower time course than that induced by capsaicin [91]. Similar difference in time course seems to occur at the level of the sensory receptors. In the cat, the Bezold-Jarisch cardiorespiratory vagal reflex triad (pulmonary chemoreflex) to intravenous injection of RTX develops much slower and lasts much longer than that evoked by capsaicin [75]. It is even more remarkable that in the rat long term blocking the function of these pulmonary sensors to the stimulatory effects of capsaicin or phenyldiguanide was achieved by RTX without an initial activation of the reflex (Figure 2A).

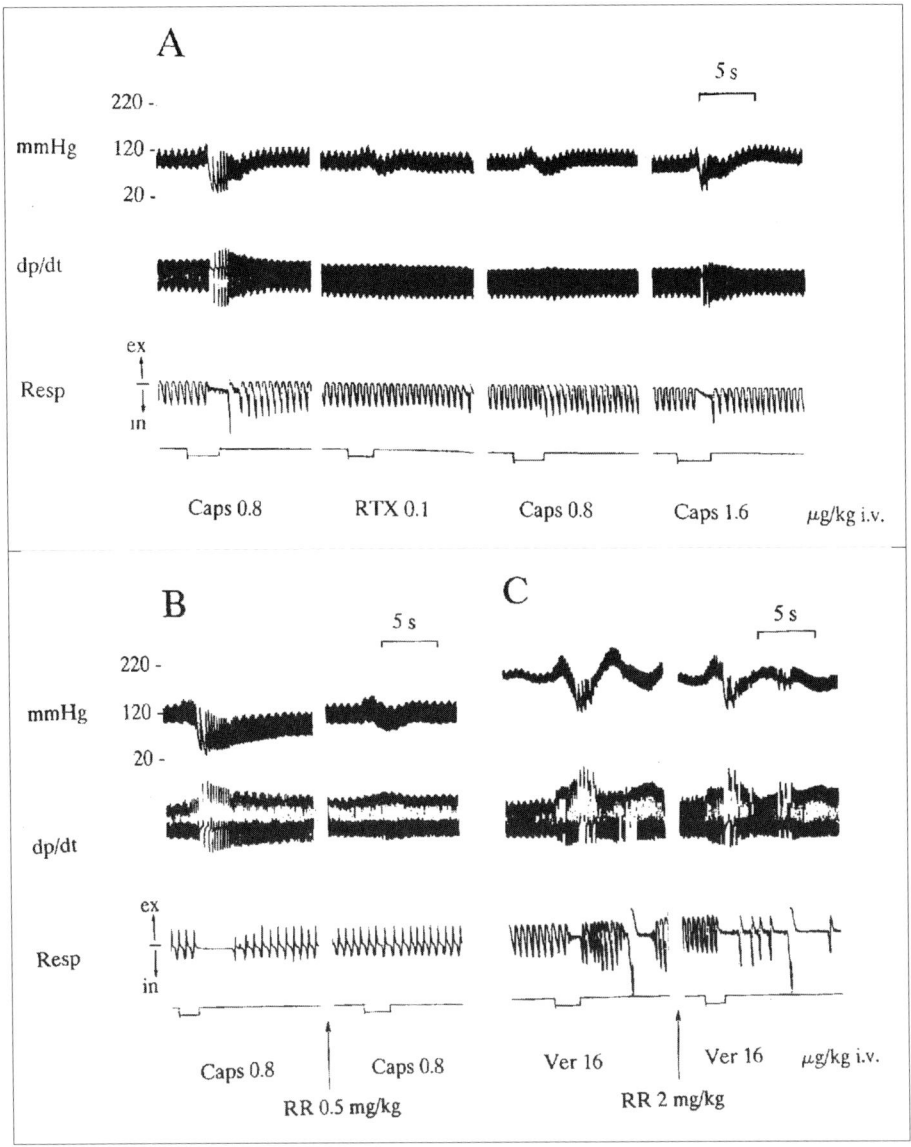

Figure 2. Effect of resiniferatoxin (RTX on panel A) and ruthenium red (RR on panel B, C) on the pulmonary chemoreflex elicited by capsaicin (Caps) and veratidine (Ver) in three rats (A, B, C) anesthetized by 1.0-1.2 g/kg s.c. urethane. In each panel, upper records : blood pressure ; dp/dt : heart contractility ; lowest records : respiratory movements. Note that RTX inhibited the capsaicin-induced response without provoking the reflex (A) and RR inhibited the effect of capsaicin but not the veratridine-induced reflex.

RR antagonized the action of capsaicin, but not that of veratridine (Figure 2B,C). In the guinea pig RR aerosol also attenuated the capsaicin or RTX evoked neural bronchoconstrictor response and calcitonin gene-related peptide release but not that induced by nicotine, bradykinin or histamine [43]. Veratridine opens the tetrodotoxin-sensitive fast sodium channels on the regenerative region of the nerve fiber [60]. The observation that activation of the regenerative region in this way (Figure 3) was not inhibited by RR indicates that interaction between capsaicin and RR does not affect the regenerative spike generation, or axonal spike propagation. It has been suggested [76, 84] that the principal site of action of capsaicin, RR and RTX is at the generative region of the sensory receptors (Figure 3). Capsaicin operated cation channels of the terminal axon seems to be less accessible to these drugs because they are within Schwann cell envelope. In fact, it has been shown that ultrastructural changes induced by capsaicin in terminal part of nerve fibers in the rat's cornea was conspious only in these «free nerve endings» and in the partly uncovered sites of the terminal axon [79]. Similar «free» axonal beads of the terminal portion of unmyelinated sensory fibers have been described in other parts of the body [20]. Therefore they could serve as multiple transduction sites to chemical nociceptive or other stimuli. Moreover it has already been described that intra-arterial injection of capsaicin to the rabbit ear elicited after a burst of discharges functional blockade of the C-polymodal nociceptors to one or another type of stimuli. For example abolition of the mechanical responsiveness of a single unit could match with unchanged responsiveness to noxious heating and *vice versa* [73, 76]. On one hand, this is indicative for a blockade of one sensory transducer without affecting the other one at the same unit. Considering the relatively simple membrane effects of capsaicin, this observation forms the first experimental evidence that a C-polymodal nociceptive unit might in fact consist of an axon with multiple sets of single modal generator regions at the nerve terminal arborization. On the other hand, the remained responsiveness to one kind of natural stimulus suggests that in the case of close arterial injection blockade of axonal conduction [54] or a site of action on the regenerative region (Figure 3) is of secondary importance.

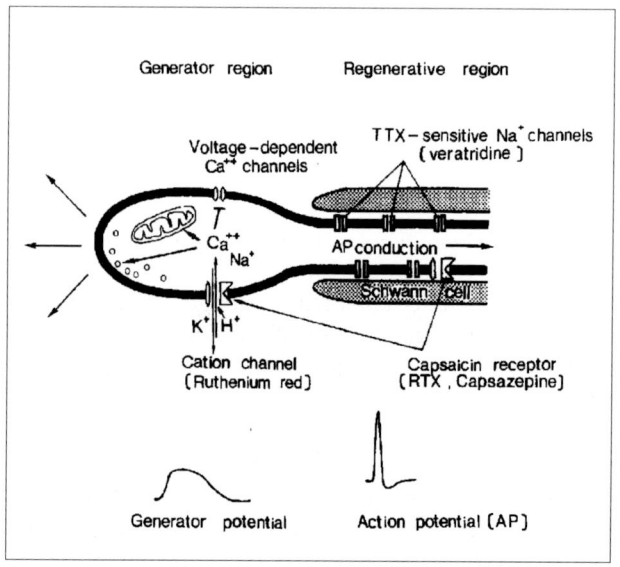

Figure 3. Schematic representation of the site and mode of action of capsaicin, resiniferatoxin and their antagonists of capsazepine and ruthenium red on the polymodal nociceptor. Three arrows on the left indicate the release of mediators (tachykinins, calcitonin gene-related peptide, somatostatin) which elicit effector responses (dual sensory-efferent function). (Modified from [84].) For more details *see* text.

Drugs as the veratrum alkaloids or volatile anaesthetics which act on the regenerative region of mechanoreceptors sensitize the receptors without lowering the threshold to their natural stimuli [60]. On the contrary, topical application of capsaicin to the skin elicits a pronounced lowering of the thermal threshold of the nociceptors and in the human skin allodynia develops to mild warm temperature or to gentle stroking [68]. Again, in the rat noxious heat threshold is lower for a few hours after systemic capsaicin application [75]. These observations point again to a site of action of capsaicin at the generator region of the nociceptors. It is worthy to mention that in an *in vitro* rat's skin preparation bradykinin and low pH (6.1) induced a decrease in threshold of C-polymodal nociceptors to thermal and mechanical stimuli, respectively [37, 66]. The prediction of Paintal for the primary importance of the regenerative region in excitation induced by drugs was based mainly on experimental results on mechanoreceptors with myelinated fibers [4, 60]. It is tempting to assume that the physiological relevance of the capsaicin-sensitivity in a major subset of primary afferent neurons resides on their characteristic chemoceptive generator regions at the receptors. The capsaicin-operated cation channels respond to low shift of pH and protons released from the surrounding tissues might be a common stimulus for them. Furthermore, involvement of the capsaicin-gated cation channel in the transduction process to noxious heating is also indicated by the following ground. Systemic application of RR (4 mg/kg s.c.) in the rat induced a significant increase in noxious heat threshold by $2.3 \pm 0.2°C$ ($n=10$) for several hours [85]. This polar molecule apparently does not penetrate through the blood brain barrier [3], and local application of RR also antagonizes excitation of nociceptors by capsaicin or thermal stimuli [1, 2, 65]. Nociceptor function of pulmonary capsaicin-sensitive receptors is indicated by the observation that in humans the immediate sensation elicited by intravenous injection of capsaicin is substernal burning pain [90].

Mechanism of capsaicin-induced sensory blockade

Long-lasting unresponsiveness of polymodal nociceptors and other capsaicin-sensitive receptors develops after initial activation evoked by high doses of capsaicin. No lasting blockade ensued on the capsaicin-insensitive neural population in studies where unit recordings were made either from single afferent fibers or from cell bodies of isolated neurons of sensory or sympathetic ganglia. The function of various autonomic neuroeffectors remained also unimpaired [24, 50, 51, 75-77]. It has been suggested that the initial mechanism for the sensory blockade or neurotoxicity are the same as those for stimulation. Prolonged influx of Ca2+ into the sensors at the terminal (Figure 3) and «free beads» of terminal axon [86] or into the cell induce intracellular damage probably by impairment of mitochondria and activation of Ca2+-dependent enzymes.

Furthermore, influx of Na+ through the capsaicin-activated channels is accompanied by passive Cl- ion and water uptake producing in this way a damage by osmotic swelling. [7]. Neuroselective osmotic swelling with damaged mitochondria («high-amplitude» swelling) of the cell body develops within 5 min in 10 μM capsaicin solution under *in vitro* conditions [54]. Instillation of capsaicin (33 mM) into the eye of the rat induces similar ultrastructural changes for at least 24 hours in some «free nerve endings» of the cornea [79]. It has been suggested [72, 75, 77] that at the cellular level there are four stages in responses depending on the degree of agonism induced by capsaicin-type agents.

Stage 1

It is the sensory excitation, which is reproducible when near threshold concentrations of capsaicin are used under a given experimental condition. Excitation is accompanied by release of neuropeptide mediators (tachykinins, calcitonin gene-related peptide, somatostatin) from the sensory receptors or central terminals of primary afferent neurons in a tetrodotoxin-insensitive manner (Figure 3).

Stage 2

It is the sensory neuron blocking effect with decreased or no responses of the sensors to natural stimuli. The release of sensory neuropeptides is also abolished, but it could occur without evidence of depletion. Ultrastructural changes and the loss of function are reversible.

Stage 3

It is the degenerative neurotoxic effect when nerve terminals of the capsaicin-sensitive primary afferent neurons undergo degeneration with loss of axons, particularly at their terminal portion in the periphery [14] or in the dorsal horn [61]. The effect is irreversible although there are signs of a partial functional recovery [82]. Cell body of B-cells of cranial or dorsal root ganglia show similar ultrastructural changes as observed after acute *in vitro* capsaicin exposure. These morphological signs in the somata last for more than two months - in line with the impaired function - after systemic pretreatment of rats and mice [12, 35, 76, 77, 79].

Stage 4

It is the irreversible cell destruction, which is characteristic for systemic pretreatment of rats and mice in the neonatal age [21, 30, 32, 40, 59]. Cell destruction ensued within 20 min causing a more rapid degeneration of C-terminals than during transganglionic degeneration after peripheral nerve transection [22, 30]. These acute effects of capsaicin in the neonatal age are probably restricted to the capsaicin-sensitive subset of primary afferent neurons. C-polymodal nociceptors seem to be mature in the newborn rats in respect of their responsiveness to natural stimuli [16]. Activation of capsaicin/RTX-gated cation channels in cultured neurons from the dorsal root ganglia of the neonatal or adult rat were also similar [91].

It has been claimed that an exceptionally high first dose of capsaicin (100 mg/kg s.c.) could produce within a few hours complete cell destruction of a subset of B-cells in the adult rat [31, 32]. The ultrastructural picture of these damaged somata, however, strikingly resembles to the surviving neurons observed several weeks after the treatment [12, 35]. Neurofilament accumulation, neuronal cell fissure and fragmentation with altered satellite cells surrounding degenerating neurons described after neonatal treatment [21] were not reported in rats treated in the adult age. Furthermore, after systemic treatment when 90% of all axons degenerate in the ureter no appreciable degeneration in dorsal root was seen [13]. These data cast some doubts about the evidence for complete cell destruction after systemic capsaicin treatment in the adult rat [75].

Qualitative differences between the effect of neonatal and adult treatments in the rat and mice

There are versatile ways to block the function of capsaicin-sensitive primary afferents in mature mammals by high doses of the drug. Topical application to the receptive field (*e.g.* to the blister base, or skin on humans, instillation into the eye of rodents), close arterial injections and perfusions, systemic treatments (rat, mouse, guinea-pig, rabbit, cat), *in vitro* uses on isolated organs and tissue culture, periaxonal treatments (rat, guinea-pig), intrathecal, intracysternal or intracerebroventricular injections have been effective in this respect. The reader is referred to description of details of these treatments in recent reviews [24, 25, 75-77].

Under various conditions in different mammalian species the impaired subset of sensors are identical to that which is excited by low concentration ranges. Significant differences occur in the induced severity of impairment depending mainly on the degree of agonism and the site(s) of the neurons and their processes which are exposed to the drug. The evidence obtained from single unit studies suggests that the loss of function is due to both stage 2 and stage 3 degree of impairment within the capsaicin-sensitive neuron population of the same animal [75-77]. Signs of stage 1 excitation should be considered after systemic application for several hours [75] and the reversible nonselective axonal blockade after local treatments in high concentrations might be a source of misinterpretation [77].

Newborn rats treated with capsaicin are usually tested in the adult age to decide the role of capsaicin-sensitive afferents in various experimental conditions. Single unit recordings, from cutaneous nerves of these animals revealed, however, that there is no selective loss of polymodal nociceptors, in striking contrast to that obtained in rats treated with capsaicin in the adult age [46, 82, 89]. The profound reduction of C- and A-delta fibers is due to an indiscriminate loss of functionally identified units. The spectrum of destructed primary afferent neurons depends on the dose [59]. Selective degeneration of C afferents has been observed within the range of 20-30 mg/kg, but with higher doses loss of myelinated fibers (18% loss at 50 mg/kg) and a significant elimination of large light, monoclonal antibody RT96 labelled A-type sensory neurons (34% loss after 85 mg/kg) was described [40]. On the other hand, the remained C-polymodal nociceptors react to capsaicin or natural stimuli as that of the untreated controls [46, 75, 89].

After a systemic dose of 50 mg/kg s.c. degeneration of both B-type and A-type sensory neurons was observed also in the newborn mice. This study [21] revealed an important difference in the time course. B-type neurons showed rapid degeneration already 5 hours after the treatment, while A-type neurons started to degenerate about three days later. The effects were attributed to a direct action of capsaicin on the former and secondary changes on the latter type of neurons.

After neonatal treatment secondary changes with reorganization in sensory pathway, particularly in the dorsal horn, are striking [11, 52, 58, 63, 88]. There are also marked developmental alterations in nociceptive threshold, immunoreactive calcitonin gene-related peptide and substance P in the dorsal horn [19]. Furthermore, in the periphery tissue concentrations of histamine and 5-hydroxy- tryptamine are increased, innervation density of sympathetic neurons is increased [25]. Urinary excretion is impaired in neonatal, but not in the adult treated rats [53] and in contrast to the present findings the Bezold Jarisch reflex is not inhibited after neonatal capsaicin pretreatment [56].

Taking into consideration the profound readjustments after neonatal capsaicin treatments, it is almost impossible to differentiate between the participation of primary and secondary events in nociception and regulatory responses if testings are made in the adult age. It is also questionable on this ground that practically all sensory neuropeptides supposed to be depleted by capsaicin are real markers for the capsaicin-sensitive subset of primary afferent neurons [24, 25]. There are convincing data in adult rodents that tachykinins, calcitonin gene-related peptide (CGRP), and somatostatin are depleted and fluoride resistant acid phosphatase is also diminished after the treatment. Convincing evidence is lacking, however, for cholecystokinin (CCK), vasoactive intestinal polypeptide (VIP), arginine vasopressin, bombesin, or galanin. Many assessments were made in respect of CCK or VIP, and for example after intrathecal injection - when pronounced analgesia was observed - neither immunohistochemistry nor radioimmunoassay showed any effect of capsaicin-type agents [34, 57]. In fact, expression of CCK messenger RNA is not present in the dorsal root ganglia of the rat [64].

There is no evidence for depletion of VIP in the adult rat and several negative results have been reported in respect of the guinea-pig [24, 25]. Both species are similarly sensitive to capsaicin [75] and the occurrence of VIP immunostained ganglion cells in the trigeminal, nodose and spinal ganglia are similar [44]. As far as I know the only report on a capsaicin-induced decrease of VIP-like immunoreactive fibers in adult treated rats ($n=2$) was described in the trachea [38], which is a variance of that found on the same tissue of the guinea-pig [45]. In the light of these data in adult rodents B-type sensory neurons and their terminals containing VIP-like immunoreactivity seem not to be sensitive to capsaicin. Conclusive evidence suggests, however, that capsaicin induces VIP release from the human gut although a direct on VIP-containing neurons needs further investigations [49].

Function of polymodal nociceptors and other capsaicin-sensitive receptors

Studies with capsaicin in animals and human beings provided evidence for activation of polymodal nociceptors without the intervention of low threshold mechanoreceptors and A-delta mechanonociceptors to produce sensory pain and nociception. The versatile ways of its application and the unique selective blockade of a nociceptor population is a powerful pharmacological means in this research field. Furthermore, it has opened a new trend of research to develop drugs acting on nociceptors. The capsaicin-sensitive afferentiation comprises about half of the population of primary afferent neurons. With the aid of capsaicin new aspects of the functional role of this neural system have emerged, besides its pivotal role in nociception and pain. These new aspects have been discussed in recent [76, 77, 86, 92] and earlier reviews [23, 47, 71, 74]. Therefore the major conclusions of these results are only briefly summarized here. It has been suggested that polymodal nociceptors are nerve terminals with multiple sensory-efferent functions [76, 86]. Effector response as increase in microcirculation develops at threshold stimulation which may occur below the level of signalling pain or nociception. Ultra-violet irradiation is a type of stimulation which induces sparse activity (*e.g.* 6 impulses/min) without preceeding high frequency activation to produce sensitization [73]. Stimulation with higher intensities elicits nociception and the released tachykinins induce local inflammation. Axon reflexes are not obligatory arrangements to mediate these effector responses [78]. The tetrodotoxin-resistant terminal (Figure 3) or axonal varicosities are the sites of both the sensory transduction and mediator releasing processes. Mediators released from capsaicin-sensitive interoceptors with thin fibers evoke various effector responses in internal organs (vasodilatation, inflammation, bronchoconstriction, motility changes in the gastrointestinal and urinary tract, increase in heart rate, etc.). Some mediators are released to act on distant parts of the body producing an anti-inflammatory effect [62, 76]. In respect of the afferent function besides pain and nociception elicited from both exteroceptive and interoceptive areas [90] capsaicin evokes also warmth and itch sensation from the skin, sneezing and coughing from the respiratory airways. Furthermore, the chemoceptive nature of the capsaicin-sensitive interoceptors might participate in regulation of the inner chemical environment [75]. These functions might be related to subpopulations of capsaicin-sensitive receptors, but the possibility of more than one afferent function for the same neuron population should also be considered.

Acknowledgements

This work was supported by research grants OTKA No 307 and TKT T-563.

References

1. Amann R, Donnerer J, Lembeck F. Activation of primary afferent neurons by thermal stimulation. Influence of ruthenium red. *Naunyn-Schmiedeberg's Arch Pharmacol* 1990 ; 341 : 108-13.
2. Amann R, Lembeck F. Ruthenium red selectively prevents capsaicin-induced nociceptor stimulation. *Eur J Pharmacol* 1989 ; 161 : 227-9.
3. Amann R, Maggi CA. Ruthenium red as a capsaicin antagonist. *Life Sci* 1991 ; 49 : 849-56.
4. Anand A, Paintal AS. Possible role of capillary permeability in the excitation of sensory receptors by chemical substances. *Prog Brain Res* 1988 ; 74 : 337-40.
5. Baumann TK, Simone DA, Shain CN, LaMotte RH. Neurogenic hyperalgesia : the search for the primary cutaneous afferent fibers that contribute to capsaicin-induced pain and hyperalgesia. *J Neurophysiol* 1991 ; 66 : 212-27.
6. Belmonte C, Gallar J, Pozo MA, Rebollo I. Excitation by irritant chemical substances of sensory afferent units in the cats cornea. *J Physiol* 1991 ; 437 : 709-25.
7. Bevan S, Szolcsányi J. Sensory neurone-specific actions of capsaicin : mechanisms and applications. *Trends Pharmacol Sci* 1990 ; 11 : 330-3.
8. Bevan S, Yeats J. Protons activate a cation conductance in a sub-population of rat dorsal root ganglion neurones. *J Physiol* 1991 ; 433 : 145-61.
9. Bevan S, Hothi S, Hughes G, James JF, Rang HP, Shah K, Walpole CSJ, Yeats JC. Capsazepine : a competitive antagonist of the sensory neurone excitant capsaicin. *Br J Pharmacol* 1992 ; 107 : 544-52.
10. Carter RB. Topical capsaicin in the treatment of cutaneous disorders. *Drug Dev Res* 1991 ; 22 : 9-123.
11. Cervero F, Plenderleith MB. Spinal cord sensory systems after neonatal capsaicin. *Acta Physiol Hung* 1987 ; 69 : 393-401.
12. Chiba T, Masuka S, Kawano H. Correlation of mitochondrial swelling after capsaicin treatment and substance P and somatostatin immunoreactivity in small neurons of dorsal root ganglion in the rat. *Neurosci Lett* 1986 ; 64 : 311-6.
13. Chung K, Schwen RJ, Coggeshall RE. Ureteral axon damage following subcutaneous administration of capsaicin in adult rats. *Neurosci Lett* 1985 ; 64 : 311-6.
14. Chung K, Klein CM, Coggeshall RE. The receptive part of the primary afferent axon is most vulnerable to systemic capsaicin in adult rats. *Neurosci Lett* 1990 ; 53 : 221-6.
15. Dickenson AH, Dray A. Selective antagonism of capsaicin by capsazepine : evidence for a spinal receptor site in capsaicin-induced antinociception. *Br J Pharmacol* 1991 ; 104 : 1045-9.
16. Fitzgerald M. Cutaneous primary afferent properties in the hind limb of the neonatal rat. *J Physiol* 1987 ; 383 : 79-92.
17. Foster RW, Ramage AG. The action of some chemical irritants on somatosensory receptors of the cat. *Neuropharmacol* 1981 ; 20 : 191-8.
18. Gamse R, Molnar A, Lembeck F. Substance P release from spinal cord slices by capsaicin. *Life Sci* 1979 ; 35 : 629-36.
19. Hammond DL, Ruda MA. Developmental alterations in nociceptive threshold, immunoreactive calcitonin gene-related peptide and substance P, and fluoride-resistant acid phosphatase in neonatally capsaicin-treated rats. *J Comp Neurol* 1991 ; 312 : 436-50.

20. Heppelmann B, Messlinger K, Neiss WF, Schmidt RF. Ultrastructural three-dimensional reconstruction of Group III and Group IV sensory nerve endings («free nerve endings») in the knee joint capsule of the cat : evidence for multiple receptive sites. *J Comp Neurol* 1990 ; 292 : 103-16.
21. Hiura A, Ishizuka H. Changes in features of degenerating primary sensory neurons with time after capsaicin treatment. *Acta Neuropathol* 1989 ; 78 : 35-46.
22. Hiura A, Vilalobos EL, Ishizuka H. The action of capsaicin on primary afferent central terminals in the superficial dorsal horn of newborn mice. *Arch Histol Cytol* 1990 ; 53 : 455-66.
23. Holzer P. The local effector function of capsaicin-sensitive sensory nerve endings : involvement of tachykinins, and other neuropeptides. *Neuroscience* 1988 ; 24 : 739-68.
24. Holzer P. Capsaicin : cellular targets, mechanism of action, and selectivity for thin sensory neurons. *Pharmacol Rev* 1991 ; 43 : 143-201.
25. Holzer P. Capsaicin : selective toxicity for thin primary sensory neurons. In : Selective neurotoxicity. Herken H, Hucho F, eds. *Handbook of Experimental Pharmacology*. Berlin : Springer Verlag, 1992 ; 107 : 419-81.
26. Hôgyes A. Beitrage zur physiologischen Wirkung des Bestandteile des Capsicum annuum. *Arch Exp Pathol Pharmakol* 1878 ; 9 : 117-30.
27. Jancsó N. *Speicherung. Stoffanreicherung in Reticuloendothel und in der Niere.* Budapest : Akadémiai Kiadó, 1955.
28. Jancsó N, Jancsó-Gábor A, Szolcsányi J. Direct evidence for neurogenic inflammation and its prevention by denervation and by pretreatment with capsaicin. *Br J Pharmacol* 1967 ; 31 : 138-51.
29. Jancsó N, Jancsó-Gábor A, Szolcsányi J. The role of sensory nerve endings in neurogenic inflammation induced in human skin and in the eye and paw of the rat. *Br J Pharmacol* 1968 ; 33 : 32-41.
30. Jancsó G, Kiraly E, Jancsó-Gábor A. Pharmacologically induced selective degeneration of chemosensitive primary sensory neurone. *Nature* 1977 ; 270 : 741-3.
31. Jancsó G, Kiraly E, Joó I, Such G, Nagy A. Selective degeneration by capsaicin of a subpopulation of primary sensory neurons in the adult rat. *Neurosci Lett* 1985 ; 59 : 200-14.
32. Jancsó G, Kiraly E, Such G, Joó F, Nagy A. Neurotoxic effect of capsaicin in mammals. *Acta Physiol Hung* 1987 ; 69 : 259-313.
33. Jessell TM, Iversen,LL, Cuello AC. Capsaicin-induced depletion of substance P from primary sensory neurones. *Brain Res* 1978 ; 152 : 183-8.
34. Jhamandas K, Yaksh TL, Harty G, Szolcsányi J, Go VLW. Action of intrathecal capsaicin and its structural analogues on the content and release of spinal substance P : selective action and relationship to analgesia. *Brain Res* 1984 ; 306 : 215-25.
35. Joó F, Szolcsányi J, Jancsó-Gábor A. Mitochondrial alterations in the spinal ganglion cells of the rat accompanying the long-lasting sensory disturbance induced by capsaicin. *Life Sci* 1969 ; 8 : 621-6.
36. Kenins P. Responses of single nerve fibers to capsaicin applied to the skin. *Neurosci Lett* 1982 ; 29 : 83-8.
37. Koltzenburg M, Kress M, Reeh PW. The nociceptor sensitization by bradykinin does not depend on sympathetic neurons. *Neuroscience* 1992 ; 46 : 465-73.
38. Kolubi B, Yamano M, Ohhata K, Matsunaga T, Tohyama M. Presence of VIP fibers of sensory origin in the rat trachea. *Brain Res* 1990 ; 522 : 107-11.
39. Konietzny F, Hensel H. The effect of capsaicin on the response characteristic of human C-polymodal nociceptors. *J Therm Biol* 1983 ; 8 : 213-5.
40. Lawson SN. The morphological consequences of neonatal treatment with capsaicin on primary afferent neurons in adult rats. *Acta Physiol Hung* 1987 ; 69 : 315-21.

41. Lembeck F. Columbus, capsicum and capsaicin : past, present and future. *Acta Physiol Hung* 1987 ; 69 : 295-313.
42. Lembeck F. Substance P : from extract to excitement. *Acta Physiol Scand* 1988 ; 133 : 435-54.
43. Lou YP, Karlsson JA, Franco-Cereceda A, Lundberg JM. Selectivity of ruthenium red in inhibiting bronchoconstriction and CGRP release induced by afferent C-fiber activation in the guinea-pig lung. *Acta Physiol Scand* 1991 ; 142 : 191-9.
44. Lundberg JM, Martling CR, Hökfelt T. Airways, oral cavity and salivary glands : classical transmitters and peptides in sensory and autonomic motor neurons. Björklund A, Hökfelt T, Owman C, eds. *Handbook of chemical neuroanatomy. The peripheral nervous system.* 1988 ; Vol. 6 : 391-444.
45. Luts A, Widmark E, Ekman R, Waldeck B, Sundler F. Neuropeptides in guinea pig trachea : distribution and evidence for the release of CGRP into tracheal lumen. *Peptides* 1990 ; 11 : 1211-6.
46. Lynn B. Capsaicin : action on nociceptive C-fibers and therapeutic potential. *Pain* 1990 ; 41 : 61-9.
47. Maggi CA, Meli A. The sensory-efferent function of capsaicin-sensitive sensory neurons. *Gen Pharmacol* 1988 ; 19 : 1-43.
48. Maggi CA, Patacchini R, Tramontana M, Amann R, Giuliani S, Santicioli P. Similarities and differences in the action of resiniferatoxin and capsaicin on central and peripheral endings of primary sensory neurons. *Neuroscience* 1990 ; 37 : 531-9.
49. Maggi CA, Giuliani S, Santicioli P, Patacchini R, Said SJ, Theodorsson E, Turini D, Barbanti G, Giachetti A, Meli A. Direct evidence for the involvement of vasoactive intestinal polypeptide in the motor response of the human isolated ileum to capsaicin. *Eur J Pharmacol* 1990 ; 185 : 169-78.
50. Maggi CA. The pharmacology of the efferent function of sensory nerves. *J Auton Pharmacol* 1991 ; 11 : 173-208.
51. Maggi CA. Capsaicin and primary afferent neurons : from basic science to human therapy ? *J Auton Nerv Syst* 1991 ; 33 : 1-14.
52. Marlier L, Rajaofetra N, Poulat P, Privat A. Modification of serotonergic innervation of the rat spinal cord dorsal horn after neonatal capsaicin treatment. *J Neurosci Res* 1990 ; 25 : 112-8.
53. Manzini S, Bacciarelli C, Perfumi M, Massi M. Impairment of renal urinary excretion in neonatal, but not in adult capsaicin-pretreated rat. *Neurosci Lett* 1992 ; 135 : 1-4.
54. Marsh SJ, Stansfeld CE, Brown DA, Davey R, McCarthy D. The mechanism of action of capsaicin on sensory C-type neurons and their axons *in vitro. Neuroscience* 1987 ; 23 : 275-89.
55. Martin HA, Basbaum AJ, Kwiat GC, Goetzl EJ, Levine JD. Leukotrine and prostaglandin sensitization of cutaneous high-threshold C and A-delta mechanociceptors in the hairy skin of rat hindlimbs. *Neuroscience* 1987 ; 22 : 651-9, 399-406.
56. Meller ST, Lewis SJ, Ness TJ, Brody MJ, Gebhart GF. Neonatal capsaicin treatment abolishes the nociceptive responses to intravenous 5- HT in the rat. *Brain Res* 1991 ; 542 : 212-8.
57. Micevych PE, Yaksh TL, Szolcsányi J. Effect of intrathecal capsaicin analogues on the immunofluorescence of peptides and serotonin in the dorsal horn in rats. *Neuroscience* 1983 ; 8 : 23-131.
58. Nagy JI, Hunt SP. The termination of primary afferents within the rat dorsal horn : evidence for rearrangement following capsaicin treatment. *J Comp Neurol* 1983 ; 218 : 145-58.
59. Nagy JI, Iversen LL, Goedert M, Chapman D, Hunt SP. Dose dependent effects of capsaicin on primary sensory neurons in the neonatal rat. *J Neurosci* 1983 ; 3 : 399-406.
60. Paintal AS. Effects of drugs on vertebrate mechanoreceptors. *Pharmacol Rev* 1964 ; 16 : 341-80.
61. Palermo NN, Brown HK, Smith DL. Selective neurotoxic action of capsaicin on glomerular C-type terminals in rat substantia gelatinosa. *Brain Res* 1981 ; 208 : 506-10.

62. Pintér E, Szolcsányi J. Inflammatory and antiinflammatory effects of antidromic stimulation of dorsal roots in the rat. *Agents Actions* 1988 ; 25 : 240-2.
63. Réthelyi M, Salim MZ, Jancsó G. Altered distribution of dorsal root fibers in the rat following neonatal capsaicin treatment. *Neuroscience* 1986 ; 18 : 749-62.
64. Seroogy KB, Mohapatra NK, Lund PK, Réthelyi M, McGehee DS, Perl ER. *Mol Brain Res* 1990 ; 7 : 171-6.
65. Staszewska-Woolley J, Woolley G. Effects of neuropeptides, ruthenium red and neuraminidase on chemoreflexes mediated by afferents in the dog epicardium. *J Physiol* 1991 ; 436 : 1-13.
66. Steen KH, Reeh PW, Anton F, Handwerker HO. Protons selectively induce lasting excitation and sensitization to mechanical stimulation of nociceptors in rat skin, *in vitro. J Neurosci* 1992 ; 12 : 86-95.
67. Szállási A, Blumberg PM. Resiniferatoxin and its analogs provide novel insights into the pharmacology of the vanilloid (capsaicin) receptor. *Life Sci* 1990 ; 47 : 1399-408.
68. Szolcsányi J. A pharmacological approach to elucidation of the role of different nerve fibers and receptor endings in mediation of pain. *J Physiol Paris* 1977 ; 73 : 251-9.
69. Szolcsányi J. Effect of pain-producing chemical agents on the activity of slowly conducting afferent fibers. *Acta Physiol Hung* 1980 ; 56 : 86.
70. Szolcsányi J. Capsaicin-type pungent agents producing pyrexia. In : Milton AS ed. *Handbook of experimental pharmacology, pyretics and antipyretics*. Berlin : Springer-Verlag, 1982 ; Vol 60 : 437-78.
71. Szolcsányi J. Capsaicin-sensitive chemoceptive neural system with dual sensory-efferent function. In : Chahl LA, Szolcsányi J, Lembeck F, eds. *Antidromic vasodilatation and neurogenic inflammation*. Budapest : Akadémiai Kiadó, 1984 : 27-56.
72. Szolcsányi J. Sensory receptors and the antinociceptive effects of capsaicin. In : Hakanson R, Sundler F, eds. *Tachykinin antagonists*. Amsterdam : Elsevier, 1985 : 45-54.
73. Szolcsányi J. Selective responsiveness of polymodal nociceptors of the rabbit ear to capsaicin, bradykinin and ultraviolet irradiation. *J Physiol* 1987 ; 388 : 9-23.
74; Szolcsányi J. Antidromic vasodilatation and neurogenic inflammation. *Agents Actions* 1988 ; 23 : 4-11.
75. Szolcsányi J. Capsaicin, irritation and desensitization. Neurophysiological basis and future perspectives. In : Green BG, Mason JR, Kare MR, eds. *Chemical senses : irritation*. New York : Marcel Dekker, 1990 ; Vol 2 : 141-68.
76. Szolcsányi J. Perspectives of capsaicin-type agents in pain therapy and research. In : Parris WCV, ed. *Contemporary issues in chronic pain management*. Boston : Kluwer Academic Publ, 1991 : 97-122.
77. Szolcsányi J. Action of capsaicin on sensory receptors. In : Wood JN, ed. *Capsaicin in the study of pain*. London : Academic Press, 1994 : in press.
78. Szolcsányi J, Jancsó-Gábor A. Sensory effects of capsaicin congeners. I. Relationship between chemical structure and pain producing potency of pungent agents. *Arzneim Forsch (Drug Res)* 1975 ; 25 : 1877-81.
79. Szolcsányi J, Jancsó-Gábor A, Joó F. Functional and fine structural characteristics of the sensory neuron blocking effect of capsaicin. *Naunyn-Schmiedeberg's Arch Pharmacol* 1975 ; 287 : 157-69.
80. Szolcsányi J, Jancsó-Gábor A. Sensory effect of capsaicin congeners II. Importance of chemical structure and pungency in desensitizing activity of capsaicin-type compounds. *Arzneim Forsch (Drug Res)* 1976 ; 26 : 33-7.
81. Szolcsányi J, Sann H, Pierau FK. Nociception in pigeons is not impaired by capsaicin. *Pain* 1986 ; 27 : 247-60.
82; Szolcsányi J, Anton F, Reeh PW, Handwerker HO. Selective excitation by capsaicin of mechano-heat sensitive nociceptors in rat skin. *Brain Res* 1988 ; 446 : 262-8.

83. Szolcsányi J, Szállási A, Joó F, Blumberg PM. Resiniferatoxin : an ultrapotent selective modulator of capsaicin-sensitive primary afferent neurons. *J Pharmacol Exp Ther* 1990 ; 255 : 923-8.
84. Szolcsányi J, Barthó L, Pethô G. Capsaicin-sensitive bronchopulmonary receptors with dual sensory-efferent function : mode of action of capsaicin antagonists. *Acta Physiol Hung* 1991 ; 77 : 293-304.
85. Szolcsányi J, Nagy J, Pethô G. Effects of CP-96,345 a non-peptide substance P antagonist, capsaicin, resiniferatoxin and ruthenium red on nociception. *Regul Pept* 1992 ; Suppl. 1 : S153.
86. Szolcsányi J, Pintér E, Pethô G. Role of unmyelinated afferents in regulation of microcirculation and its chronic distorsion after trauma and damage. In : Jänig W, Schmidt RF, eds. *Reflex sympathetic dystrophy. Pathophysiological mechanisms and clinical implications.* VCH Weinheim 1992 : 245-61.
87. Thériault E, Otsuka M, Jessell T. Capsaicin-evoked release of substance P from primary sensory neurons. *Brain Res* 1979 ; 170 : 209-13.
88. Wall PD, Fitzgerald M, Nussbaumer JC, Van der Loos H, Devor M. Somatotopic maps are disorganized in adult rodents treated neonatally with capsaicin. *Nature* 1982 ; 295 : 691-3.
89. Welk E, Fleischer E, Petsche U, Handwerker HO. Afferent C-fibers in rats after neonatal capsaicin treatment. *Pflugers Arch* 1984 ; 400 : 66-71.
90. Winning AJ, Hamilton RD, Shea SA, Guz A. Respiratory and cardiovascular effects of central and peripheral intravenous injections of capsaicin in man : evidence for pulmonary chemosensitivity. *Clin Sci* 1986 ; 71 : 519-26.
91. Winter J, Dray A, Word JN, Yeats JC, Bevan S. Cellular mechanism of action of resiniferatoxin : a potent sensory neuron excitotoxin. *Brain Res* 1990 ; 520 : 131-40.
92. Wood JN. *Capsaicin in the study of pain.* London : Academic Press, 1994 ; in press.
93. Wood JN, Winter J, James IF, Rang MP, Yeats J, Bevan S. Capsaicin-induced ion fluxes in dorsal root ganglion cells in culture. *J Neurosci* 1988 ; 8 : 3208-20.
94. Yaksh TL, Farb D, Leeman S, Jessel T. Intrathecal capsaicin depletes substance P in the rat spinal cord and produces prolonged thermal analgesia. *Science* 1979 ; 206 : 481-3.

9

Studies on the release of CGRP into the skin blister base

T.H.M. MIRZAI, T.L. YAKSH

Department of Anesthesiology, University of California, San Diego, USA.

Calcitonin gene related peptide (CGRP) was measured in the media placed in a cup over a blister formed on the plantar surface of the hind paw of the anesthetized rat. Antidromic stimulation (3hz) of the sciatic nerve at high, but not low intensities or application of capsaicin and bradykinin resulted in a concentration dependent (1-100 µM) increase in CGRP in the blister base media. Capsaicin pretreatment blocked release. Deletion of Ca and addition of EGTA blocked evoked release. TTX treatment blocked antidromic but not capsaicin or bradykinin-evoked release. Indomethacin blocked bradykinin, but not antidromic or capsaicin-evoked release. Column elution reveals CGRP immunoreactivity coelutes with authentic CGRP. These results demonstrate that modest physiological stimuli and autocoids that can excite primary afferent terminals can evoke prominent extracellular movement of a C fiber neuropeptide.

Orthodromic action potentials in primary afferents are generated when an appropriate stimulus is applied to the peripheral nerve ending. Such stimuli, by an interaction with specific receptors, will evoke a local generator potential that spreads to the axon where voltage sensitive sodium channels are activated, leading to a regenerative potential. In the case of small primary afferents, the effective stimuli may include specific chemical products such as elevated hydrogen ion concentrations (low pH), bradykinin, a variety of cytokines as well as protaglandins [21, 26, 30] and the homovanillic acid derivative, capsaicin [32]. While it is common to consider the spinopetal conduction of afferent potentials and the subsequent release of neuropeptides from the central terminals as the common mode of function for such axons, there is a long history indicating that the peripheral afferent terminals themselves may function to mediate a local effect through the release of active factors. The earliest studies by Bayliss [1, 2], demonstrating a peripheral dilatation induced by antidromic stimulation, were clear indications of the likely release of active factors from these terminals. Subsequent work revealed these effects were abolished by the action of capsaicin [18] and this strongly implicated the role of small unmyelinated afferents. The demonstration of substance P and later calcitonin gene related peptide (CGRP) in type B ganglion cells and in unmyelinated afferents [7, 8, 12], and the demonstration that these peptides could evoke significant vasodilation and plasma extravasation [6, 13, 16] made it likely that these products were released from the terminals of the C fibers and that this event accounted for the observed physiological effects of antidromic stimulation [22]. Such release into the extra vascular-extracellular milieu of C fiber terminal contents, such as substance P and/or CGRP, has in fact been shown in a number of innervated tissues, including the knee joint [34, 35], pia-arachnoid [24], eye [4] skin [11, 33, 35], ureter [17] and trachea [15].

While antidromic vasodilation can evoke the release of neuropeptide, it is also reasonable that agents which are known to depolarize the C fiber terminal may similarly evoke the release of the terminal contents. The use of local peptide release thus permits a mechanism whereby the receptor pharmacology of the terminal may be identified. As noted above, several classes of agents may in fact excite the terminal and would correspondingly serve to release the contents of the terminal. Consideration of the effects of such agents on release would serve to provide insight on (1) the relationship between terminal depolarization and release and (2) serve to characterize properties of the terminal which lead to its release of bioactive peptides. We have employed several models, including the knee joint [34] and trachea [15]. However, the present report will briefly describe work carried out examining the release from the nerve endings exposed in a blister base model.

Methods

Model

A cutaneous blister was induced on the hind paw of a halothane anesthetized (1.5%) male Sprague Dawley rat (300-350 gr). GAs was delivered in a $50\%O_2$/air mixture. The blister was created by placing each hind paw of the animal on a 60C surface for 4 min. Blisters were allowed to develop over the ensuing 3.5 hr interval. At this time, rats were again anesthetized with halothane (1.5%) delivered by mask. With the rat in a prone position, the blisters on the hind paw were then surrounded by a barrier formed by a length of 30 ga malleable wire inside a length of PE50 tubing. The barrier was held in place by cyano-acrylate applied around the perimeter of the blister. The raised skin of the blister was then carefully cut away. This formed a reservoir of about 0.25-0.35

ml volume. To collect release, 0.25 ml of Krebs buffer was placed in the blister cup. (6.91 g/ml NaCl ; 0.35 mg/ml KCl ; 0.28 mg/ml $CaCl_2$; 0.16 mg/ml KH_2PO_4 ; 0.30 $MgSO_4$; 2.10 mg/ml $NaHCO_3$, bubbled with 95% O_2/5% CO_2).

The Krebs buffer was removed and replaced every 20 min and the collected samples were assayed for CGRP. After the final samples, the rat was euthanized by an overdose of sodium pentobarbital.

To antidromically stimulate the sciatic nerve, the sciatic nerve was exposed just central to the politeal fossa. A bipolar tubular electrode was placed around the nerve and vegetable oil filled the incision. With each experiment, the stimulation intensity that evoked a minor motor twitch was defined (the minimum motor threshold, MMT). For large afferent stimulation, 2x MMT intensities were employed. For C fiber stimulation, 20 xMMT intensities were employed. Typically frequencies of 3 Hz and pulse widths of 3 msec were employed. To apply drugs, agents were mixed such that the final concentration was delivered in the appropriate sample into the blister base cup.

Drugs

Agents applied into the blister base, included capsacin, bradykin triacetate ; (Sigma), tetrodotoxin ; Hydroxy-propyl -β-cyclodextrin (RBI) ; morphine (Merck). Capsaicin was mixed in 5% cyclodextrin and saline. All other agents were mixed in saline (0.9%).

Assays

All samples were assayed for CGRP-LI by competitive radioimmunoassay using goat antibody No G987 (1:84,000) and 125 I Tyr-CGRP. The absolute sensitivity of the assay for CGRP was 7 pg/tube. The CGRP assay shows 100% cross reactivity with rat and human CGRP. For the CGRP fragments CGRP 23-37, CGRP 28-37 and calcitonin, cross reactivity was not observed at doses up to 10 pmol/ml.

The levels of sP-LI was measured in a number of samples in the early phases of these studies and these data are reported. These levels were too low to permit routine assay and subsequent studies were carried out measuring CGRP alone.

Column identification of immunoreactivity

Several release samples were purified using a SepPak C18 column, dried and reconstituted in solution A (0.1% trifluroaceitic acid in ddH20). Standards or samples (fluid released by capsaicin -100uM stimulation in rats) was injected on to a μ-Bondapak, C18 column (3.9 x 30 cm), using 5 min 100%, 30 min linear gradient, 5 min 100% solution B (0.1% TFA in acetonitile) at a flow rate of 1 ml/min. One min fractions were dried, reconstituted in assay buffer and assayed for CGRP-LI.

Results

Resting levels

Measurement of CGRP-LI in the blister base fluid collected at the opening of the blister revealed levels of 585 ± 105 pg. Examining the levels of CGRP over the ensuing several periods of collection revealed a progressive, though modest, reduction in CGRP levels (Figure 1). In the initial blister base samples, sP levels were measured and found to be considerably lower (13.9 ± 9.3 pg/ 20 min, N = 28). Levels of sP and CGRP measured concurrently in the resting blister base fluid covaried, with the regression slope being 0.016 ± 0.0026, p <0.05).

Evoked release

The resting levels of CGRP-LI in the blister base were elevated in a stimulation dependent fashion by the addition of capsaicin (Figure 2) and bradykinin to the blister base. This elevation by either agent was concentration dependent over a range of 0.1-100 μM for capsaicin and (1-10 μM) for bradykinin (Figure 3).

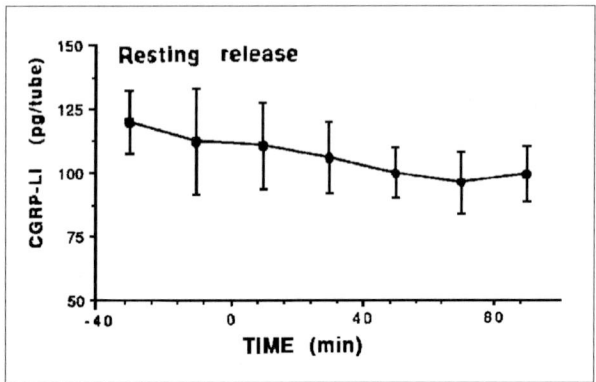

Figure 1. Resting levels of CGRP-LI (pg/tube) in blister base samples taken at 20 min intervals. Line presents the means and S.E.M. of 8 rats.

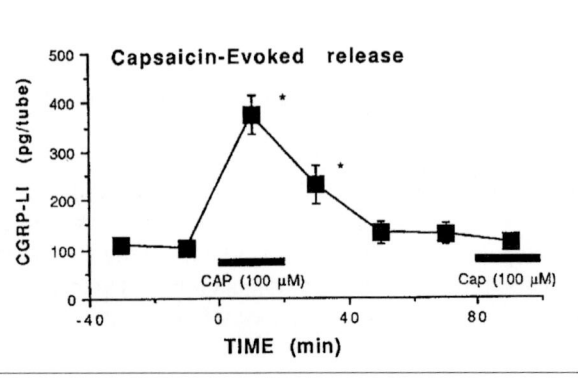

Figure 2. Levels (pg/tube) of CGRP-LI in the blister base expressed as a function of time after the administration of CAP into the blister base media. Capsaicin was administered twice, as indicated by the black bars. Note that the second application was without effect. Line presents the mean ± S.E.M of 5 rats.

Antidromic stimulation of the sciatic nerve at 20 times but not 2 times the minimum motor threshold at a frequency of 1 Hz resulted in a stimulus dependent increase in the levels of CGRP-LI. (Figure 4).

Effects of capsaicin desensitization on evoked release

The treatment of the blister base with capsaicin (100 µM) 60 min prior to stimulation abolished the release evoked by antidromic nerve stimulation or by either capsaicin, or bradykinin applied to the blister base (Figure 1 and Figure 5). In contrast, treatment with vehicle did not alter the release evoked by these three modalities at this later time.

Effects of sodium channel blockade

Addition of TTX (10 µM) to the blister base 60 min prior to the stimulation had no effect upon resting release, but served to block the release evoked by antidromic

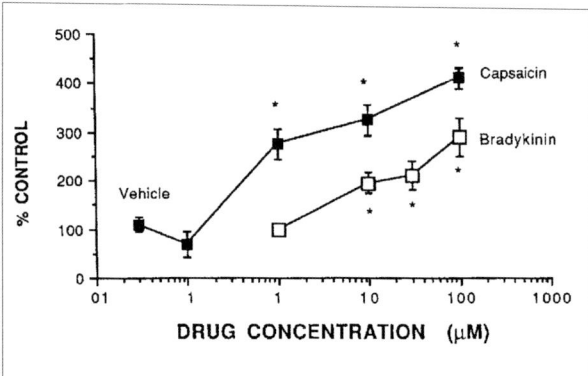

Figure 3. Increase in CGRP-LI in blister base, expressed as percent of prestimulation control, plotted *versus* the concentration of capsaicin or bradykinin administered into the blister base. Each point has 3-5 rats. Both concentration response curves show a statistically significant increase (1 way ANOVA, $p < 0.01$).

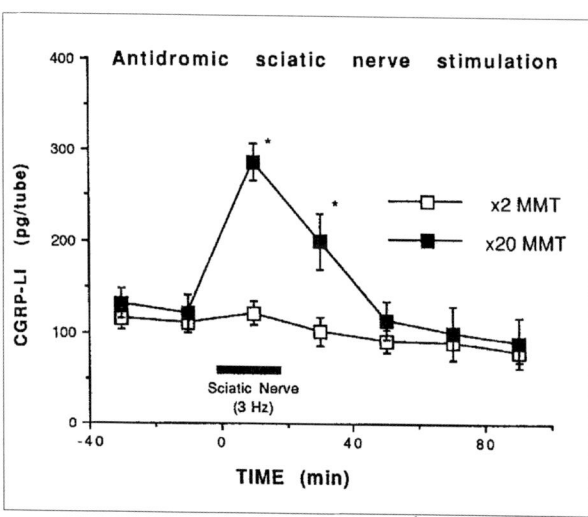

Figure 4. Levels (pg/tube) of CGRP-LI before and after antidromic stimulation of the sciatic nerve at stimulation intensities which were x2 and x20 of the minimum motor threshold (MMT) at 3 Hz. Each line presents the mean and S.E.M. of 3 and 4 rats, respectively.
* $p < 0.05$ as compared to prestimulation control.

stimulation, but did not affect the release evoked by bradykinin (10 μM) or capsaicin (100 μM) (Figure 6).

Calcium dependency of CGRP-LI release

To define the Ca^{2+} dependency of the CGRP-LI release, CaY^{2+} was deleted from the Krebs buffer and 3 mM EGTA was added (Figure 7). This treatment led to a significant reduction in the levels of CGRP-IR otherwise evoked by the application of capsaicin (100 μM) (276 ± 29 versus 157 ± 36 pg/ tube ; N = 3 and 4, respectively) or antidromic stimulation (3 Hz, 20xMMT) (195 ± 32 versus 74 ± 36 pg/tube, respectively, N = 5 and 4, respectively).

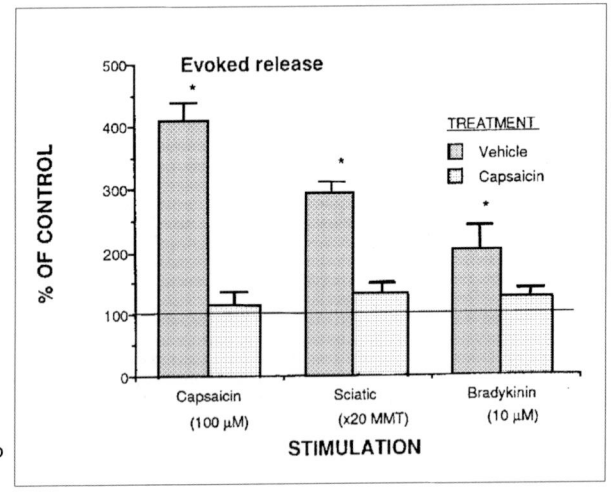

Figure 5. Histogram displays the levels of CGRP-LI in blister base as a percent of prestimulation control following the capsaicin (100 μM), bradykinin (30 μM) or after antidromic stimulation of the sciatic nerve (3 Hz, x20 MMT), in rats examined 60 min after the application of vehicle (cyclodextrin) or capsaicin (100 μM).
* p< 0.05 as compared to prestimulation sample.

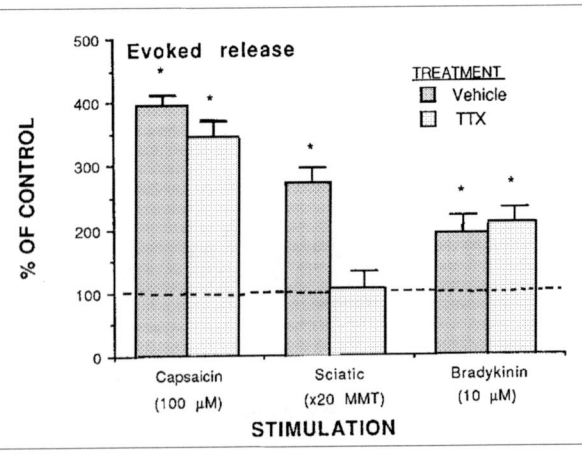

Figure 6. Histogram displays the levels of release of CGRP-LI from the blister base as a percent of prestimulation control following the application of capsaicin (100 μM), antidromic nerve stimulation (3Hz, 20 x MMT) or bradykinin (10 μM) where stimulation was carried out 60 min after the application of tetrodotoxin (TTX) into the blister base. * p < 0.05 as compared to prestimulation levels.

Effects of indomethacin on evoked release

The addition of indomethacin (10 μM) to the perfusate had no effect upon the release evoked by antidromic nerve stimulation or capsaicin, but abolished the release evoked by bradykinin (Figure 7).

Identification of CGRP-LI

Elution of pooled samples obtained during capsaicin stimulation revealed that the immunoreactivity coeluted with the authentic rat CGRP standard (Figure 8).

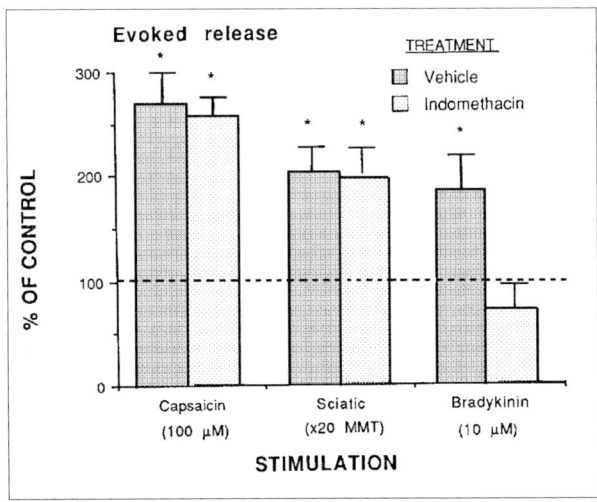

Figure 7. Histogram displays the levels of release of CGRP-LI from the blister base as a percent of prestimulation control following the application of capsaicin (100 μM), antidromic nerve stimulation (3Hz, 20x MMT) or bradykinin (10 μM) where stimulation was carried out 60 min after the application in to the blister base of Indomethacin (10 μM).
* $p < 0.05$ as compared to prestimulation levels.

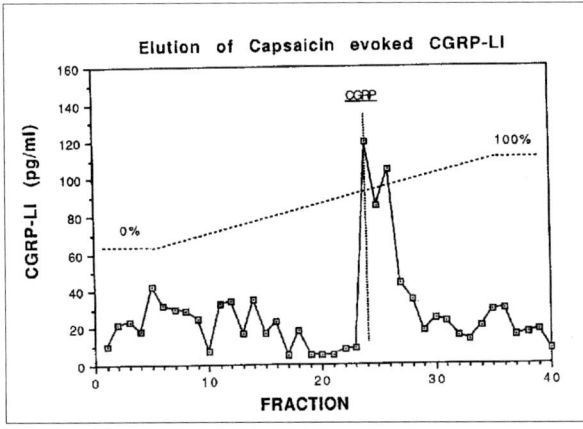

Figure 8. Profile of elution of CGRP-LI immunoreactivity obtained from the blister base during the administration of local capsaicin (100 μM). *See* text for details. Dashed line indicates the linear acetonitrile gradient. The vertical dashed line indicates the sample in which the authentic CGRP standard was observed to elute.

Discussion

Immunohistochemical studies have revealed the presence of small diameter, unmyelinated sensory axons forming part of a subpapillary network terminating in the intraepithelium of the skin. These axons contain several neuropeptides, including CGRP and sP [20]. Such peripheral sensory terminals, likely representing those fibers classified as free nerve endings, have been shown to possess vesicles and mitochondria [10] indicating a probable physical substrate for exocytotic secretion. The location of these peptides along with the ability of these agents to have effects upon local vascular beds similar to that produced by antidromic stimulation of sensory afferents supports the hypothesis that neurohormones released from these peripheral afferent terminals mediate the observed physiological actions.

Release of CGRP from peripheral terminals

The present studies have demonstrated that the levels of sP and CGRP can be measured in blister fluid. These results suggest that these materials may be secreted into the extracellular space from the peripheral terminal and suggest that the afferent stores of these peptides represent a releasable pool. The identification of the CGRP immunoreactivity as a substance that coelutes on a reverse phase column with authentic CGRP provides confirmation that the radioimmunoassay indeed reveals the presence of CGRP in the blister base fluid. These observations showing a significant extracellular release of CGRP are consistent with previous reports on peripheral sP release in a variety of tissues including the eye, skin, ureter, trachea, pial vasculature and synovial joint (*see* introduction for references).

The low levels of sP in the present study precluded a systematic examination of the release of this material, though it was measurable in the initial blister base sample, suggesting that it can accumulate after the injury. The low levels of sP relative to CGRP may reflect upon several variables. First, net levels of CGRP and the number of CGRP-positive dorsal root ganglion cells exceed those by several fold ([7, 22]. Secondly, sP may be more sensitive to peptidase inactivation [23, 25]. In preliminary studies, however, we have noted that the addition of neutral endopeptidase inhibitors did not significantly elevate these low levels (Mirzai and Yaksh, unpublished observations). Thus, it is plausible that the low levels are consistent with the smaller releasable pools of sP.

Origin of blister base CGRP

The presence of CGRP in small primary afferents suggests this to be a likely source of CGRP in the blister base. This association is further supported by several observations :
- CGRP levels are elevated by the local application of capsaicin, an agent known to have significant selectivity for activating C fiber terminals and ganglion cells [3],

- CGRP levels are not elevated by stimulation intensities that preferentially activate large diameter myelinated, but not small diameter unmyelinated axons,
- desensitization of the terminals by the pre-application of capsaicin was shown to abolish the release of CGRP otherwise evoked by antidromic stimulation or by bradykinin.

These data strongly support the thesis that the extracellular CGRP collected in the blister base originated at least in part from small primary afferents. CGRP-LI is found in motor horn cells [19]. Thus, it is also possible that release from the peripheral motor terminal might account for some portion of this release. As the blister base reveals a superficial aspect of the skin above the intact fascia of the underlying musculature, this seems an unlikely source. In addition, CGRP release was not evoked when sciatic stimulation was carried out at an intensity that activated large axons alone. While not absolute, it appears reasonable that were a significant proportion of the activity to derive from motor axons, a measurable increase would have been evoked by the low threshold stimulation. Finally, treatment with TTX blocked the ability of antidromic stimulation to increase blister CGRP levels. This treatment did not block the motor movement that was typically evoked by this stimulation. This observation thus also excludes the possibility that the increased levels were secondary to simple motor activity. In short, we believe the data support that the collected immunoreactivity was derived from the terminals of small primary afferents.

The afferent terminal as a releasing system

In the present studies, it has been shown that the levels of CGRP-LI can be elevated by stimuli which are known to acutely activate the free nerve endings (C fibers), *e.g.* antidromic electrical stimulation, capsaicin and bradykinin. This release appears to possess many of the properties expected from a terminal releasing systems, including Ca-dependency. Similar results have been reported in other peripheral terminal releasing systems including the trachea [15].

The mechanism whereby terminal depolarization is evoked reflects upon the complexity of the local periterminal environment. Thus, treatment with TTX prevents the release evoked by antidromic stimulation of the sciatic nerve. In contrast, the effects of bradykinin and capsaicin were unaffected. This indicates that these agents exerted their effects at a site distal to the voltage / TTX - sensitive sodium channels of the axon. A further subdivision in mechanism is revealed by the observation that treatment with indomethacin blocked the effects of bradykinin, but had no effect upon the release evoked by capsaicin. This observation is consistent with a number of studies in which it has been shown that the effects of bradykinin are mediated by the release of cycloxygenase products. In trachea, the effects of bradykinin on CGRP release are similarly blocked by indomethacin. In this regard, the application of several prostanoids will evoke the release of CGRP in that preparation [14]. Work with capsaicin has largely confirmed that its actions are mediated by a binding site that is located on the C fiber terminal [3]. Thus, there are at least three mechanisms where by an increase in peripheral terminal depolarization can be evoked : antidromic invasion, indirect stimulation through the release of prostaglandins and a direct stimulatory effect upon the terminal. This is clearly not an exhaustive listing, but suggests that a variety of mechanisms may impact upon the local secretory activity of the afferent terminal.

Significance of the release from the peripheral terminal

The potent effects of antidromic stimulation on local vasomotor tone and capillary permeability have been well described. Functionally, Szolcsanyi has shown that even modest antidromic stimulation rates can produce powerful and long lasting physiological effects [31]. Systematic studies on the frequency dependency of release has provided corroborating data in that frequencies no higher that 3 Hz can evoke very significant increase in the extracellular levels of neuropeptides in the skin (present study) and in the trachea [15]. Measurement of release requires the collection of sufficient material to measure and this typically limits the sensitivity with which we can assess terminal secretory activity. Yet, given the ability of various autocoids to produce release, it is probable that even mild depolarization of the terminal may evoke a local generator potential adequate to produce release at a level that might have biological significance and not be measurable by current techniques. In that sense, the local release may serve a trophic function modulating local tissue function viz capillary permeability, and vasomotor tone. While it is clear that the presence of autocoids can be established and that such autocoids can evoke terminal release, the possibility of «natural» antidromic activity cannot be excluded. Recent studies by Carlton (personal communication) have shown that the magnitude of the local inflammatory response in the knee joint can be reduced by root section central to the associated sensory ganglion. Moreover, they have also demonstrated small afferent antidromic activity on the dorsal roots following peripheral stimulation, *i.e.* dorsal root reflexes. Under these circumstances, it is possible that a local stimulus would evoke homosegmental antidromic activity that would release terminal contents in the vicinity of the original stimulus. While the role of the axon reflex is established for certain physiological endpoints, the relevance of these systems to various pain states is less clear. It might be speculated that antidromic activity might serve to sensitize the peripheral sensory terminal. Reeh and colleagues [29] did not observe such a facilitation. However, Ochoa in a series of systematic human investigations has suggested a syndrome he has termed the «ABC» (angry-backfiring-C fiber) syndrome [27, 28]. In this work, selective block data and recording form peripheral fascicles have led to the suggestion that certain states of hyperalgesia may depend upon antidromic activity in small afferents. Such observations instill further relevance to understanding the releasing properties of the peripheral terminal of small unmyelinated fibers.

Acknowledgment

This work was supported by funds from AI26249 (TLY) and a University of California President's undergraduate fellowship (THMM).

References

1. Bayliss WM. On the origen from the spinal cord of the vasodilator fibers of the hindlimb and on the nature of these fibers. *J Physiol* 1901 ; 26 : 173-209.
2. Bayliss WM. Further researches on the antidromic nerve impulse *J Physiol* 1902 ; 28 : 276-99.
3. Bevan S, Szolcsanyi J. Sensory neuron-specific actions of capsaicin : mechanisms and applications. *Pharmacol Sci* 1990 ; 11 : 330-3.
4. Bill A, Stjernschantz J, Mandahl A, Brodin E, Nilsson G. Substance P : release on trigeminal nerve stimulation, effects in the eye. *Acta Physiol Scand* 1979 ; 106 : 371-3.
5. Cesselin F. Enkephalinase is involved in the degradation of endogenous substance P released from slices of rat substantia nigra. *J Pharmacol Exp Ther* 1987 ; 243 : 674-80.
6. Gamse R, Saria A. Potentiation of tachykinin-induced plasma protein extravasation by Calcitonin gene-related peptide. *Eur J Pharmacol* 1985 ; 114 : 61-6.
7. Gibbins IL, Furness JB, Costa M, MacIntyre I, Hillyard CJ, Girgis S. Co-localization of calcitonin gene-related peptide-like immunoreactivity with substance P in cutaneous, vascular and visceral sensory neurons of guinea pigs. *Neurosci Lett* 1985 ; 57 : 125-30.
8. Gulbenkian S, Merighi A, Wharton J, Varndell IM, Polak JM. Ultrastructural evidence for the coexistence of calcitonin gene-related peptide and substance P in secretory vesicles of peripheral nerves in the guinea pig. *J Neurocytol* 1986 ; 15 : 535-42.
9. Handwerker HO, Reeh PW. Nociceptors : chemo pain and inflammation. *Pain Res Clin Man* 1991 ; 4 : 59-70.
10. Hanesch U, Heppelmann B, Messlinger K, Schmiddt RF. Nociception in normal and arthitic joints : Structural and functional aspects. In : Willis WD, ed. *Hyperalgesia and allodynia.* 1992 : 81-106.
11. Helme RD, Koschorke GM, Zimmermann M. Immunoreactive substance P release from skin nerves in the rat by noxious thermal stimulation. *Neurosci Lett* 1986 ; 63 : 295-9.
12. Hokfelt T, Kellerth JO, Nilsson G, Pernow B. Experimental immunohistochemical studies on the localization and distribution of substance P in cat primary sensory neurons. *Br Res* 1975 ; 100 : 235-52.
13. Holzer P. Local effector functions of capsaicin-sensitive sensory nerve endings : involvement of tachykinins, calcitonin gene-related peptide and other neuropeptides. *Neuroscience* 1988 ; 24 : 739-68.
14. Hua XY, Yaksh TL. Pharmacology of the effects of bradykinin, serotonin, and histamine on the release of calcitonin gene-related peptide from C-fiber terminals in the rat trachea. *J Neurosci* 1993 ; 13 : 1947-53.
15. Hua XY, Yaksh TL. Release of calcitonin gene-related peptide and tachykinins from the rat trachea. *Peptides* 1992 ; 13 : 113-20.
16. Hua XY. Tachykinins and calcitonin gene-related peptide in relation to peripheral functions of capsaicin-sensitive sensory neurons. *Acta Physiol Scand (Suppl.)* 1986 ; 551 : 1-45.
17. Hua XY, Saria A, Gamse R, Theodorsson-Norheim E, Brodin E, Lundberg JM. Capsaicin induced release of multiple tachykinins (substance P, neurokinin A and eledoisin-like material) from guinea-pig spinal cord and ureter. *Neuroscience* 1986 ; 19 : 313-9.
18. Jancso N, Jancso-Gabor A, Szolcsanyi J. Direct evidence for neurogenic inflammation and its revention by denervation and by pretreatment with capsaicin. *Br J Pharmacol* 1967 ; 1 : 138-51.
19. Kar S, Gibson SJ, Rees RG, Jura WG, Brewerton DA, Polak JM. Increased calcitonin gene-related peptide (CGRP), substance P, and enkephalin immunoreactivities in dorsal spinal cord and loss of CGRP-immunoreactive motoneurons in arthritic rats depend on intact peripheral nerve supply. *J Mol Neurosci* 1991 ; 3 : 718.

20. Kruger L, Silverman JD, Mantyh PW, Sternini C, Brecha NC. Peripheral patterns of calcitonin-gene-related peptide general somatic sensory innervation : cutaneous and deep terminations. *J Comp Neurol* 1989 ; 280 : 291-302.
21. Lang E, Novak A, Reeh PW, Handwerker HO. Chemosensitivity of fine afferents from rat skin in vitro. *J Neurophysiol* 1990 ; 63 : 887-901.
22. Levine JD, Fields HL, Basbaum AI. Peptides and the primary afferent nociceptor. *J Neurosci* 1993 ; 13 : 2273-86.
23. Mauborgne A, Bourgoin S, Benoliel JJ, Hirsch M, Berthier JL, Hamon M, Moskowitz MA, Brody M, Liu-Chen LY. *In vitro* release of immunoreactive substance P from putative afferent nerve endings in bovine pia arachnoid. *Neuroscience* 1983 ; 9 : 809-14.
24. Nadel JA. Membrane-bound peptidases : endocrine, paracrine, and autocrine effects. *Am J Resp Cell Mol Biol* 1992 ; 7 : 469-70.
25. Neugebauer V, Schaible HG, Schmidt RF. Sensitization of articular afferents to mechanical stimuli by bradykinin. *Pflugers Arch* 1989 ; 415 : 330-5.
26. Ochoa JL. The newly recognized painful ABC syndrome ; thermographic aspects. *Thermol* 1986 ; 2 : 65-107.
27. Ochoa JL, Yarnitsky D. Mechanical hyperalgesias in neuropathic pain patients : dynamic and static subtypes. *Ann Neurol* 1993 ; 33 : 465-72.
28. Reeh PW, Kocher L, Jung S. Does neurogenic inflammation alter the sensitivity of unmyelinated nociceptors in the rat ? *Brain Res* 1986 ; 384 : 42-50.
29. Steen KH, Reeh PW, Anton F, Handwerker HO. Protons selectively induce lasting excitation and sensitization to mechanical stimulation of nociceptors in rat skin, *in vitro*. *J Neurosci* 1992 ; 12 : 86-95.
30. Szolcsanyi J. Antidromic vasodilatation and neurogenic inflammation. *Agents Actions* 1988 ; 23 : 4-11.
31. Szolcsanyi J, Anton F, Reeh PW, Handwerker HO. Selective excitation by capsaicin of mechano-heat sensitive nociceptors in rat skin. *Brain Res* 1988 ; 446 : 262-8.
32. White DM, Helme RD. Release of substance P from peripheral nerve terminals following electrical stimulation of the sciatic nerve. *Brain Res* 1985 ; 336 : 27-31.
33. Yaksh TL. Substance P release from knee joint afferent terminals : modulation by opioids. *Brain Res* 1988 ; 458 : 319-24.
34. Yaksh TL, Bailey J, Roddy DR, Harty GJ. Peripheral release of substance P from primary afferents. In : Dubner R, Gebhart GF, Bond MR, eds. Proceedings of the Vth World Congress on Pain, Elsevier Science Publishers BV 1988 : 51-4.

10

Peripheral aspects of opioid activity : studies in animals

V. KAYSER, G. GUILBAUD

Unité de Recherches de Physiopharmacologie du Système Nerveux, INSERM U161, Paris, France.

There is increasing evidence supporting a peripheral antinociceptive site of action for opioids in hyperalgesic inflammatory conditions in animals. In this paper, studies providing evidence for an antinociceptive effect of opioids agonists administered peripherally in rat models of inflammatory pain, then studies providing evidence for the contribution of a peripheral component to the antinociceptive effect of systemically administered opioid agonists in inflammatory states will be considered in turn. We will see that several difficulties were encountered in these studies, essentially due to the problem of the selectivity of the opioid agonists and antagonists available and to the major problem of antagonist reversibility. For these reasons, a lot of questions were not completely resolved.

The antinociceptive effects of exogenous as well as endogenous opioids are traditionally associated with activation of opioid receptors located in the central nervous system. Indeed, although widely distributed in the central nervous system, mu, delta, and kappa opioid receptors as well as receptor selective opioid peptides, are concentrated in several sites that have been implicated in the regulation of nociceptive messages [3].

Recently, however, attention has also focussed on the role of the opioid receptors located on peripheral terminals of the primary afferent neurons [10, 24, 40, 41, 45].

While previous data on peripheral antinociceptive effects of opioid agonists in normal conditions remains controversial [17, 25, 29, 35], there is increasing evidence supporting a peripheral antinociceptive site of action for opioids in hyperalgesic inflammatory conditions in animals.

In this paper, we will first consider animal studies providing evidence for a clear antinociceptive effect of opioid agonists administered peripherally in rat models of inflammatory pain. In the second section we will consider animal studies providing evidence for the contribution of a peripheral component to the antinociceptive effect of systemically administered opioid agonists in inflammatory states.

We will see that several difficulties are encountered in these studies, and this was essentially due to two reasons. Firstly, the problem of the selectivity of the opioid agonists and antagonists available. Secondly, the major problem of antagonist reversibility, especially for naloxone. Indeed, attempts to antagonize the observed effects with naloxone have generated conflicting results, due to the fact that to avoid central actions of the antagonist resulting from an enhanced leakage into the systemic circulation, especially in inflammatory conditions, only extremely low doses of local naloxone could be used to reverse the action of the agonist. Due to the complexity of the effects of naloxone according to the dose used, especially in inflammatory states, and in particular with low doses, there was also the possibility that naloxone would produce marked-antinociceptive effects when injected either i.v. [19] or locally [9, 31]. Such antinociceptive effects could obviously mask antagonism of the antinociceptive effect of the agonists.

For these reasons, it will be seen that a lot of questions were not completely resolved.

Studies providing evidence for an antinociceptive effect of peripherally administered opioids in rat models of peripheral inflammation / hyperalgesia

Evidence has accumulated suggesting that peripherally administered opioids can produce powerful antinociceptive effects in inflammatory conditions. These effects were described both in rats with a short duration inflammatory response induced by the intraplantar injection of formalin as well as in rats with a more prolonged nociceptive response ranging from a few hours with prostaglandin or carrageenan inflammation to few days with unilateral Freund's adjuvant-induced inflammation.

In this part of the paper, we will consider successively studies performed in prostaglandin- and carrageenan-injected rats [9, 12, 15], then in rats with a unilateral painful inflammation produced by the local injection of Freund's adjuvant [39, 40], and finally in animals with formalin-evoked cutaneous pain [11] (Table I).

Studies in prostaglandin- and carrageenan-injected rats

Morphine and met-enkephalin

Fereirra and Nakamura first suggested in 1979 that morphine and met-enkephalin administered locally into the rat paw could have a peripheral antinociceptive activity in rats with prostaglandin- or carrageenan induced hyperalgesia (Table I).

Table I. Antinociceptive effects of locally administered opioids in animal models of peripheral inflammation/hyperalgesia.

Authors	Model	Treatment	Test	Antagonism	Dose
Fereirra and Nakamura [9]	Pg	Morphine Met-enkephalin	PWT	Naloxone	7 µg
Joris et al. [15]	Cg	Fentanyl EKC Levorphanol	PWL	Lacking	
Hargreaves et al. [12]	Cg	EKC Levorphanol	PWL	Lacking	
Stein et al. [38]	FA	Fentanyl	PWT	Naloxone	1.2 µg
Stein et al. [38]	FA	DAMGO	PWT	Naloxone CTAP	1-4 µg
		DPDPE		Naloxone ICI 174,864	10-40 µg
		U-50, 488H		Naloxone Nor-BNI	2-6 µg
Electrophysiological study					
Haley et al. [11]	Formalin	U-50,488H	Nociceptive neurons	Naloxone 12 min before formalin	100 µg

Pg = Prostaglandin ; Cg = Carrageenin ; FA = Freund's adjuvant ;
EKC = Ethylketocyclazocine ; Nor-BNI = Norbinaltorphimine ;
PWT = Paw withdrawal threshold to noxious pressure ;
PWL = Paw withdrawal latency to radiant heat stimulation.

In these experiments, using the paw withdrawal threshold to noxious pressure (PWT), Fereirra and Nakamura showed that the intraplantar injection of morphine (10 µg) greatly reduced the intensity of prostaglandin-hyperalgesia for two and a half hours. The local injection of met-enkephalin (50 µg) had a similar effect but of shorter duration. Both drugs produced similar localized antinociceptive effects in rats with an intraplantar injection of carrageenan. Since in the two models the effect of the drugs was restricted to the injected paws, the authors suggested that the action of locally administered opioids was peripheral and not due to systemic absorption of the drugs. One explanation for this action would have been a simple local anaesthetic effect, however, it was demonstrated that local morphine and met-enkephalin were 50-100 times more potent than the local anaesthetic lidocaine.

To further characterize this peripheral site of action, Fereirra and Nakamura investigated the effects of the intraplantar injection of naloxone on antinociception produced by morphine (10 µg) administered locally into the paw of prostaglandin-hyperalgesic rats. However, the local dose of naloxone (7 µg i.pl.) used produced antinociceptive effects in prostaglandin-hyperalgesic rats and as reported by the authors, the «maximum effect to was reached sooner and intensity was greater with the mixture of the two drugs than with each substance given separately». The antagonism of the morphine effect could be masked, and the authors concluded that the peripheral analgesic effect of morphine on prostaglandin-hyperalgesia could be due to an inhibition of adenylate-cyclase activity.

Thus, in this study from Fereirra and Nakamura, a peripheral analgesic action of opioid agonists (morphine and met-enkephalin) administered locally into the rat hyperalgesic paw was demonstrated for the first time. However, the dose of local naloxone (7 µg i.pl.) chosen to reverse the effect of morphine produced analgesic effects in prostaglandin-hyperalgesic rats. Since lower doses of the antagonist were not used, it was concluded that naloxone did not antagonize the effect of morphine at this peripheral site, suggesting that opioid receptors were not involved.

Fentanyl and ethylketocyclazocine

Joris et al. [15] and Hargreaves et al. [12] using paw-withdrawal latency (PWL) to radiant heat nociceptive stimulation in rats which had received an intraplantar injection of carrageenan in both hindpaws, confirmed that opioids (fentanyl and ethylketocyclazocine) administered locally into a site of inflammation at doses which have no systemic effect produce peripheral effects restricted to the injected area. However, in these studies also, antagonist-reversibility was not tested «because of naloxone's reported agonist-like effects in this model of inflammation [12, 15] (Table I).

As an example, Figure 1 illustrates the effect of the mu-agonist fentanyl administered locally in carrageenin-injected rats : the injection of carrageenan into both hinpaws followed by saline (SAL) resulted in a profound decrease in paw withdrawal latency ($P < 0.01$) as compared to the control group receiving saline for all injection. In rats injected with carrageenan followed by opioid, the inflamed paws injected with 0.3 µg fentanyl were significantly less hyperalgesic ($P < 0.001$) than the contralateral inflamed paws injected with saline. This effect persisted for more than 2 hours. In sharp contrast, 0.3 µg fentanyl administered systemically (sc : FENTANYL) had no effect on carrageenan-hyperalgesia.

Comparable prolonged effects lasting for more than 2 hours (not shown here) were obtained after peripheral administration of a kappa-agonist, ethylketocyclazocine (10 µg i.pl.) in carrageenin-injected rats.

In additional experiments, it was shown that levorphanol (20 to 60 µg), another mu-receptor agonist, produced a dose-related blockade of carrageenan-induced hyperalgesia while in contrast, its dextrorotary isomer, dextrorphan, was inactive.

These experiments demonstrating significant blockade of carrageenan-induced hyperalgesia after peripheral, but not systemic application of equivalent doses of the agonists provide evidence for a peripherally located site of action. The fact that these

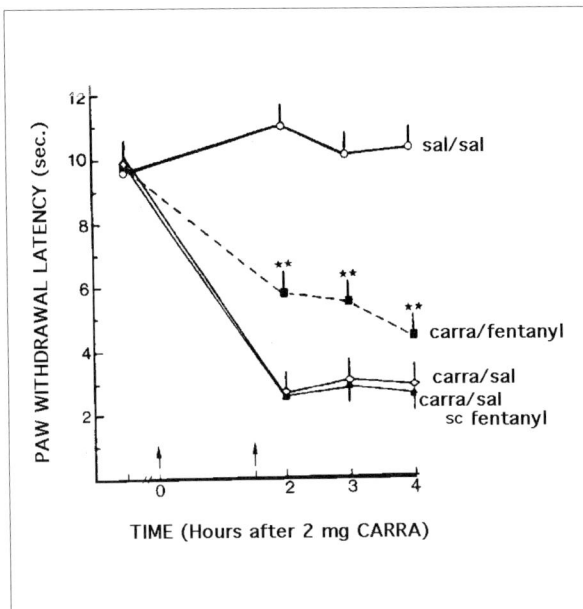

Figure 1. Peripheral effect of fentanyl (0.3 μg). A first group of rats received an initial injection of saline (SAL) into the plantar surface of both hind paws at time 0 (first arrow), and 90 min later (second arrow) received injections of SAL into both hind paws and subcutaneously (s.c.) into the neck (SAL/SAL, open circles). The three groups received initial injections of carrageenan (CARRA). Ninety min later, one CARRA group received a sc injection of SAL into the neck and FEN (0.3 μg) into one inflamed paw (CARRA/FENTANYL, filled squares). Another CARRA group received SAL into both paws and FEN (0.3 μg) into the neck (CARRA/SAL sc : FENTANYL, filled triangles). The last CARRA group received SAL into the paws and the neck (CARRA/SAL, open diamonds). (Modified from [15].)

effects (at least those of levorphanol) were dose-dependent and stereospecific may indicate an opioid receptor-specific mechanism of action. Nevertheless, considerable controversy persisted over whether these effects were truly mediated through opioid receptors since in these studies, antagonist reversibility was not unequivocally demonstrated. Furthermore, the multiplicity of opioid receptor types involved in such peripheral effects was questioned.

Further studies performed by Stein et al. [38, 39] in rats with a Freund's adjuvant-induced unilateral painful inflammation provided evidence for antagonist reversibility and specificity.

Studies in rats with a Freund's adjuvant-induced unilateral painful inflammation

Fentanyl

Stein et al. [38], using the paw withdrawal threshold (PWT) to noxious pressure in rats with a unilateral painful inflammation produced by the injection of Freund's adjuvant into the paw, examined first the possible peripheral site of action of opioids, using the mu-agonist fentanyl (Table I).

They demonstrated clearly that the intraplantar injection of fentanyl at doses of 0.1-1.2 μg, doses inactive when given systemically, resulted in a significant increase of paw pressure withdrawal thresholds in inflamed, but not in non-inflamed paws of the Freund's adjuvant-induced arthritic rats. This effect was dose-dependent and in this case, it was reversed by the intraplantar injection of naloxone at a dose (1.2 μg) which given alone was devoided of action. The naloxone-antagonism was stereospecific since (+) naloxone was ineffective in antagonizing the peripheral effect of fentanyl.

These data clearly showed that the mu-agonist fentanyl can modify the response to noxious pressure in inflamed but not non-inflamed paws *via* a peripheral site of action. Stereospecific reversibility by naloxone as well as dose dependency strongly indicated an opioid mechanism of action, suggesting a possible role for peripherally located opioid receptors in the modulation of nociception in inflamed tissue.

A further study performed in the same model by Stein *et al.* [40] suggested that peripheral mu, delta and kappa opioid receptors may mediate antinociception in inflammation.

DAMGO, DPDPE and U-50,488H

These experiments were designed to investigate :
- the antinociceptive effects of peripherally, compared with systemically applied mu, delta and kappa selective opioid agonists in unilateral hindpaw inflammation,
- whether these effects were dose-dependent, stereospecific and naloxone reversible,
- whether these effects were mediated by distinguishable receptor populations, using specific antagonists.

Using the paw withdrawal threshold (PWT) to noxious pressure (Figure 2), it was first demonstrated that the intraplantar injection of both the selective mu-agonist DAMGO (1 to 8 μg), delta-agonist DPDPE (20 to 80 μg) and kappa-agonist U-50,488 H (20 to 100 μg) produced marked antinociceptive effects in rats with a unilateral painful inflammation produced by Freund's adjuvant injection, restricted to the inflamed paw. Equivalent doses were ineffective when administered systemically, suggesting thus that all three agonists have a peripheral site of action in inflamed tissue. The antinociceptive effect of the peripherally applied opioid agonists was stereospecific and dose-dependent as shown in Figure 2. In addition, the time-course of the effects was similar to that occuring after intrathecal application of the agonists, although the effect of DAMGO appears to dissipate relatively fast.

It was clearly demonstrated in further experiments that the effects of DAMGO, DPDPE and U-50,488 H in inflamed paws could be reversed by peripherally applied naloxone (Figure 3). Moreover, this antagonism was dose-dependent and stereospecific, suggesting thus strongly that peripherally applied mu, delta and kappa agonists elicit opioid receptor-specific antinociceptive effects in inflamed paws. It should be noted, however, that doses of naloxone seven-fold higher (20 and 40 μg i.pl.) than those used for DAMGO and U-50,488 H were needed to reverse the effect of the delta agonist DPDPE (Figure 3).

In order to clarify whether DAMGO, DPDPE and U-50,488 H interact with separate receptor populations in the periphery mu, delta and kappa selective antagonists were applied in a final part of this study. The results demonstrated that the antinociceptive effect of each agonist can be reversed by its respective antagonist exclusively (Figure 4).

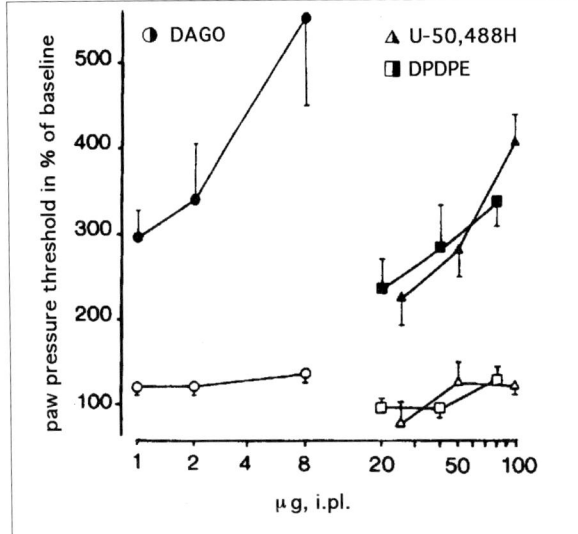

Figure 2. Dose-response relationships of effects of i.pl. DAGO, DPDPE and U-50, 488 H upon paw pressure withdrawal thresholds of rats with unilateral hindpaw inflammation. Measurements were conducted at the time of the peak effect, 5 min after drug injection. Closed symbols, inflamed paw; open symbols, non inflamed paw. n = 5-6 rats per dose. (Modified from [40].)

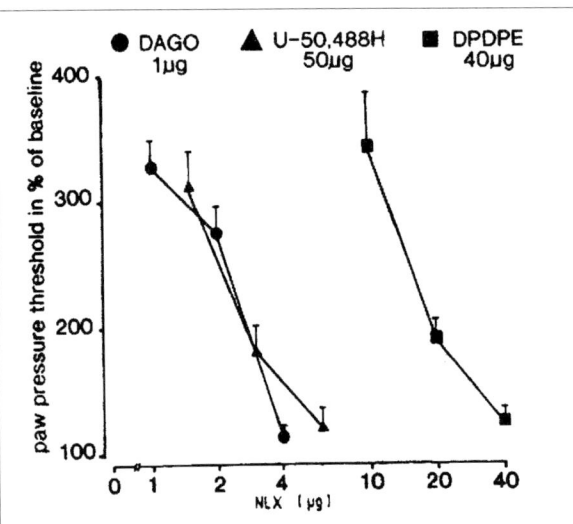

Figure 3. Dose-response relationships of effects of i.pl. stereoisomers of naloxone (NLX) upon paw pressure withdrawal thresholds elevation induced by DAGO, DPDPE and U-50, 488 H in inflamed paws. Measurements 5 min after drug injection are depicted. Closed symbols, (-)-naloxone; open symbols, (+)-naloxone. n = 5-6 rats per dose. (Modified from [40].)

Combined with experiments suggesting that different ranges of naloxone are required to antagonize the effects of the different agonists, these data strongly indicate that the three agonists interact with three heterogeneous opioid receptor populations.

These observations suggest that peripheral opioid antinociception (at least against noxious pressure) in hyperalgesic inflammatory conditions is mediated through mu, delta as well as kappa receptors.

One exception, however, is an electrophysiological study with formalin where kappa- but not mu- or delta-agonists administered i.pl. possessed peripheral antinociceptive actions.

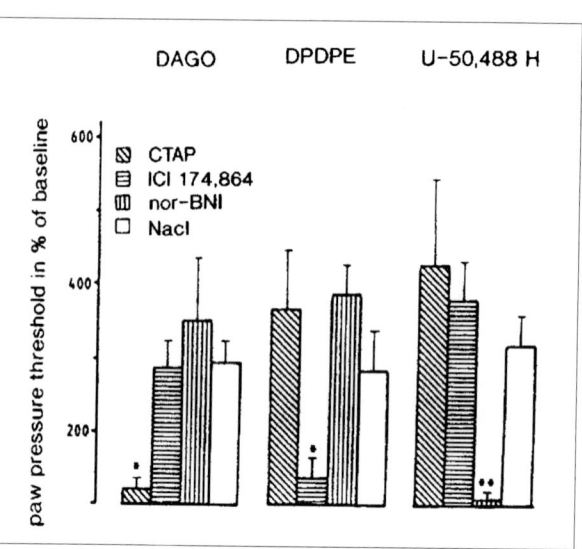

Figure 4. Effects of i.pl. CTAP, ICI 174,864, nor-BNI and NaCl upon paw pressure withdrawal threshold elevation induced by i.pl. DAGO, DPDPE and U-50,488 H in inflamed paws. Measurements were performed at peak effect (5 min after drug injection). n = 6-7 rats per dose. Significance of differences between NaCl and antagonist groups : * p< 0.05, ** p< 0.01- (Mann-Whitney test). (Modified from [40].)

Studies in formalin-injected rats

The formalin test for the identification of antinociceptive agents is widely used in behavioural studies in rodents as it produces two distinct phases of pain-related behaviour over about one hour [8, 13, 44]. The early phase of this chemically induced response is thought to result from direct peripheral activation by formalin of the sensory fibers whilst the late phase results from a peripheral inflammatory reaction involving the generation of bradykinin and prostaglandins [11, 13, 36].

An electrophysiological model of this test has been developed in the halothane anaesthetized rat : it has been demonstrated that the s.c. injection of formalin directly into the center of the receptive field of dorsal horn nociceptive neurones resulted in two peaks of neuronal firing over a period of 60 min [7] which coincide almost exactly with the time course of the licking behaviour.

Haley et al. [11] demonstrated recently that administration of the kappa-agonist U-50, 488 H (25-100 μg) directly into the receptive field of these neurones 10 min prior to formalin, resulted in a dose-related reduction of both the first and second peaks of the response. By contrast, neither morphine (100 μg) nor the delta-agonist DSTBULET (100 μg), administered as a pretreatment directly into the site of formalin injection, had any significant effect on either peak of the formalin response.

The inhibition of formalin evoked activity by the kappa-agonist apparently resulted from a local, peripheral action of U-50, 488 H since administration of 100 μg U-50, 488 H into the contralateral, non-inflamed paw had no influence upon the formalin response. In addition, the effects of U-50, 488 H were clearly reversed by naloxone (100 μg) injected directly into the plantar region of the paw 12 min prior to formalin, indicating thus that these effects result from an opioid action. Naloxone alone (100 μg) administered either i.p. or intraplantarly had no effect on either phase of the formalin response.

These results clearly indicate that the formalin response in rats could be modulated by peripherally administered kappa- but not mu- or delta-opioid agonists. This suggests that the profile of inhibition of this short duration inflammatory response by peripherally administered opioids differs markedly from that seen above in more prolonged inflammatory states.

As indicated by the authors [11], this suggests that changes over time occur in the proportions of opioid receptor subtypes present or active at the peripheral terminals. Indeed, the rapid onset of the formalin response (within a few seconds) and the ability of U-50, 488 H to inhibit all phases of activity suggest that the receptor mediating this inhibitory action must already be present in an active form. It could be thus hypothesized that the mu- and delta-receptors mediating inhibition in more prolonged inflammatory states take time to either become active or to be synthetized and transported along the axon to reach their peripheral site of action [45]. However, the variable profile of peripheral opioid inhibition may therefore simply reflect the different peripheral stimuli present.

In agreement with these results from Haley et al. [11], recent behavioural experiments showed that the intraplantar injection of a kappa-opioid agonist with limited access to the central nervous system, GR94839 (30-100 μg), selectively inhibited the second phase of the rat formalin-induced licking test [32], an inhibition which was reversed by naltrexone (0.3 mg/kg s.c.).

In conclusion, behavioural evidence has accumulated, suggesting that peripherally applied opioid agonists can produce antinociceptive effects in hyperalgesic inflammatory states. It appears from the last study from Stein et al. [40] performed in rats with a unilateral painful inflammation lasting from 4 to 6 days, that three different populations of receptors could mediate these effects.

Taken together, these results suggest that in hyperalgesic inflammatory conditions peripherally located opioid receptors become functionally active and may be of significance in the modulation of nociception by endogenous as well as exogenous opioids.

The contribution of this peripheral effect to the overall antinociceptive action of opioid agonists when administered systemically in hyperalgesic inflammatory conditions could thus be questioned. Series of experiments were designed by several groups including ours, in an attempt to evaluate the contribution of this peripheral effect to the overall antinociceptive action of systemically applied opioids.

In a second part of this paper, we will thus consider successively studies performed in formalin, then in rats with a localized inflammation, carrageenan and Freund's adjuvant-injected animals (Table II).

Table II. Antinociceptive effect of systemically administered opioids in animal models of localized inflammatory pain.

Authors	Model	Treatment	Test	Antagonist	Dose
Abbott [1]	Formalin (Rat)	Morphine EKC	Spontaneous pain	Naloxone Methylbromide	10mg/kg
Oluyomi et al. [28]	Formalin (Mice)	Morphine Methylmorphine	Paw Licking	Naloxone Methylnaloxone	2mg/kg 10mg/kg
Rogers et al. [32]	Formalin (Rat)	GR94839	Paw Licking	Naltrexone Nor-BNI	1µg 100µg
Kayser et al. [22]	Cg	Morphine	VT	Naloxone	0.25-1µg
Stein et al. [38]	FA	Morphine U-50,488H	PWT	Naloxone	1-3µg 5-15µg

Cg = Carrageenan ;
EKC = Ethylketocyclazocine ;
VT = Vocalization threshold to paw pressure ;
PWT = Paw withdrawal threshold to noxious pressure.
FA = Freund's adjuvant ;
Nor-BNI = Norbinaltorphimine ;

Studies providing evidence for a peripheral component in the antinociceptive effect of systemically administered opioids in animal models of peripheral inflammation

Studies in formalin-injected rat and mice

It has been stated that both early and late phases of the formalin response can be centrally modulated by opioids [7, 8, 36]. Recent studies, however, have indicated that the antinociceptive effects of systemic opioid agonists in the late phase of the formalin test may result of summation of central and peripheral actions.

Peripheral antinociceptive actions of systemic ethylketocyclazocine in the rat formalin test

In an initial study from Abbott [1], the antinociceptive actions of ethylketocyclazocine (a non-selective kappa- and mu-agonist), and morphine were examined in rats using a thermal nociceptive test (tail immersion) and the paw formalin test (nociceptive scores of spontaneous pain). In this latter case, drug injections were timed so that testing could be carried out 30-40 min after formalin, thereby in the late phase of the formalin-evoked pain behaviour.

In the formalin test, the antinociceptive effects of high doses of ethylketocyclazocine (0.4 to 0.8 mg/kg s.c.), but not morphine (2.5 to 10mg/kg s.c.), were attenuated by the peripherally acting antagonist naloxone methylbromide (10 mg/kg s.c.). By contrast, naloxone methylbromide had no effect on antinociception produced by ethylketocyclazocine in the tail-immersion test.

When ethylketocyclazocine was injected intraventricularly, only partial antinociception was observed in the formalin test. Conversely, naloxone given intraventricularly only partially attenuated the antinociception produced by ethylketocyclazocine given systemically.

These data suggest that the non-specific mu- and kappa-opioid agonist ethylketocyclazocine administered systemically produces centrally mediated antinociception at low doses in the formalin test while at high doses, an additional peripheral effect is recruited.

Since no peripheral effects were observed in the tail-immersion test, this suggests that opioid mechanisms may be involved in the inflammatory reaction to formalin injection. By contrast, morphine antinociception reaches a ceiling at doses that are devoid of such peripheral actions in the formalin test. These results could be related to the electrophysiological study of Haley *et al.* [11] described above, indicating that the formalin response in rats could be modulated by peripherally administered kappa- but not mu- or delta-opioid agonists.

Although the peripheral effects were obtained in the present study only at high doses, with a non-specific agonist and although selective opioid antagonists could not be used, these results indicate clearly that systemic opioid agonists could have an additional peripheral antinociceptive effect in inflammatory states, but not in normal conditions.

Oluyomi *et al.* [28] have examined whether the activity of systemic morphine in the mouse formalin test involves peripheral opioid receptors using a quaternary analogue which does not enter the central nervous system after systemic administration, methylmorphine and its specific antagonist, methylnaloxone.

Differential antinociceptive effects of systemic morphine and methylmorphine in the mouse formalin test

In this study from Oluyomi *et al.* [28], the antinociceptive activities of morphine, and its quaternary analogue methylmorphine, were compared after intraperitoneal administrations in the mouse paw formalin test (licking or biting of the formalin injected hindpaw).

In these experiments, as in the preceeding study from Abbott [1], it was demonstrated that systemic morphine (2.5 to 10 mg/kg i.p.) produced a dose-dependent inhibition of both the early and late phases of the formalin-induced response and these antinociceptive effects were antagonized by systemic naloxone (2 mg/kg i.p.). This confirms that a centrally acting opioid agonist, when administered systemically, suppresses both phases of the licking response to formalin.

In contrast, when methylmorphine (10 to 80 mg/kg i.p.) was administered systemically, only the late phase of the response was inhibited. Methylmorphine has reduced lipophilicity and does not enter the central nervous system after systemic administration. The effect of systemic methylmorphine was blocked by pretreatment with methylnaloxone (10 mg/kg i.p.).

This suggests that the early phase of the response to formalin in the mouse may be inhibited by stimulation of central opioid receptors, whilst stimulation of peripheral opioid receptors results in a reduction in the second phase, suggesting again that inhibition of the late phase may involve both peripheral and central opioid receptors.

Peripheral antinociceptive effect of systemic GR94839,
a peripherally selective kappa agonist in the rat formalin test

In this study from Rogers *et al.* [32], the antinociceptive activity of GR94839 (a kappa-opioid agonist with limited access to the central nervous system) was examined in rats using the paw formalin test (licking of the formalin injected paw).

In these experiments, it was demonstrated that systemic GR94839 (1-10mg/kg s.c.) inhibited the second phase of the rat formalin response at doses seven fold lower than those required to inhibit the first phase. By contrast, GR103545 (a centrally-penetrating kappa-agonist) was equieffective against both phases.

Intraplantar administration of the opioid antagonists, naltrexone (1 μg) (a non-selective opioid antagonist) or norbinaltorphimine (100 μg) (a kappa-selective antagonist), reversed the antinociceptive effect of systemic GR94839 (3 mg/kg s.c.) against the second phase of the formalin response. Injection of the antagonists alone into the formalin-injected paw had no effect on the duration of licking in the late phase, and injection of antagonist into the contralateral paw did not reverse the antinociceptive effects of systemic GR94839.

The present findings are in agreement with previous studies [1, 11] where a peripheral inhibition of the formalin response by kappa-opioids was demonstrated.

These results obtained with formalin argue for the participation of a peripheral component to the antinociceptive effects of opioids administered systemically in inflammatory conditions. However, it is difficult to determine the exact contribution of this peripheral effect to the overall antinociceptive effect produced by the systemically administered opioid agonists in these inflammatory conditions.

Studies performed in models of more prolonged inflammatory pain and using mechanical noxious stimuli (paw withdrawal threshold and vocalization threshold to noxious pressure) have attempted to determine the contribution of this peripheral effect to the antinociceptive effect of systemic opioids in inflammatory states.

Studies in rats with carrageenan- and Freund's adjuvant-induced unilateral painful inflammation

Various forms of prolonged experimental painful inflammation in animals have been associated with an enhanced antinociceptive effect of systemically administered opioid agonists [2, 6, 16, 19, 20, 26, 27, 30, 37]. As an example, in Freund's adjuvant-induced polyarthritic rats used as a model of experimental pain, using a centrally integrated test, the vocalization threshold to paw pressure, we showed that low doses of systemic opioid agonists, including morphine, induced a more potent and prolonged antinociceptive effect than in normal animals [6, 19, 20, 27] and this could be related to clinical evidence suggesting that responses to opioids may differ in subjects experiencing chronic pain [42, 43]. One interpretation of these findings was that prolonged painful inflammation results in an alteration of endogenous opioid systems in the central nervous system of the animals and consequently, in an altered response to exogenously applied opioids. Indeed, numerous biochemical studies have provided evidence that a variety of inflammatory states are associated with elevated levels of opioid gene transcripts and peptides in the spinal cord ; however no significant changes in mu, delta or kappa receptor binding have been found [4, 5, 14, 26, 33].

An alternative interpretation is that changes in sensitivity to opioid agonists are occuring in the periphery, *i.e.* in the inflamed paws, and thus contribute to the potent antinociceptive effects of opioid agonists applied systemically in rat models of inflammatory pain.

This hypothesis was tested in rats with a unilateral carrageenan- [22] and Freund's adjuvant-induced inflammatory pain [39].

Studies in carrageenan-injected rats

We investigated the possible contribution of a peripheral component in the enhanced antinociceptive effect of a low dose of systemic morphine in the modulation of the response to noxious pressure on inflamed paws, using rats with a unilateral painful inflammation produced by carrageenan and a supraspinally integrated test, the measure of the vocalization threshold to paw pressure. Previous experiments performed in our laboratory have shown that this test was particularly sensitive to low doses of opioid compounds in the same range as those used in therapeutic [19, 27].

The effects of a relatively low dose of morphine (1 mg/kg i.v.) which produces potent antinociceptive effects in other models of inflammatory pain [19], and then the effects of escalating low doses of naloxone (0.25-1 μg injected i.v., or locally into the inflamed paw) on the antinociceptive effect of morphine, were thus analyzed in rats injected with carrageenin 4 h previously. At this time, the carrageenin-injected rats exhibited a significant decrease in the vocalization threshold to paw pressure, by comparison with the pre-carrageenin-control values [18].

We demonstrated that the injection of the relatively low dose of 1 mg/kg i.v. morphine produced a more potent and long-lasting antinociceptive effect on the inflamed than on the contralateral hindpaw (Figure 5A). The overall antinociceptive effect of morphine was about two times greater on the inflamed paw than on the non-inflamed paw. These antinociceptive effects of morphine were almost abolished by a relatively high dose of naloxone (ten times lower than that of morphine : 0.1 mg/kg) administered i.v. (Figure 5B). These data are in agreement with previous studies on opioids, where enhanced antinociceptive effects were observed in hyperalgesic inflammatory conditions in rat models of inflammation [9, 12, 16, 19, 20, 27, 38, 40].

In agreement with some of the studies mentioned above [38, 40], we were able to reverse the antinociceptive effect of morphine on the inflamed paw by a local injection

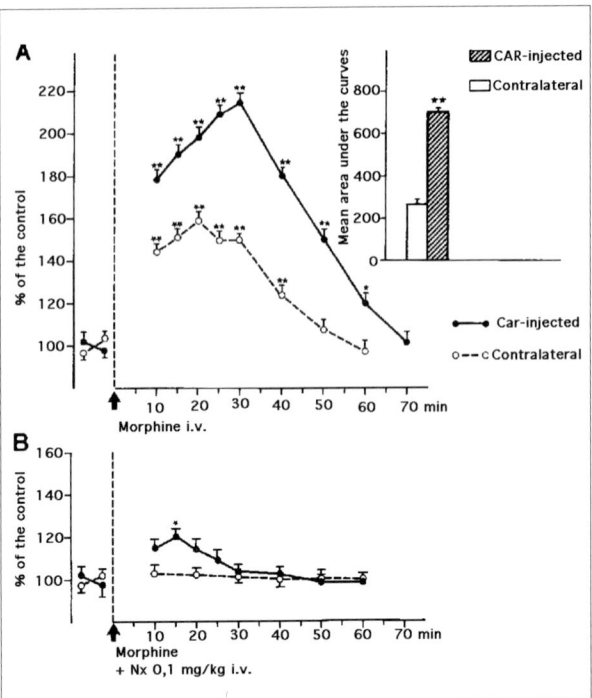

Figure 5. A : Mean curves for the effects of 1 mg/kg i.v. morphine on the thresholds for vocalization (± S.E.M.) determined from the inflamed and the non-inflamed paw of rats injected with carrageenin. Each value is expressed as a percentage of the threshold value obtained before the injection of morphine. $n = 9$ rats. *$P< 0.05$, **$P< 0.01$, Dunnett's t-test with vocalization threshold expressed in grams. On the right : a comparison between the mean areas under the curves obtained for each paw after injection of 1 mg/kg i.v. morphine, as illustrated in A.
** $P< 0.01$,Wilcoxon-signed rank test.
B : Mean curves for the effects of 0.1 mg/kgi.v. naloxone, on the antinociceptive effect of 1 mg/kg i.v. morphine in rats injected with carrageenin. Each value is expressed as a percentage of baseline threshold ± S.E.M., $n = 6$ rats,
* $P< 0.05$, Dunnett's t-test.

of extremely low doses of naloxone, ineffective when injected i.v., and this effect was strictly restricted to the inflamed area (Figure 6 and Figure 7). The antagonistic effect of local naloxone was obtained with a dose as low as 0.5 µg and was significantly enhanced when the dose of 1 µg was used (Figure 6 and Figure 7). Naloxone alone (1 µg in a volume of 0.1 ml) injected into the inflamed paw of carrageenin-injected rats which had received an acute injection of saline instead of morphine, induced only a slight tendency to a non-significant antinociceptive effect (mean vocalization threshold was 18 ± 2 % at 15 min after the injection, n= 9). In contrast to other studies [38, 40], higher doses of local naloxone were not used to reverse the effect of morphine and thus the exact contribution of this peripheral action to the enhanced effect of morphine could not be determined. Indeed, in previous experiments using low doses of fentanyl administered into the rat brachial plexus sheath, we have shown that the dose of 2.5 µg naloxone injected locally into the paw appears to have central effects in normal rats [21]. It can be presumed that in inflammatory conditions the systemic diffusion of naloxone would be enhanced.

Results obtained in our study strongly suggest the participation of a peripheral opioid receptor mechanism in the antinociceptive effect of morphine given systemically at relatively low doses in rat models of inflammatory pain.

They offer a possible explanation for the previous observation of an enhanced antinociceptive action of systemic morphine in rats subjected to inflammatory conditions : a synergism of peripheral and central actions may result in the augmented potency of morphine in these animals.

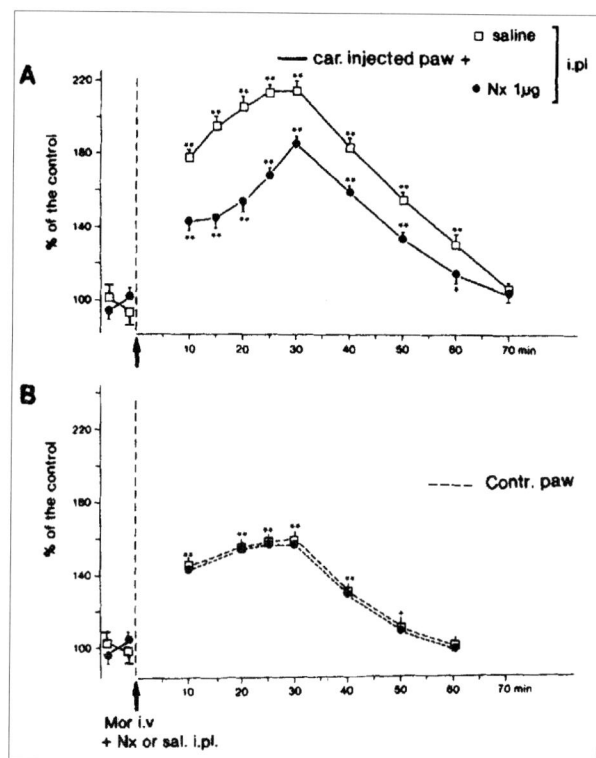

Figure 6. Mean curves for the effects of a low dose of naloxone (1 µg in a volume of 0.1 ml) or saline administered locally into the inflamed paw, on the antinociceptive effect of 1 mg/kg i.v. morphine in rats injected with carrageenin. Each value is expressed as a percentage of baseline threshold ± S.E.M.
A : Carrageenan (Car.)-injected paw- B : Contralateral paw.

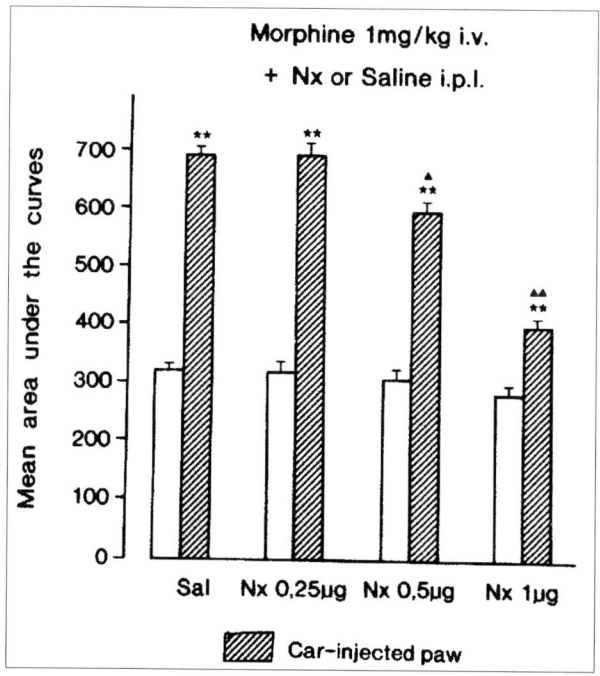

Figure 7. Comparison between the mean areas under the curves obtained for each paw after injection of a combination of morphine 1 mg/kg i.v. and naloxone (0.25, 0.5 and 1 µg) or saline administered locally into the inflamed paw in a volume of 0.1 ml, as illustrated in Figure 5. Area values are expressed as arbitrary units ± S.E.M. Wilcoxon signed rank test was used for statistical analysis.
** $P < 0.01$, inflamed compared to non-inflamed paw ;
$P < 0.05$, $P < 0.01$, naloxone compared to saline.

Due to the fact that higher doses of local naloxone were not used to avoid complications *via* central and peripheral effects [9, 19, 20, 31], the exact contribution of this peripheral action in the enhanced effect of morphine could not be determined in the present study. In addition, the peripheral opioid receptor specific mechanism involved was not determined, although the extremely low doses of local naloxone (0.5 and 1 μg i.pl.) able to significantly reverse the effect of systemic morphine strongly suggest the intervention of a peripheral mu-type receptor.

This aspect was investigated by Stein *et al.* [39] using different opioid agonists in another model of unilateral inflammatory pain.

Studies in Freund's adjuvant-injected rats

In this study performed in rats with a unilateral hindpaw inflammation produced by Freund's adjuvant-induced injection, and using the paw withdrawal threshold to noxious pressure, Stein *et al.* [39] demonstrated that the antinociceptive potency of both morphine (0.65 to 2 mg/kg), and the kappa-opioid agonist U-50, 488 H (2.5 to 20 mg/kg), administered subcutaneously, was markedly enhanced in the inflamed paws compared to that in contralateral, non-inflamed paws. The analgesic efficacy of both agonists against paw pressure in the non-inflamed paws of animals treated with Freund's adjuvant was not different from that of normal animals. Moreover, the antinociceptive effect of each agonist against pressure exerted on the tail was not different between treated and control animals.

The enhanced antinociceptive effect of both agonists could be antagonized by low doses of naloxone (1 to 3 μg for morphine, 5 to 15 μg for the kappa-agonist) injected directly into the paw, but not by the equivalent doses of naloxone administered systemically. Moreover, this antagonism was stereospecific and dose-dependent.

These findings strongly support the contention that both morphine and U-50, 488 H elicit opioid receptor-specific effects *via* a peripheral site of action in inflamed tissue and that these effects account for their observed increased antinociceptive potency.

The effects of morphine were reversed by extremely low doses of local naloxone (1 to 3 μg), comparable to that used in our study. By contrast, i.pl. naloxone was less potent at blocking the kappa agonist. This finding supports the concept that peripheral morphine and U-50, 488 H antinociception are mediated by two separate opioid receptor populations. It should be noted, however, that the doses of naloxone (5 to 15 μg i.pl.) needed to reverse the peripheral effect of U-50, 488 H are in the range of those able to diffuse into the systemic circulation [21].

As a general conclusion, recent evidence indicates that exogenous opioids can produce localized opioid receptor-mediated antinociception in peripheral inflamed tissue, suggesting thus that local application of small doses of conventional opiates or the development of opioid agonists unable to cross the blood-brain barrier may provide a new perspective for pain management by producing analgesia without central side effects such as respiratory depression, sedation, or dependence (cf Stein, this volume). Several studies were even able to differentiate the types of peripheral opioid receptors involved. However, the physiological significance of these receptors has not been yet elucidated. In particular, the question arises as to what are the endogenous ligands for these receptors and what stimuli bring them into play. Recent studies from Stein *et al.* [41] that will be not reported here showed that activation of endogenous opioids by a cold water swim in rats with hind paw inflammation results in a similar local antinociceptive effect but suggested that pituitary-adrenal opioid pools are not directly involved in producing this effect. Further studies showed increased amounts of opioid peptides in immune cells infiltrating the inflamed tissue and immunoreactive opioid receptors on peripheral terminals of sensory neurons [41]. In addition, the local administration of antibodies against opioid peptides or receptors or systemic pretreatment with the immunosuppressant cyclosporine blocks cold water swim-induced antinociception. These findings suggest that antinociception in inflammation can be brought about by endogenous opioids from immune cells interacting with opioid receptors on peripheral sensory nerves. These results could be related to other studies performed in rats with unilateral Freund's adjuvant-induced inflammation, showing that capsaicin-sensitive C-fiber afferents are essential for the increased antinociceptive effect of systemic morphine in the inflamed tissue [2].

However, even if data on peripheral antinociceptive effects of opioids in normal tissue remains controversial [17, 25, 35], inflammatory states may not be unique, and such peripheral effects could occur in other conditions. Indeed, we have demonstrated potent and long lasting antinociceptive effects after injection of low doses of fentanyl into the normal rat brachial plexus sheath, which were reversed by low doses of locally administered naloxone, suggesting the involvement of a peripheral site of action of the opioid in this particular case [21]. Moreover, it appears from recent experiments [23] that peripheral antinociceptive effects of systemic morphine could also be revealed in a model of persistent non-inflammatory pain where peripheral nerve fibers have been damaged by loose ligature. In these conditions, the peripheral opioid effects could be related to changes of opioid receptors located on degenerating and/or regenerating fibers.

Acknowledgements

The authors wish to thank Dr AH Dickenson for the English revision and Mr G Corvalan for the photography.

References

1. Abbott FV. Peripheral and central antinociceptive actions of ethylketocyclazocine in the formalin test. *Eur J Pharmacol* 1988 ; 152 : 93-100.
2. Bartho L, Stein C, Herz A. Involvement of capsaicin-sensitive neurones in hyperalgesia and enhanced opioid antinociception in inflammation. *Naun Schmied Arch Pharmacol* 1990 ; 242: 666-70.

3. Besson JM, Chaouch A. Peripheral and spinal mechanisms of nociception. *Physiol Rev* 1987 ; 67 : 67-186.
4. Cesselin F, Montastruc JL, Gros C, Bourgoin S, Hamon M. Met-enkephalin levels and opiate receptors in the spinal cord of chronic suffering rats. *Brain Res* 1980 ; 191 : 289-93.
5. Delay-Goyet P, Kayser V, Zajac JM, Guilbaud G, Besson JM, Roques BP. Lack of significant changes in μ, δ opioid binding sites and neutral endopeptidase EC 3.4.24.11 in the brain and spinal cord of arthritic rats. *Neuropharmacology* 1989 ; 28 : 1341-6.
6. Desmeules JA, Kayser V, Gacel G, Guilbaud G, Roques BP. The highly selective δ agonist BUBU induces an analgesic effect in normal and arthritic rat and this action is not affected by repeated administration of low doses of morphine. *Brain Res* 1993 ; 611 :243-8.
7. Dickenson AH, Sullivan AF. Subcutaneous formalin-induced activity of dorsal horn neurones in the rat : differential response to an intrathecal opiate administered pre or post formalin. *Pain* 1987 ; 30 : 349-60.
8. Dubuisson D, Dennis SG. The formalin test : a quantitative study of the analgesic effect of morphine, meperidine, and brain stem stimulation in rats and cats. *Pain* 1977 ; 4 : 161-5.
9. Fereirra SH, Nakamura M. Prostaglandin hyperalgesia : the peripheral analgesic activity of morphine, enkephalins and opioid antagonists. *Prostaglandins* 1979 ; 18 : 191-200.
10. Fields H, Emson PC, Leigh BK, Gilbert RFT, Iversen LL. Multiple opiate receptor site on primary afferent fibers. *Nature* 1980 ; 284 : 351-3.
11. Haley J, Ketchum S, Dickenson A. Peripheral k-opioid modulation of the formalin response : an electrophysiological study in the rat. *Eur J Pharmacol* 1990 ; 191 : 437-46.
12. Hargreaves KM, Dubner R, Joris J. Peripheral actions of opiates in the blockade of carrageenin-induced inflammation. In : Dubner R, Gebhart GF, Bond MR, eds. Proceeding. Vth World Congress on Pai.n. Amsterdam : Elsevier Science Publishers, 1988 : 55-60.
13. Hunskaar S, Hole K. The formalin test in mice : dissociation between inflammatory and non-inflammatory pain. *Pain* 1987 ; 30 : 103-14.
14. Iadarola MJ, Brady LS, Draisci G, Dubner R. Enhancement of dynorphin gene expression in spinal cord following experimental inflammation : stimulus specificity, behavioural parameters and opioid receptor binding. *Pain* 1988 ; 35 : 313-26.
15. Joris JL, Dubner R, Hargreaves KM. Opioid analgesia at peripheral sites : a target for opioids released during stress and inflammation ? *Anesth Analg* 1987 ; 66 : 1277-81.
16. Joris J, Costello A, Dubner R, Hargreaves K. Opiates supress carrageenan-induced oedema and hyperthermia at doses that inhibit hyperalgesia. *Pain* 1990 ; 43 : 95-103.
17. Jurna I, Grosman W. The effect of morphine on mammalian nerve fibers. *Eur J Pharmacol* 1977 ; 44 : 338-40.
18. Kayser V, Guilbaud G. Local and remote modifications of nociceptive sensitivity during carrageenin-induced inflammation in the rat. *Pain* 1987 ; 28 : 99-107.
19. Kayser V. The reactivity of arthritic rat to acute and chronic administration of various opioid substances. In : Besson JM, Guilbaud G, eds. *The arthritic rat as a model of clinical pain* ? Amsterdam : Elsevier Science Publisher, 1988 : 111-38.
20. Kayser V, Guilbaud G. Differential effects of various doses of morphine and naloxone on two nociceptive test thresholds in arthritic and normal rats. *Pain* 1990 ; 41 : 353-63.
21. Kayser V, Gobeaux D, Lombard MC, Guilbaud G, Besson JM. Potent and long lasting antinociceptive effects after injection of low doses of a mu-opioid receptor agonist, fentanyl, into the brachial plexus sheath of the rat. *Pain* 1990 ; 42 : 215-25.
22. Kayser V, Chen YL, Guilbaud G. Behavioural evidence for a peripheral component in the enhanced antinociceptive effect of a low dose of systemic morphine in carrageenin-induced hyperalgesic rats. *Brain Res* 1991 ; 560 : 237-44.
23. Kayser V, Lee SH, Guilbaud G. Evidence for a peripheral component in the antinociceptive effect of systemic morphine in rats with peripheral mononeuropathy.*Neurosci* 1994 : in press.

24. Laduron P. Axonal transport of opiate receptors in the capsaicin sensitive neurones. *Brain Res* 1984 ; 294 : 157-60.
25. Lim RKS, Guzman F, Rodgers DW, Goto K, Braun C, Dickerson GD, Engle RJ. Site of action of narcotic and non-narcotic analgesics determined by blocking bradykinin-evoked visceral pain. *Arch Int Pharmacodyn* 1964 ; 152 : 25-58.
26. Millan MJ, Czlonkowski A, Morris B, Stein C, Arendt R, Huber A, Höllt V, Herz A. Inflammation of the hind limb as a model of unilateral, localized pain : influence on multiple opioid systems in the spinal cord of the rat. *Pain* 1988 ; 35 : 299-312.
27. Neil A, Kayser V, Gacel G, Besson JM, Guilbaud G. Opioid receptor types and antinociceptive activity in chronic inflammation : both κ- and μ-opiate agonist effects are enhanced in arthritic rats. *Eur J Pharmacol* 1986 ; 130 : 203-8.
28. Oluyomi AO, Hart SL, Smith TW. Differential antinociceptive effects of morphine and methylmorphine in the formalin test. *Pain* 1992 ; 49 : 415-8.
29. Raja SN, Meyer RA, Campbell JN, Khan AA. Narcotics do not alter the heat responses of unmyelinated primary afferents in monkeys. *Anesthesiology* 1986 ; 65 : 468-73.
30. Randall LO, Selitto JJ. A method for measurement of analgesic activity on inflamed tissue. *Arch Int Pharmacodyn* 1957 ; 4 : 409-19.
31. Rios L, Jacob JC. Local inhibition of inflammatory pain by naloxone and its N-methyl quaternary analogue. *Eur J Pharmacol* 1983 ; 96 : 277-83.
32. Rogers H, Birch PJ, Harisson SM, Palmer E, Manchee GR, Judd DB, Naylor A, Scopes DIC, Hayes AG. GR94839, a κ-opioid agonist with limited access to the central nervous system, has antinociceptive activity. *Br J Pharmacol* 1992 ; 106 : 783-9.
33. Ruda MA, Iadarola MJ, Cohen LV, Young WS. In situ hybridisation histochemistry and immunocytochemistry reveal an increase in spinal cord dynorphin biosynthesis in a rat model of peripheral inflammation and hyperalgesia. *Proc Natl Acad Sci USA* 1988 ; 85 : 622-6.
34. Russell NJW, Schaible HA, Schmidt RF. Opiates inhibit the discharge of fine afferent units from inflamed knee joint of the cat. *Neurosci Lett* 1987 ; 76 : 107-12.
35. Senami M, Aoki M, Kitahata LM, Collins JG, Kumeta Y, Murata K. Lack of opiate effects on cat C polymodal nociceptive fibers. *Pain* 1986 ; 27 : 81-90.
36. Shibata M, Ohkubo T, Takahashi H, Inoki R. Modified formalin test : characteristic biphasic pain response. *Pain* 1989 ; 38 : 347-50.
37. Shippenberg TS, Stein C, Huber A, Millan MJ, Herz A. Motivational effects of opioids in an animal model of prolonged inflammatory pain : alteration in the effects of κ- but not of μ-receptor agonists. *Pain* 1988 ; 35 : 179-86.
38. Stein C, Millan MJ, Shippenberg TS, Herz A. Peripheral effect of fentanyl upon nociception in inflamed tissue of the rat. *Neurosci Lett* 1988 ; 84 : 225-8.
39. Stein C, Millan MJ, Yassouridis A, Herz A. Antinociceptive effects of μ- and κ-agonists in inflammation are enhanced due to a peripheral opioid receptor-specific mechanism. *Eur J Pharmacol* 1988 ; 155 : 255-64.
40. Stein C, Millan MJ, Shippenberg TS, Peter K, Herz A. Peripheral opioid receptors mediating antinociception in inflammation. Evidence for involvement of Mu, Delta and Kappa receptors. *J Pharmacol Exp Ther* 1989 ; 248 : 1269-75.
41. Stein C, Hassan AHS, Przewlocki R, Gramsch C, Peter K, Herz A. Opioids from immunocytes interact with receptors on sensory nerves to inhibit nociception in inflammation. *Proc Natl Acad Sci USA* 1990 ; 87 : 5935-9.
42. Twycross RG. Narcotics In : Wall PD, Melzack R, eds. *Textbook of pain*. Edinburgh : Churchill Livingstone, 1984 : 514-25.
43. Walsh TD, Baster R, Bowman K, Leber R. High-dose morphine and respiratory function in chronic cancer pain. *Pain* 1981 ; Suppl 1 : 39.

44. Wheeler-Aceto H, Porreca F, Cowan A. The rat paw formalin test : comparison of noxious agents. *Pain* 1990 ; 40 : 229-38.
45. Young WS, Wamsley JK, Zarbin MA, Kuhar MJ. Opioid receptors undergo axonal flow. *Science* 1980 ; 210 : 76-8.

11

Peripheral opioid analgesia : mechanisms and therapeutic applications

C. STEIN

*Departement of Anesthesiology and Critical Care Medicine,
Johns Hopkins University, Baltimore, Maryland, USA.*

Opioid analgesia has been associated with the activation of opioid receptors in the central nervous system. Recently, however, a number of studies have demonstrated that exogenous as well as endogenous opioid agonists can elicit pronounced antinociceptive effects via activation of opioid receptors in peripheral tissues. Such effects have been shown to occur primarily in inflamed tissue and were demonstrated both in animal experiments and under clinical conditions in patients. This chapter will give an overview of experimental and clinical studies that have examined peripheral analgesic actions of opioids and will discuss mechanisms and potential therapeutic implications.

Peripheral antinociceptive effects of exogenous opioids

A fairly large number of animal studies examining peripheral antinociceptive effects of exogenous opioids has appeared (review in [2, 35]). To differentiate between peripheral and central actions, compounds that do not cross the blood-brain barrier or the local *versus* systemic application of equivalent doses of agents were used. To demonstrate that such peripheral effects were mediated by opioid receptors, reversibility by standard opioid antagonists (*e.g.* naloxone), dose-dependency or stereospecificity were examined and most of these investigations indeed support the occurrence of opioid receptor-specific effects at peripheral sites. Among agonists with differing affinities for the three types of opioid receptors, preferential mu-ligands were generally the most potent, but delta- and kappa-ligands were active as well. Thus, the prudent statement at present would be that, depending on the particular circumstances, all three receptor types can be present and functionally active in peripheral tissues (for details, see [35]).

Peripheral antinociceptive effects of endogenous opioids

A few recent studies have examined the activation of peripheral opioid receptors by endogenous opioid peptides. In these reports a model of stress (cold water swim) was chosen to activate endogenous opioid systems in rats with unilateral inflammation of the hindpaw. Following cold water swim, nociceptive thresholds increased selectively in the inflamed paw and this effect was mediated by peripheral opioid receptors [25, 36]. Moreover, this effect was abolished by mu- and delta-, but not by kappa-selective antagonists as well as by antibodies against ß-endorphin [36, 37]. These findings suggest that peripheral mu- and delta-receptors in inflamed tissue can mediate local antinociception following their activation by opioid peptides released during stress. The question as to the anatomical source of these endogenous opioids will be discussed below.

Mechanisms

Role of inflammation

Almost all experimental studies reporting peripheral antinociceptive actions of opioids have used models of inflammation. The inflammatory reaction was induced by various agents (*e.g.* prostaglandins, carrageenan, killed mycobacteria, acetic acid, formalin, bradykinin). When evaluating the effects of opioids under such circumstances, one has to bear in mind that the different agents and routes of administration produce different types of inflammation. Therefore it is conceivable that, depending on the nature and stage of the inflammatory reaction, different types of local opioid receptors become active which may partly explain why some studies found, *e.g.* peripheral antinociceptive effects of kappa-agonists and others did not. Another important fact is that studies comparing peripheral opioid actions in inflamed *versus* non inflamed tissue have unequivocally reported greater antinociceptive effects in inflammation. These observations indicate that the inflammatory process is important for the manifestation of peripheral opioid antinociceptive actions, and that one has to be critical when comparing the different models with each other or with the clinical situation (for details, see [2, 35]).

Opioid peptides in peripheral tissue

Significant amounts of ß-endorphin and met-enkephalin have been found within inflamed subcutaneous tissue. These peptides are localized in cells of the immune system, namely in T- and B-lymphocytes, monocytes and macrophages [28, 37]. *In situ* hybridization studies have revealed the presence of mRNA's encoding opioid peptide precursors in the same anatomical distribution, suggesting that opioid peptides are actually synthesized within these cells [28]. These observations are consistent with *in vitro* studies demonstrating the presence of opioid peptides in different immune cells [14, 34]. Furthermore, suppression of the immune system by cyclosporine A or irradiation abolishes stress-induced antinociception in inflamed tissue [28, 37]. Taken together, these findings suggest that endogenous opioids producing localized antinociception in inflamed tissue originate from resident immune cells.

Another conceivable source for opioid peptides in peripheral tissue is the peripheral nervous system. Prodynorphin- and/or proenkephalin-derived peptides have been detected in sensory ganglia [4, 27] and in peripheral terminals of sensory nerves [11, 39]. The functional significance of these peptides, however, has not been elucidated so far.

Opioid receptors in peripheral tissue

Opioid binding sites have been demonstrated on immune cells and opioid-mediated modulation of several of their functions (*e.g.* chemotaxis, superoxide production, mast cell degranulation) has been reported [34]. However, the rapid onset of local antinociceptive effects in animal experiments (within minutes of adminstration of the opioid agonists) argues against the notion that they are mediated indirectly by such mechanisms. On the other hand, there is abundant biochemical and electrophysiological evidence for the existence and functional significance of opioid receptors on primary afferent neurons [8, 21, 24] Recently, we have demonstrated such receptors immunocytochemically [37] and functionally [3]. Following the occupation of these receptors by an opioid agonist, an antinociceptive effect may be produced by at least two mechanisms : first, the excitability of the nociceptive input terminal may be attenuated or the propagation of action potentials may be inhibited [9, 31, 41]. Second, the release of excitatory substances (*e.g.* substance P) from central and/or peripheral endings of primary afferents may be inhibited [22, 42]. The latter effect may also account for opioid anti-inflammatory actions reported by some investigators (review in [2]). One explanation for the enhanced antinociceptive effects seen under inflammatory conditions is an increased *de novo* synthesis and peripherally directed axonal transport of opioid receptors [20, 43] which leads to an increase in their density ("upregulation") on peripheral nerve terminals [12]. On the other hand, pre-existent, but possibly inactive neuronal opioid receptors may undergo conformational changes owing to the specific milieu in inflamed tissue and thus be rendered active.

Conclusions

The following conclusions may be drawn from the available experimental data : exogenous and endogenous opioids can produce opioid receptor-specific antinociceptive effects outside the central nervous system. Depending on the particular circumstances, three different receptor types (mu, delta, kappa) can become active in peripheral tissue. Inflammatory hyperalgesic conditions appear to be especially amenable to peripheral opioid antinociceptive actions. The most likely mechanism of these actions appears to be the activation of opioid receptors located on primary afferent neurons. The endogenous ligands for these receptors are produced and contained in immune cells infiltrating the inflamed tissue.

Human studies

Several controlled studies examining the analgesic effects of opioids outside the central nervous system have appeared (Table I). These have examined the perineural or intravenous-regional application of morphine [5-7, 23, 29], the intravenous administration of a peptide unable to cross the blood-brain barrier [26], the intra-articular [1, 13, 15, 16, 19, 30, 38] or the interpleural [40] application of morphine. Most of these studies investigated postoperative pain, one examined experimental pain [26], and one did not specify the painful condition [23]. To assess pain, various direct (visual analogue scale, numerical rating scale, verbal scales) or indirect measures (supplemental analgesic consumption, pulmonary function testing, time to first supplemental analgesic requirement) were used.

The results from these investigations are not uniform : the majority demonstrate analgesic effects, but some do not [5-7, 29, 30, 40]. The majority of the latter has examined perineural (or interpleural) application of opioids which has to be distinguished from that at the nerve terminal (*e.g.* intra-articular). For instance, it is conceivable that axonal opioid receptors are functionally less efficient than receptors at the nerve terminals, especially when one considers the possible influence of peripheral inflammation (*see* above). Furthermore, the anatomical circumstances are different : axons are encased in Schwann-cells and, in the case of A-delta fibers, they are surrounded by several layers of lipoid myelin. These layers progressively disappear towards the peripheral terminals and thus, peripherally applied agents may gain access to the nerve more readily. Interestingly, animal experiments have shown that, when opioids are injected not perineurally but into the brachial plexus sheath, potent and long lasting antinociception is achieveable [18], suggesting that peripheral nerve sheaths may indeed significantly hinder the access of perineurally applied drugs. Finally, methodological shortcomings may account for some of the negative results. Studies examining postoperative pain have to be well standardized. Ideally, a single surgeon should perform operations of minimally varying type and duration on a homogeneous patient population under a standardized anesthetic regimen in a constant environment.

Table I. Studies examining peripheral analgesic effects of opioids in humans.

Pain condition	Pain assessment	Agonists	Dose (peak effect)	Further comments	Exclusion of central effects	Locus of application	References
Postoperative	VAS, VRS	Morphine	2-6 mg	no effect	Comparing left vs. right limb	Perineural	Bullingham et al. [5]
Postoperative	VAS (non shown), VRS	Morphine Buprenorphine	1-4 mg 0.12 mg	no effect	Comparing left vs. right limb	Perineural i.v. regional	Bullingham et al. [6]
Not specified	VAS, VRS	Morphine	0.04-6 mg		Local vs. i.m; application (in one group only)	Perineural	Mays et al. 23]
Postoperative	VAS	Morphine	4 mg	no effect	Local vs. epidural application	Perineural	Dahl et al. [7]
Experimental	VAS	Enkephaline Analogue	0.75-7.5 mcg/kg/min		Lipophobic peptide	Intravenous	Posner et al. [26]
Postoperative	VAS, NRS, MPQ, SAC	Morphine	0.5-1 mg (3-6 h)	Naloxone reversible	Local vs. i.v. application	Intra-articular	Stein et al. [38]
Postoperative	VAS, TFA, SAC	Morphine	5 mg	no effect	Local vs. i.m. application	Perineural	Racz et al. [29]
Postoperative	VAS, SAC	Morphine	1 mg (4-48 h)		no	Intra-articular	Khoury et al. [19]
Postoperative	VAS, NRS, MPQ, SAC, PFT	Morphine	2.5 mg 0.5 mg/h	drainage, no effect	Local vs. i.v. application	Interpleural	Welte et al. [40]
Postoperative	VAS, TFA, SAC	Morphine (Epinephrine)	6 mg	effect on TFA	no	Intra-articular	Heard et al. [13]
Postoperative	VAS, TFA, SAC	Morphine (Epinephrine)	3 mg	no effect	no	Intra-articular	Raja et al. [30]
Postoperative	VAS, TFA, SAC	Morphine	5 mg (0-12 h)	tourniquet	Plasma levels < 10ng/ml	Intra-articular	Joshi et al. [15]
Postoperative	VAS, TFA, SAC	Morphine	5 mg (2-24 h)	drainage tourniquet	no	Intra-articular	Joshi et al. [16]
Postoperative	VAS, TFA	Morphine	5 mg (1-24 h)	tourniquet	no	Intra-articular	Joshi et al. [17]

VAS : visual analogue scale ; NRS : numerical rating scale ; VRS : verbal rating scale ; MPQ : McGill pain questionnaire
TFA : time to first analgesic use ; SAC : supplemental analgesic consumption ; PFT : pulmonary function test.

Patients have to be randomly assigned to distinct groups receiving internally consistent treatments and the number of subjects should remain constant throughout the observation period.

Results after intra-articular opiate administration appear more promising : the majority of these studies has reported convincing analgesic effects of small, systemically inactive doses of morphine, administered into the knee joint of patients undergoing intra-articular surgery [1, 15-17, 19, 38]. These effects were shown to be opioid receptor-specific [38], of similar potency to those of conventional local anesthetics and surprisingly long lasting (up to 48 hours after injection) [17, 19].

Heard *et al.* [13] found no significant effect on subjective pain ratings, but did report a significantly prolonged time to first supplementary analgesic use in patients receiving intra-articular morphine. Interestingly, we found the maximum analgesic effect of intra-articular morphine to occur somewhat delayed (between 3 and 6 hours after injection) [38]. This may explain Raja's [30] failure to detect such effects, since by that time half of their subjects were lost due to discharge from the hospital. Of note, Joshi *et al.* [15-17] did not find such a delay in morphine's onset of action but they stress to keep a tourniquet inflated for 10 min after the intra-articular injection, under the assumption that blood flow to the knee joint will be inhibited and thus, the chance of morphine's rapid systemic absorption will be minimized. Also noteworthy is their finding of analgesic effects even after open knee surgery using postoperative intra-articular drainage [16].

Untoward side effects were not reported in any of those papers. To confirm a peripheral site of action, equal doses of morphine were administered systemically as a control [38] or plasma levels of morphine were measured [15]. The latter were found to be much lower than those generally accepted as necessary for central analgesic actions. The reasons for the long duration of these peripheral opioid effects are not clear so far. Possible explanations include low blood flow to the knee joint, morphine's low lipid solubility and its consequent slow absorption into the circulation and/or opioid anti-inflammatory actions (*see* also [2]).

Conclusions

The available clinical data tend to concur with the experimental findings. The number of controlled studies, however, is still small and some suffer from methodological shortcomings. Inferring from the animal studies, inflammatory hyperalgesic conditions seem to be especially amenable to peripheral opioid antinociception. Thus, the direct local application of small, systemically inactive doses of agonists in clinical situations of inflammatory pain may be particularly rewarding to study. Furthermore, opioid compounds unable to cross the blood-brain barrier [10, 32, 33] may become available and may represent a novel class of analgesic agents devoid of central side effects. Since multiple types of peripheral opioid receptors can become active, one may be able to interchange selective agonists in case tolerance should occur to one agent. The presence of endogenous opioid peptides in immune cells within inflamed tissue opens up new routes of investigation into the local activation of these innate antinociceptive substances.

In summary, peripheral opioid analgesic effects require more extensive controlled clinical studies in view of the potential avoidance of centrally mediated adverse effects such as respiratory depression, dependence, dysphoria, nausea, or sedation. The fact that several different groups have now independently reported potent and long lasting analgesic effects after intra-articular morphine is encouraging and calls for more studies examining not only acute but also chronic inflammatory painful conditions.

References

1. Amand MS, Allen GC, Lui A, Johnson DH, Heard M. Intra-articular morphine and bupivacaine for analgesia following outpatient arthroscopic knee surgery [abstract]. *Anesthesiology* 1992 ; 77 : A817.
2. Barber A, Gottschlich R. Opioid agonists and antagonists : an evaluation of their peripheral actions in inflammation. *Med Res Rev* 1992 ; 12 : 525-62.
3. Barthó L, Stein C, Herz A. Involvement of capsaicin-sensitive neurones in hyperalgesia and enhanced opioid antinociception in inflammation. *Naun Schmied Arch Pharmacol* 1990 ; 342 : 666-70.
4. Botticelli LJ, Cox BM, Goldstein A. Immunoreactive dynorphin in mammalian spinal cord and dorsal root ganglia. *Proc Natl Acad Sci USA* 1981 ; 78 : 7783-6.
5. Bullingham R, O'Sullivan G, McQuay H, Poppleton P, Rolfe M, Evans P, Moore A. Perineural injection of morphine fails to relieve postoperative pain in humans. *Anesth Analg* 1983 ; 62 : 164-7.
6. Bullingham RES, McQuay HJ, Moore RA. Studies on the peripheral action of opioids in postoperative pain in man. *Acta Anaesthiol Belg* 1984 ; 35 (Suppl) : 285-90.
7. Dahl JB, Daugaard JJ, Kristoffersen E, Johannsen HV, Dahl JA. Perineuronal morphine : a comparison with epiduralmorphine. *Anaesthesia* 1988 ; 43 : 463-5.
8. Fields HL, Emson PC, Leigh BK, Gilbert RFT, Iversen LL. Multiple opiate receptor sites on primary afferent fibers. *Nature* 1980 ; 284 : 351-3.
9. Frank GB. Stereospecific opioid receptors on excitable cell membranes. *Can J Physiol Pharmacol* 1985 ; 63 : 1023-32.
10. Hardy GW, Lowe LA, Sang PY, Simpkin DSA, Wilkinson S, Follenfant RL, Smith TW. Peripherally acting enkephalin analogues. 1. Polar pentapeptides. *J Med Chem* 1988 ; 31 : 960-6.
11. Hassan AHS, Przewlocki R, Herz A, Stein C. Dynorphin, a preferential ligand for kappa-opioid receptors, is present in nerve fibers and immune cells within inflamed tissue of the rat. *Neurosci Lett* 1992 ; 140 : 85-8.
12. Hassan AHS, Ableitner A, Stein C, Herz A. Inflammation of the rat paw enhances axonal transport of opioid receptors in the sciatic nerve and increases their density in the inflamed tissue. *Neuroscience* 1993 ; in press.
13. Heard SO, Edwards WT, Ferrari D, Hanna D, Wong PD, Liland A, Willock MW. Analgesic effect of intra-articular bupivacaine or morphine after arthroscopic knee surgery : a randomized, prospective, double-blind study. *Anesth Analg* 1992 ; 74 : 822-6.
14. Heijnen CJ, Kavelaars A, Ballieux RE. ß-endorphin : cytokine and neuropeptide. *Immunol Rev* 1991 ; 119 : 41-63.

15. Joshi GP, McCarroll SM, Cooney CM, Blunnie WP, O'Brien TM, Lawrence AJ. Intra-articular morphine for pain relief after knee arthroscopy. *J Bone Joint Surg* 1992 ; 74-B : 749-51.
16. Joshi GP, McCarroll SM, Brady OH, Hurson BJ, Walsh G. Intra-articular morphine for pain relief after anterior cruciate ligament repair. *Br J Anaesth* 1993 ; 70 : 87-8.
17. Joshi GP, McCarroll SM, O'Brien TM, Lenane P. Intra-articular analgesia following knee arthroscopy. *Anesth Analg* 1993 ; 76 : 333-6.
18. Kayser V, Gobeaux D, Lombard MC, Guilbaud G, Besson JM. Potent and long lasting antinociceptive effects after injection of low doses of a mu-opioid receptor agonist, fentanyl, into the brachial plexus sheath of the rat. *Pain* 1990 ; 42 : 215-25.
19. Khoury GF, Chen ACN, Garland DE, Stein C. Intra articular morphine, bupivacaine and morphine/bupivacaine for pain control after knee videoarthroscopy. *Anesthesiology* 1992 ; 77 : 263-6.
20. Laduron P. Axonal transport of opiate receptors in capsaicin sensitive neurones. *Brain Res* 1984 ; 294 : 157-60.
21. LaMotte C, Pert CB, Snyder SH. Opiate receptor binding in primate spinal cord : distribution and changes after dorsal root section. *Brain Res* 1976 ; 112 : 407-12.
22. Lembeck F, Donnerer J. Opioid control of the function of primary afferent substance P fibers. *Eur J Pharmacol* 1985 ; 114 : 241-6.
23. Mays KS, Lipmann JJ, Schnapp M. Local analgesia without anesthesia using peripheral perineural morphine injections. *Anesth Analg* 1987 ; 66 : 417-20.
24. Ninkovic M, Hunt SP, Gleave JRW. Localization of opiate and histamine H1-receptors in the primary sensory ganglia and spinal cord. *Brain Res* 1982 ; 241 : 197-206.
25. Parsons CG, Czlonkowski A, Stein C, Herz A. Peripheral opioid receptors mediating antinociception in inflammation. Activation by endogenous opioids and role of the pituitary-adrenal axis. *Pain* 1990 ; 41 : 81-93.
26. Posner J, Moody SG, Peck AW, Rutter D, Telekes A. Analgesic, central, cardiovascular and endocrine effects of the enkephalin analogue Tyr-D.Arg-Gly-Phe(4N02)-Pro-NH2 (443C81) in healthy volunteers. *Eur J Clin Pharmacol* 1990 ; 38 : 213-8.
27. Przewlocki R, Gramsch C, Pasi A, Herz A. Characterization and localization of immunoreactive dynorphin, alpha-neoendorphin, met-enkephalin and substance P in human spinal cord. *Brain Res* 1983 ; 280 : 95-103.
28. Przewlocki R, Hassan AHS, Lason W, Epplen C, Herz A, Stein C. Gene expression and localization of opioid peptides in immune cells of inflamed tissue. Functional role in antinociception. *Neuroscience* 1992 ; 48 : 491-500.
29. Racz H, Gunning K, Della Santa D, Forster A. Evaluation of the effect of perineuronal morphine on the quality of postoperative analgesia after axillary plexus block : a randomized double-blind study. *Anesth Analg* 1991 ; 72 : 769-72.
30. Raja SN, Dickstein RE, Johnson CA. Comparison of postoperative analgesic effects of intra-articular bupivacaine and morphine following arthroscopic knee surgery. *Anesthesiology* 1992 ; 77 :1143-7.
31. Russell NJW, Schaible HG, Schmidt RF. Opiates inhibit the discharges of fine afferent units from inflamed knee joint of the cat. *Neurosci Lett* 1987 ; 76 : 107-12.
32. Schiller PW, Nguyen TMD, Chung NN, Dionne G, Martel R. Peripheral antinociceptive effect of an extremely mu-selective polar dermophin analog (DALDA). In : Quirion R, Jhamandas K, Gianoulakis C, eds. International narcotics research conference. New York : AR Liss, 1990 : 53-6.
33. Shaw JS, Caroll JA, Alcock P, Main BG. ICI 204448 : a kappa-opioid agonist with limited access to the CNS. *Br J Pharmacol* 1989 ; 96 : 986-92.
34. Sibinga NES, Goldstein A. Opioid peptides and opioid receptors in cells of the immune system. *Annu Rev Immunol* 1988 ; 6 : 219-49.

35. Stein C. Peripheral mechanisms of opioid analgesia. *Anesth Analg* 1993 ; 76 : 182-91.
36. Stein C, Gramsch C, Herz A. Intrinsic mechanisms of antinociception in inflammation. Local opioid receptors and ß-endorphin. *J Neurosci* 1990 ; 10 : 1292-8.
37. Stein C, Hassan AHS, Przewlocki R, Gramsch C, Peter K, Herz A. Opioids from immunocytes interact with receptors on sensory nerves to inhibit nociception in inflammation. *Proc Natl Acad Sci USA* 1990 ; 87 : 5935-9.
38. Stein C, Comisel K, Haimerl E, Lehrberger K, Yassouridis A, Herz A, Peter K. Analgesic effect of intra-articular morphine after arthroscopic knee surgery [see comments]. *N Engl J Med* 1991 ; 325 : 1123-6. Comment in : *N Engl J Med* 1991 ; 325 : 1168-9.
39. Weihe E, Hartschuh W, Weber E. Prodynorphin opioid peptides in small somatosensory primary afferents of guinea pig. *Neurosci Lett* 1985 ; 58 : 347-52.
40. Welte M, Haimerl E, Groh J, Briegel J, Sunder-Plassmann L, Herz A, Peter K, Stein C. Effect of interpleural morphine on postoperative pain and pulmonary function after thoracotomy. *Br J Anaesth* 1992 ; 69 : 637-9.
41. Werz MA, Macdonald RL. Heterogeneous sensitivity of cultured dorsal root ganglion neurones to opioid peptides selective for mu- and delta-opiate receptors. *Nature* 1982 ; 299 : 730-3.
42. Yaksh TL. Substance P release from knee joint afferent terminals : modulation by opioids. *Brain Res* 1988 ; 458 : 319-24.
43. Young III WS, Wamsley JK, Zarbin MA, Kuhar MJ. Opioid receptors undergo axonal flow. *Science* 1980 ; 210 : 76-7.

12

Strategies for the design of a peripherally acting analgesic drug

R.G. HILL

Merck, Sharp and Dohme Research Laboratories, Neuroscience Research Centre, Terlings Park, Harlow, UK.

The concept of an analgesic working on peripheral targets is not a new one, but in the recent literature new, putative approaches to this objective have been revealed. Our greater understanding of neurotransmission, of the factors leading to neuronal activation and of the nociceptive process allows a mechanistic approach to this target by exploiting knowledge of the receptors at which algogenic substances act, of the ion channels which permit impulse transmission in the sensory nerve fibers and of the enzymes which are involved in the synthesis of algogens and potentiating agents.

Some of the expedients which are now open to us are completely novel, having been recently discovered, and others are refinements of existing strategies. The overall thrust of peripheral therapy is to achieve pain relief without the side effects associated with potent centrally acting analgesics (typified by opioids such as morphine). The possibility of topical or regional therapy is also raised, further increasing the specificity of treatment and avoiding the medication of areas of the body that are unaffected by the disease process giving rise to the pain. It remains to be established, however, that a peripheral treatment is capable of producing the profound relief of severe pain that can be achieved with centrally acting opioids.

In terms of specific expedients that can be adopted to ensure a peripheral locus of action, then the range of options is somewhat limited. The most obvious is exploitation of a system that is not present in the central nervous system, and this is becoming increasingly difficult, for as our knowledge of the neural transduction processes improves, we are realising that more and more systems are represented in both the peripheral and central nervous systems. This will be discussed with particular reference to the NSAID drugs and cyclo-oxygenase enzyme systems. It is also germane to reflect that the sensory fibers carrying nociceptive messages into the central nervous system are pseudo-unipolar fibers with cell bodies in the dorsal root ganglia and in the main these fibers are peptide containing (*see* [102]). The peptide content is manufactured in the cell body for transport to and release from both central and peripheral terminals on activation of the fiber, thus there is no operational differentiation of central or peripheral activity, although the pathophysiological consequences of release at the two sites may be very different.

The second possibility is exploit a system that is present both in the central nervous system and in the periphery but to use a drug that is excluded from the central locus, so as to target the peripheral site. Although theoretically attractive this strategy is far from simple to achieve in practice. The pharmaceutical principles are outside the scope of the current chapter but suffice it to say that those physicochemical properties that produce brain penetration are also frequently the properties that aid transport of drug across other biological barriers, such as the gut wall and in particular across the cell membrane, where penetration is necessary for a drug such as an enzyme inhibitor with an intracellular site of action. The opioid drugs will be used as examples here.

The third and most novel possibility is to exploit a system that is only turned on (*i.e.* induced) during the nociceptive process so that, although the underlying mechanism may be ubiquitous, the therapy can be selective because it is only active in a particular region (*i.e.* the drug is present throughout the body tissues but only acts where it is needed). The bradykinin receptor, cyclo-oxygenase and nitric oxide synthase systems will be used to exemplify this approach.

Mechanisms of nociception

In order to attack the pain producing machinery with new therapeutic entities, it is necessary to have a clear understanding of the mechanisms leading to the activation of nociceptor fibers but, as a large part of this volume is given over to consideration of such matters, only a cursory treatment of basic mechanisms will be given here and the reader is referred especially to the chapters by Handwerker, Torebjork, Schmidt, Gebhart and Dray.

The principal transducing elements in pain perception are the unmyelinated C-fibers and the smallest group of myelinated fibers the A-δ, and although other functionalities are exhibited by these small fiber types, the preponderant role is one of nociception. For example, a recent study in the rat foot revealed that in sural nerve 44% of C-fibers and 68% of A-δ fibers were nociceptors with 77% of C-fibers and all the A-δ fibers sampled in plantar nerve being nociceptive [64]. Under pathological conditions A-β fibers may assume a nociceptive role and this may be related to the central re-programming that takes place in neuropathic conditions [21], as it has been demonstrated that in the ligature neuropathy model as early as one day post ligature the spinal cord dorsal horn is bombarded with high level input from the spontaneous discharge of A-δ and A-β fibers in the injured nerve [56]. It is now realized that many nociceptors are silent under normal conditions and only become active after tissue damage or inflammation (*see* for example [75]). Although most investigations on nociceptors have concerned somatic systems, it seems likely that similar mechanisms obtain for the viscera with their noxious events being handled by a mixture of high threshold afferents, silent nociceptors and other intensity coding fibers [20]. An important concept for consideration before one starts to investigate the pharmacology of nociception is acceptance that the properties of nociception change considerably in the presence of tissue damage or direct nerve injury such that fine primary afferent fibers innervate a wider area of superficial dorsal horn after peripheral axotomy [17], and damaged nerves have the capacity to stimulate neurite outgrowth [8] indicating the active secretion of trophic factors. In the case of tissue inflammation neurogenic processes have a special role and the development of arthritis may depend in part on the transmission of impulses in peptidergic fibers to the contralateral homotopic point of the initial inflammatory event [61] and, paradoxically, denervation may be a sufficient stimulus to produce inflammation of a different character to that produced by nerve stimulation [68]. Immediate early gene induction is a feature of intense and maintained stimulation of nociceptor fibers [13] leading to a cascade of protein expression that alters the biochemistry of peripheral and central targets of nociceptive afferents [51] including changes in neuropeptide content [32]. The provoking stimulus can be cutaneous [63], visceral [11] or as a result of joint inflammation [1]. These and related considerations suggest that it may be unhelpful to evaluate novel, potential therapeutic agents using tests in physiologically normal animals, such as have been used in the past for the study of centrally acting opioid drugs (for further discussion of this point, *see* [118]).

A variety of substances have the capacity to activate nociceptors and are therefore termed algogens, but it is not possible to give an exhaustive treatment here. It is possible to select particular candidates that constitute attractive targets for drug discovery and these include the proton (which may share a receptor with capsaicin) [108], bradykinin [31], 5-HT [100, 114], the interleukins [38] and excitatory amino acids acting at the kainate site [4]. Apart from bradykinin, few peptides are directly algogenic but many are contained within nociceptive afferents and are released into peripheral tissues when these fibers are activated. This leads to neurogenic inflammation (*see* [9]) and/or changes in blood flow or as yet uncharacterised effects depending on the peptide released. Those peptides of particular interest include substance P and related tachykinins [10], calcitonin gene related peptide (CGRP ; [48]), galanin [120] and cholecystokinin [117].

Ion channel blockers

The activation of nociceptor fibers involves entry of Na^+ and, probably, Ca^{2+} through voltage dependent channels and the expression of ion channels is enhanced in the presence of nerve damage both in the nerve trunk and also in the dorsal root ganglion cell where K^+ channels become important in sustaining abnormal discharges [56]. The infiltration of local anaesthetic agents to produce pain relief by blocking Na^+ channels is well established, but more recently it has been found that intravenous lignocaine is of use in the treatment of chronic pain [111] and that orally active agents capable of blocking fast inward sodium currents such as mexiletine, tocainide and flecainide will also produce pain relief, particularly in neuralgias and neuropathies [26, 33, 70]. Some Ca^{2+} channel blockers such as nifedipine and diltiazem have also been found useful in treatment of sympathetically maintained pain and peripheral neuropathies [96] as have a number of anticonvulsant drugs that are capable of blocking multiple cation channels [74, 95]. One recent report has shown that nimodipine can ameliorate existing experimental diabetic neuropathy in both young and adult animals [58]. As our knowledge of the molecular biology of ion channels grows, the possibility of new and more selective therapeutic agents increases [107, 110]. It must be remembered that actions on blood vessels and also central effects will contribute to the overall effects of ion channel blocking drugs and in some pain states, such as vascular headache, it will be difficult to determine the precise mechanism until more selective drugs are available (*see* [46]).

Bradykinin receptor antagonists

This topic has recently been reviewed in detail [31] but, briefly, bradykinin is a peptide produced as a result of tissue damage which causes acute pain when exogenous peptide is applied, for example, to a blister base and which is believed to have a pathophysiological role in nociceptor activation. It now appears that there are two receptors that are important in the pain and inflammation producing effects of bradykinin. The first of these is called the B_2 receptor and bradykinin itself is the preferred agonist. This receptor is probably the most important in transducing the acute effects of bradykinin following injury. The second receptor (B_1) is more sensitive to a metabolite of bradykinin, (des-ARG^9) BK, than to bradykinin itself and this site appears to be more important in transducing the effects of prolonged inflammation as the receptor is only expressed in significant amounts in inflamed or damaged tissue. Peptide analogues of bradykinin have been synthesized, which act as antagonists at either B_1 or B_2 receptors and useful information on the role of these receptors has been gained in studies using these substances as tools (*see* [31]), but so far no non-peptide antagonists suitable for clinical evaluation have appeared in the literature. Experiments with peptide antagonists have demonstrated convincingly that blockade of B_2 receptors produces antinociception in a variety of rodent behavioural tests and in the human blister base. They will also reduce the oedema produced by inflammatory agents such as carrageenan [14]. Newer agents, such as Hoe 140, are very potent and sufficiently stable to metabolic enzymes to have a long duration of action *in vivo* [121]. There are as yet no B_1 antagonists of comparable potency to Hoe 140, but nevertheless using the weak B_1 antagonist (des-ARG^9-LEU^8) BK. Perkins and his colleagues [92] were able to show reversal of the hyperalgesia produced by either ultraviolet irradiation of the rat paw or injection of Freund's adjuvant into the rat knee joint. There is abundant evidence for interaction of bradykinin with many of the substances that will be discussed later, for instance cytokines such as IL-1-β may be released from macrophages following activation of a B_1 receptor and in turn may increase expression of B_1 sites [31] and activation of sensory fibers by bradykinin leads to release of the neuropeptides neurokinins and CGRP (for example, a neurokinin receptor antagonist will protect against bradykinin induced bronchoconstriction in asthmatics [53]). The blockade of receptor mediated actions of bradykinin is thus an attractive strategy towards a novel peripherally acting analgesic and the inducible nature of the B_1 receptor makes this a target with low side effect potential.

Peptides released from nociceptive afferents

The activation of nociceptive afferents causes peptide release from their peripheral terminals leading to plasma extravasation (*see* introduction) and damage to these nerve fibers causes transient loss of extravasation which is restored on re-innervation [9]. A variety of peptides are capable of causing such an inflammatory response although the receptor pharmacology of some is at present incompletely characterised. The expression of cholecystokinin in primary sensory neurones is enhanced following nerve injury [117] and galanin, also contained in sensory nerves, may be capable of exerting an endogenous antinociceptive role after nerve injury [120]. The inflammatory disease arthritis is a major reason for the use of analgesic medication and therefore much effort has been invested in development of animal models of inflamed joints. Recently it has been observed that, following injection of Freund's adjuvant or other irritant stimulus to one knee joint of a rat, an increase in substance P, neurokinin A, and CGRP levels was detected in perfusate from the synovial capsule on the injected side and also from the non-injected knee [10] supporting the suggestion that peptide containing primary afferents have a special role in the aetiology of symmetrical arthritis [61]. As inflammation develops, it has been noted that the proportion of dorsal root ganglion cells containing immunoreactivity for CGRP increases but that this change is not mirrored on the non-inflamed side [48].

Stimulation of the sciatic nerve produces a neurogenic inflammation of the hind paw that can be readily quantified by measurement of extravasation using an appropriate plasma marker. This response can readily be antagonised with a blocker of neurokinin-1 (NK_1) receptors such as CP-96,345 [65] or RP-67580 [84, 104]. CGRP appears to act by modulating the inflammatory oedema produced by substance P rather than exerting a direct inflammatory action [87] and although both peptides are released following sciatic nerve stimulation, it is noteworthy that the extravasation is completely abolished following blockade of NK_1 receptors [65] whereas it is necessary to block CGRP receptors (using the antagonist peptide CGRP 8-37) in order to reduce neurogenic blood flow increases in the rat hind paw (Tan et al., unpublished observations).

It has been proposed that neurogenic inflammation within cranial tissues is a component of the pathogenesis of migraine headache (see [83]). Those ergot alkaloids which are clinically effective in aborting a migraine attack have been shown to reduce extravasation into dural tissues following electrical stimulation of the trigeminal ganglion in the rat [101] and the selective $5-HT_1$ receptor agonist sumatriptan, recently introduced for treatment of migraine, has been shown to share this property [15], suggested to be attributable to an inhibition of neuropeptide release from the perivascular terminals of trigeminal fibers. The NK_1 receptor antagonist RP-67580 has recently been shown to produce an enantioselective reduction in dural extravasation following trigeminal ganglion stimulation [105] suggesting that as in the paw the major component of this inflammatory response is operated by substance P acting at NK_1 receptors. The dilator response following trigeminal stimulation is likely to be operated mainly through CGRP as this can be blocked by CGRP 8-37 [44] and it is interesting that CGRP is elevated in jugular vein blood during a migraine attack in man and that this elevation is reduced if the headache is aborted with sumatriptan [43]. There appear to be differences between the responses of the separate tissues innervated by the trigeminal nerve and the extravasation seen in conjunctiva, eyelid and lip, for instance, is less sensitive to blockade by NK_1 antagonists than that in the dura [105] and the blood flow increases in nasal mucosa are reduced by NK_1 receptor antagonists [93]. It is difficult to establish that blockade of neurogenic extravasation per se would produce an analgesic action in man but it is noteworthy that sumatriptan has been claimed to reduce c-fos expression in trigeminal nucleus caudalis following noxious stimulation of the meninges [88] and this non-brain penetrant agent is clinically effective against the pain of migraine, although it does not have any general antinociceptive actions in standard animal tests [36].

Capsaicin

The mechanism of action and the potential for analgesic development of capsaicin have recently been reviewed in detail [25, 30, 76, 98] but briefly this pungent factor isolated from peppers of the capsicum family has the ability to stimulate nociceptive afferent neurones in a selective manner and thereby causes pain. Its initial action is to release the neuropeptides that these fibers contain and this can lead to depletion. It has a desensitising action [72] which means that the initial stimulation of nociceptors is followed by analgesia, and this has been exploited in the use of topical preparations containing capsaicin for the treatment of post-herpetic neuralgia [98]. Other natural products such as shogaol and resiniferatoxin have a chemically distinct structure but similar pharmacology [89, 112]. The widespread use of capsaicin for pain relief is, of course, limited by its initial pain producing action and the development of agents that would exert an antinociceptive action without this effect has provided a major advance. The first such agent, olvanil [27], was shown to be effective in both behavioural and electrophysiological antinociceptive tests, but was claimed to have a central rather than a peripheral site of action. More recently, an antagonist at the capsaicin receptor, capsazepine, has been discovered and found to block the stimulant actions of capsaicin both *in vitro* and *in vivo*, including blockade of the antinociceptive actions [91], but capsazepine itself showed no antinociceptive actions. This led to an assumption that block of the actions of the presumed endogenous ligand for the capsaicin receptor would not be an appropriate strategy for producing analgesia, but recently it has been shown that capsazepine will inhibit the release of CGRP from sensory fibers in guinea pig heart by low pH or lactate [39] suggesting that under appropriate circumstances blocking capsaicin receptors may be an effective way of preventing nociceptor fiber activation. Some patients with persistent pain states show an altered sensitivity to topical capsaicin [66].

Peripheral actions of opioids

Paradoxically, there is now a body of evidence that the architypical central analgesics, the opioids, have a significant antinociceptive action at the level of the peripheral nociceptor fibers. The theoretical basis of this topic is dealt with in detail in the chapters in this volume by Kayser, Besson and Stein and it has also been reviewed by Junien and Wettstein [54]. The action of opioids is greater in inflamed tissues and in animals pretreated with capsaicin to deplete primary afferent peptides this enhanced action is lost [6]. Significant amounts of met-enkephalin and β-endorphin are found in rat tissues inflamed with Freund's adjuvant [109] and these opioids are in macrophages and other immunocytes invading the area of inflammation. Subsequently it has been shown that mRNAs encoding pro-enkephalin and pro-opiomelanocortin are only present in the tissues when inflamed [97]. Dynorphin has also been shown to be present in immunocytes of inflamed tissues and additionally to be present in sensory nerve fibers within the tissues [50]. Peripheral opioid mechanisms are also turned on in rats subjected to cold water swim stress [90]. All three opioid receptor types (μ, κ and δ) are present in inflamed tissue and it has been shown that the selective κ agonist U-50488 will attenuate the response of a dorsal horn neurone to injection of formalin into its receptive field on one hind paw, when the opioid is injected directly into the same paw at a dose too low to have a systemic effect [47]. GR-94839, a κ-opioid designed to have limited access to the central nervous system, has been shown to have anti-nociceptive activity but only in the presence of inflammation unless doses large enough to have central effects (such as locomotor impairment) were given [99]. Agonists at κ and δ receptors but not at μ receptors inhibit extravasation produced in the rat knee joint by injection of bradykinin [45] and although κ and δ opioids retained a normal antinociceptive potency in mice rendered diabetic with streptozotocin, these animals became hyporesponsive to the μ agonist morphine [57]. In normal rats, intradermal morphine was found to dose dependently inhibit PGE_2 induced hyperalgesia without a change in the baseline mechanical nociceptive threshold of the injected paw [67]. Attempts have already been made to exploit peripheral opioid receptors in the treatment of clinical pain, for instance after arthroscopic procedures on the knee [59] by intra-articular administration of morphine. Although results are encouraging, it will be necessary to produce an opioid with tailor made characteristics for this application (in that it will stay within the tissues to which it is injected and not penetrate the blood brain barrier) before the real clinical utility can be evaluated. The possible benefits are large if opioid levels of pain relief can be achieved without central nervous system side effects.

Peripheral monoamine mechanisms

It is known that a number of intractable pain states in man respond to chemical or surgical sympathectomy when other treatments have failed and it has been suggested that sympathetic nerve terminals contain substances that enhance plasma extravasation (although noradrenaline itself is associated with reduced extravasation but increased tissue damage) [7]. In rats in which experimental neuromas had been produced by sciatic nerve section and avulsion of the distal stumps, there was a massive sprouting of sympathetic terminals and an increase in tissue noradrenaline content [106] and following ligature of sciatic nerve in the rat noradrenergic perivascular nerves were found to sprout into the dorsal root ganglia [73] such that sympathetic stimulation would then excite sensory neurones. In an independent series of experiments nerve damage was found to produce sensitivity to stimulation of the sympathetic system such that its activation produced excitation of a population of C-fiber nociceptors in the rabbit ear that was blocked by selective α_2 receptor antagonists [103]. The pharmacology of these sympathetic effects is complex and the extravasation into arthritic joints caused by bradykinin infusion has been found to be attenuated by the β_2 agonist salbutamol or by the α_2 antagonist yohimbine [24]. The exploitation of this knowledge in the clinical treatment of pain depends on the design of highly selective ligands for the particular adrenoceptors involved and their targeted drug delivery to the affected peripheral site.

Peripheral excitatory amino acid receptors

Much interest has been generated by the role of NMDA receptors in the central sensitisation phenomena associated with tissue injury (e.g. *see* [22, 23]) and the NMDA receptor ion channel blocker MK-801 has been shown to reduce nociceptive behaviours in rats with experimental mononeuropathy [78]. These actions are all likely to be central however and it has recently been shown that intrathecal administration of the competitive NMDA receptor antagonist CPP abolished wind up pain in a patient with a severe and intractable neurogenic pain but pain relief was followed by the production of psychotomimetic side effects [62]. Such psychotomimetic actions are likely to limit the clinical utility of NMDA receptor antagonists in the treatment of pain, so it was of particular interest when Ault and Hildebrand [4] reported that nociceptive reflexes could be activated by the stimulation of peripheral kainate receptors. Using the isolated tail attached spinal cord preparation, they were able to demonstrate depolarisation of ventral roots following kainate or domoate to the tail, the response size being comparable to that produced by bradykinin and blocked by the selective kainate receptor antagonist DNQX (ibid). This new study puts into context the earlier work by Agrawal and Evans [2] and Evans et al. [35] which showed that only C-fibers in primary afferent nerves were depolarised by kainate. Should these observations extrapolate into man, then a peripherally acting kainate receptor antagonist is an attractive target for a novel analgesic. There is a distinct regional distribution of excitatory amino acid receptor subtypes associated with spinal sensory neurones and as molecular biology continues to discover further permutations of the receptor subunits, it is likely that multiple antinociceptive targets will emerge from an improved knowledge of this complex receptor family [41].

Growth factors

Nerve growth factor (NGF) and other trophic factors are known to be necessary for the successful development and maintenance of function in both peripheral and central nervous systems [49]. Experiments in which animals were immunised against NGF showed that the collateral reinnervation of the skin that takes place after nerve section depends on the presence and action of NGF [29] and it has been suggested that NGF is needed for the development of myelinated nociceptors [69]. NGF is now known to be a member of a family of factors collectively known as the neurotrophins and other members of this family, in particular BDNF and NT-3, have also been associated with primary afferent function. Although there is some overlap, it appears that separate populations of primary afferent fibers are capable of transporting NGF, BDNF or NT-3 from peripheral sites of injection retrogradely to the dorsal root ganglia [28]. These factors are likely to be important for function at both peripheral and central ends of sensory fibers and it is noteworthy that a specific tyrosine kinase, trkB, that is believed to be the receptor for the neurotrophin BDNF, is increased in both rat and cat spinal cord after injury [40]. Neurocytokines are also found in sensory nerves, and ciliary neuronotrophic factor (CNTF) is reduced in nerves from diabetic rats [16] and its action on normal sensory nerves indicate that synthesis of substance P and CGRP is stimulated by its presence [3]. Smaller molecules also have a trophic on peripheral nerves and for example, the ACTH analogue ORG 2766 has been shown to enhance regrowth of sciatic nerve axons after a nerve crush injury [115] whereas, paradoxically perhaps, the amino terminal octapeptide of NGF has been claimed to induce hyperalgesia in the rat [113]. Neuropathies as a consequence of nerve damage produce some of the most intractable of pains and the possibility of facilitating repair of such damage by the use of growth factors is a real therapeutic possibility. The delivery of such large molecules to their intended site of action may present problems, but for some this may be solved by retrograde transport systems [28]. It is also possible that antagonists of growth factor action may also be useful in analgesic therapy if this enables reduction in the synthesis of peptide neurotransmitters without inducing an unacceptable level of side effects.

Cytokines

The role of cytokines in inflammation is complex and outside the limited scope of this chapter, but an accessible introduction to this topic can be found in Whicher and Evans [119]. The release of interleukins (primarily IL-1-β) and the prostanoids as a result of macrophage activation and tissue damage can cause pain both by direct nociceptor activation and by sensitisation to the effects of algogens such as bradykinin (qv earlier). Experimental studies in the rat showed that in the presence of an appropriate sensitising stimulus (such as prostaglandin E_2-PGE_2) the intraplantar injection of IL-1-β would cause a persistent hyperalgesic state [37]. The hyperalgesic effects of IL-1-β have been shown to be blocked by co-administration of small peptides related to α-melanocyte stimulating hormone (α-MSH) and at least part of this interaction may be due to these peptides activating peripheral κ-opioid receptors (qv above, [94]).

Cyclo-oxygenase inhibitors

It is now accepted that non-steroidal anti-inflammatory drugs (NSAIDs) are useful in many painful conditions, including post operative pain, and in addition to their intrinsic analgesic action they may exert a beneficial opioid sparing effect [85]. This mechanism of action carries a risk of side effects, such as stomach ulceration and clotting disorders, which may well have been over estimated as a risk factor (ibid) and new evidence raises a possibility of effective analgesia with minimal side effects.

It has been demonstrated that NSAIDs can act centrally [77] or peripherally [81] to produce antinociception, and that these agents are effective when applied topically to the painful site (*e.g.* tooth socket, [81]). Cyclo-oxygenase has been shown to exist in multiple forms and, in particular, in addition to the well described constitutive form (now termed COX-1) there is an inducible enzyme (termed COX-2) which is only present after an inflammatory stimulus [52] and which is preferentially induced in human endothelial cells and monocytes by phorbol ester or lipopolysaccharide. It has been known for some time that a sub-group of NSAIDs show a mis-match between their ability to produce analgesia and to inhibit basal prostaglandin production (*see* e.g. [12]) and the existence of multiple forms of COX allows this observation to be rationalised.

Nitric oxide synthase

Another enzyme associated with pain and inflammation is nitric oxide synthase (NOS), and this enzyme has now been found to be induced in dorsal root ganglion cells of the rat following nerve section [116]. In a detailed study of rat L4/L5 ganglia it was shown that in control conditions only 1% of DRG cells express NOS but that at 14 days after axotomy 25% of DRG cells expressed the enzyme, with both large and small neurones displaying induction [19]. Preganglionic sympathetic fibers have also been shown to express NOS [82]. There may be a direct action of NO on peripheral neurones as experiments on chick ciliary ganglion cells in tissue culture show that sodium nitroprusside and L-arginine will reduce both transient and sustained calcium currents [60]. Mustard oil induced neurogenic extravasation in the skin of the rat paw is not reduced following blockade of NOS but the associated cutaneous hyperaemia is [71] and behavioural antinociception can be produced by NOS inhibition (although this may reflect both central and peripheral inhibition of the enzyme [5, 80]). It is striking that after axotomy the facilitated nociceptive flexor reflex is more sensitive to reduction by inhibitors of NOS than is the similar reflex in normal animals [116].

Aldose reductase

Aldose reductase reduces glucose to sorbitol and although part of the normal metabolism of Schwann cells, this polyol pathway appears to become activated in diabetes and has been suggested to underlie some of the defects in neuronal function seen as a consequence of this disease, and which may include painful neuropathy [18, 34]. A model of diabetes in the rat can be produced by administration of the pancreatic toxin, streptozotocin, and in such animals there is a conduction velocity reduction in peripheral sensory fibers [86] and changes in the peptide content of , in particular, perivascular fibers [79]. In general, attempts to treat diabetic neuropathy in man with aldose reductase inhibiting drugs have been disappointing, but recently animal experiments have suggested that this may have been due to using inadequate doses of drug such that complete inhibition of the enzyme was not achieved and failure to treat for an adequate period of time [18]. A recent clinical study in adult diabetics showed that after 52 weeks treatment with aldose reductase inhibitor a measurable improvement in sensory nerve function was evident, although no benefit was seen after 4 weeks treatment [42]. It should be noted that aldose reductase levels are reduced in peripheral nerve following a crush injury, and that recovery of nerve function coincides in time with partial recovery of levels of the enzyme [122] and thus it is by no means certain that inhibition of this enzyme would be beneficial in painful neuropathic conditions.

Conclusions

Although the foregoing account is far from exhaustive, it should be apparent that many avenues have now been identified for the discovery of novel, peripherally acting analgesic and anti-inflammatory drugs. As always, it will be the ratio between pain relief and the spectrum of unwanted effects produced by the new strategy that will decide whether an advance in therapeutics has been made. In this regard, the discovery that certain systems are induced only in the presence of tissue damage and inflammation is of particular relevance as inhibition of these systems should produce pain relief when the systems are active yet have minimal effect on normal physiology.

References

1. Abbadie C, Besson JM. C-fos expression in rat lumbar spinal cord following peripheral stimulation in adjuvant-induced arthritic and normal rats. *Brain Res* 1993 ; 607 : 195-204.
2. Agrawal SG, Evans RH. The primary afferent depolarizing action of kainate in the rat. *Br J Pharmacol* 1986 ; 87 : 345-55.
3. Apfel SC, Arezzo JC, Moran M, Kessler JA. Effects of administration of ciliary neurotrophic factor on normal motor and sensory peripheral nerves *in vivo. Brain Res* 1993 ; 604 : 1-6.
4. Ault B, Hildebrand LM. Activation of nociceptive reflexes by peripheral kainate receptors. *J Pharmacol Exp Ther* 1993 ; 265(2) : 927-32.
5. Babbedge RC, Wallace P, Gaffen ZA, Hart SL, Moore PK. L-N^G-nitro arginine p-nitroanilide (L-NAPNA) is anti-nociceptive in the mouse. *NeuroReport* 1993 ; 4 : 307-10.
6. Bartho L, Stein C, Herz A. Involvement of capsaicin-sensitive neurones in hyperalgesia and enhanced opioid antinociception in inflammation. *Arch Pharmacol* 1990 ; 342 : 666-70.
7. Basbaum AI, Levine JD. The contribution of the nervous system to inflammation and inflammatory disease. *Can J Physiol Pharmacol* 1990 ; 69 : 647-51.
8. Bedi KS, Winter J, Berry M, Cohen J. Adult rat dorsal root ganglion neurons extend neurites on predegenerated but not on normal peripheral nerves *in vitro. Eur J Neurosci* 1992 ; 4 : 193-200.
9. Bharali LAM, Lisney SJW. The relationship between unmyelinated afferent type and neurogenic plasma extravasation in normal and reinnervated rat skin. *Neuroscience* 1992 ; 47(3) : 703-12.
10. Bileviciute I, Lundeberg T, Ekblom A, Theodorsson E. Bilateral changes of substance P-, neurokinin A-, calcitonin gene-related peptide- and neuropeptide Y-like immunoreactivity in rat knee joint synovial fluid during acute monoarthritis. *Neurosci Lett* 1993 ; 153 : 37-40.
11. Birder LA, Roppolo JR, Iadarola MJ, de Groat WC. Electrical stimulation of visceral afferent pathways in the pelvic nerve increases c-*fos* in the rat lumbosacral spinal cord. *Neurosci Lett* 1991 ; 129 : 193-6.
12. Brune K, Beck WS, Geisslinger G, Menzel-Soglowek S, Peskar BM, Peskar BA. Aspirin-like drugs may block pain independently of prostaglandin synthesis inhibition. *Experientia* 1991 ; 47 : 257-61.
13. Bullitt E, Lee CL, Light AR, Willcockson H. The effect of stimulus duration on noxious-stimulus induced c-*fos* expression in the rodent spinal cord. *Brain Res* 1992 ; 580 : 172-9.
14. Burch RM, DeHaas C. A bradykinin antagonist inhibits carrageenan edema in rats. *Arch Pharmacol* 1990 ; 342 : 189-93.
15. Buzzi MG, Moskowitz MA. The antimigraine drug, sumatriptan (GR43175), selectively blocks neurogenic plasma extravasation from blood vessels in dura mater. *Br J Pharmacol* 1990 ; 99 : 202-6.

16. Calcutt NA, Muir D, Powell HC, Mizisin AP. Reduced ciliary neuronotrophic factor-like activity in nerves from diabetic or galactose-fed rats. *Brain Res* 1992 ; 575 : 320-4.
17. Cameron AA, Pover CM, Willis WD, Coggeshall RE. Evidence that fine primary afferent axons innervate a wider territory in the superficial dorsal horn following peripheral axotomy. *Brain Res* 1992 ; 575 : 151-4.
18. Cameron NE, Cotter MA. Dissociation between biochemical and functional effects of the aldose reductase inhibitor, ponalrestat, on peripheral nerve in diabetic rats. *Br J Pharmacol* 1992 ; 107 : 939-44.
19. Carpenter JP, Priestely J, McMahon S. Induction of the nitric oxide synthase, NADPH-diaphorase, in axotomized somatic sensory neurones in the rat. *J Physiol* 1994 ; in press.
20. Cervero F, Jänig W. Visceral nociceptors : a new world order ? *TINS* 1992 ; 15(10) : 374-8.
21. Cervero F, Laird JMA. One pain or many pains ? A new look at pain mechanisms. *NIPS* 1991 ; 6 : 268-73.
22. Coderre TJ, Melzack R. The contribution of excitatory amino acids to central sensitization and persistent nociception after formalin-induced tissue injury. *J Neurosci* 1992 ; 12(9) : 3665-70.
23. Coderre TJ, Melzack R. The role of NMDA receptor-operated calcium channels in persistent nociception after formalin-induced tissue injury. *J Neurosci* 1992 ; 12(9) : 3671-5.
24. Coderre TJ, Chan AK, Helms C, Basbaum AI, Levine JD. Increasing sympathetic nerve terminal-dependent plasma extravasation correlates with decreased arthritic joint injury in rats. *Neuroscience* 1991 ; 40(1) : 185-9.
25. Craft RM, Porreca F. Treatment parameters of desensitization to capsaicin. *Life Sci* 1992 ; 51 : 1767-75.
26. Dejgard A, Petersend P, Kastrup J. Mexiletine for the treatment of chronic painful diabetic neuropathy. *Lancet* 1988 ; i : 9-11.
27. Dickenson A, Hughes C, Rueff A, Dray A. A spinal mechanism of action is involved in the antinociception produced by the capsaicin analogue NE 19550 (olvanil). *Pain* 1990 ; 43 : 353-62.
28. DiStefano PS, Friedman B, Radziejewski C, Alexander C, Boland P, Schick CM, Lindsay RM, Wiegand SJ. The neurotrophins BDNF, NT-3 and NGF display distinct patterns of retrograde axonal transport in peripheral and central neurons. *Neuron* 1992 ; 8 : 983-93.
29. Doubleday B, Robinson PP. The role of nerve growth factor in collateral reinnervation by cutaneous C-fibers in the rat. *Brain Res* 1992 ; 593 : 179-84.
30. Dray A. Mechanism of action of capsaicin-like molecules on sensory neurons. *Life Sci* 1992 ; 51 : 1759-65.
31. Dray A, Perkins M. Bradykinin and inflammatory pain. *TINS* 1993 ; 16(3) : 99-104.
32. Dubner R, Ruda MA. Activity-dependent neuronal plasticity following tissue injury and inflammation. *TINS* 1992 ; 15(3) : 96-103.
33. Dunlop R, Davies RJ, Hockley J, Turner P. Analgesic effects of oral flecainide. *Lancet* 1988 ; i : 420-1.
34. Dyck PJ. New understanding and treatment of diabetic neuropathy. *Neuropathy* 1992 ; 326(19) : 1287-8.
35. Evans RH, Evans SJ, Pook PC, Sunter DC. A comparison of excitatory amino acid antagonists acting at primary afferent C fibers and motoneurones of the isolated spinal cord of the rat. *Br J Pharmacol* 1987 ; 91 : 531-7.
36. Feniuk W, Humphrey PPA, Connor HE. The pharmacology of sumatriptan and its mode of action in migraine. In : Olesen J, Saxena PR, eds. *5-Hydroxytryptamine mechanisms in primary headaches*. New York : Raven Press, 1992 : 213-9.
37. Ferreira SH, Lorenzetti BB, De Campos DI. Induction, blockade and restoration of a persistent hypersensitive state. *Pain* 1990 ; 42 : 365-71.
38. Follenfant RL, Nakamura-Craig M, Henderson B, Higgs GA. Inhibition by neuropeptides of

interleukin-1 β-induced, prostaglandin-independent hyperalgesia. *Br J Pharmacol* 1989 ; 98 : 41-3.
39. Franco-Cereceda A, Lundberg JM. Capsazepine inhibits low pH- and lactic acid-evoked release of calcitonin gene-related peptide from sensory nerves in guinea-pig heart. *Eur J Pharmacol* 1992 ; 221 : 183-4.
40. Frisen J, Verge VMK, Cullheim S, Persson H, Fried K, Middlemas DS, Hunter T, Hokfelt T, Risling M. Increased levels of trkB mRNA and trkB protein-like immunoreactivity in the injured rat and cat spinal cord. *Proc Natl Acad Sci USA* 1992 ; 89 : 11282-6.
41. Furuyama T, Kiyama H, Sato K, Park HT, Maeno H, Takagi H, Tohyama M. Region-specific expression of subunits of ionotropic glutamate receptors (AMPA-type, KA-type and NMDA receptors) in the rat spinal cord with special reference to nociception. *Mol Brain Res* 1993 ; 18 : 141-51.
42. Gieron MA, Malone JI, Lowitt S, Korthals JK. Improvement in peripheral nerve function after one year of Sorbinil. *NeuroReport* 1991 ; 2 : 348-50.
43. Goadsby PJ, Edvinsson L. Sumatriptan reverses the changes in calcitonin gene-related peptide seen in the headache phase of migraine. *Cephalalgia* 1991 ; 11(11) : 3-4.
44. Goadsby PJ. Inhibition of calcitonin gene-related peptide by h-CGRP(8-37) antagonizes the cerebral dilator response from nasociliary nerve stimulation in the cat. *Neurosci Lett* 1993 ; 151 : 13-6.
45. Green PG, Levine JD. δ- and κ-opioid agonists inhibit plasma extravasation induced by bradykinin in the knee joint of the rat. *Neuroscience* 1992 ; 49(1) : 129-33.
46. Greenberg DA. Ca^{++} channel blockers in migraine. *Clin Neuropharmacol* 1986 ; 9 : 311-28.
47. Haley J, Ketchum S, Dickenson A. Peripheral κ-opioid modulation of the formalin response : an electrophysiological study in the rat. *Eur J Pharmacol* 1990 ; 191 : 437-46.
48. Hanesch U, Pfrommer U, Grubb BD, Schaible HG. Acute and chronic phases of unilateral inflammation in rat's ankle are associated with an increase in the proportion of calcitonin gene-related peptide-immuno reactive dorsal root ganglion cells. *Eur J Neurosci* 1993 ; 5 : 154-61.
49. Hanley MR. Peptide regulatory factors in the nervous system. *Lancet* 1989 ; 17, June : 1373-6.
50. Hassan AHS, Przewlocki R, Herz A, Stein C. Dynorphin, a preferential ligand for κ-opioid receptors, is present in nerve fibers and immune cells within inflamed tissue of the rat. *Neurosci Lett* 1992 ; 140 : 85-8.
51. Herdegen T, Tölle TR, Bravo R, Zieglgänsberger W, Zimmermann M. Sequential expression of Jun B, Jun D and Fos B proteins in rat spinal neurons : cascade of transcriptional operations during nociception. *Neurosci Lett* 1991 ; 129 : 221-4.
52. Hla T, Neilson K. Human cyclooxygenase-2 cDNA. *Proc Natl Acad Sci USA* 1992 ; 89 : 7384-8.
53. Ichinose M, Nakajima N, Takahashi T, Yamauchi H, Inoue H, Takishima T. Protection against bradykinin-induced bronchoconstriction in asthmatic patients by neurokinin receptor antagonist. *Lancet* 1992 ; 340 : 1248-51.
54. Junien JL, Wettstein JG. Role of opioids in peripheral analgesia. *Life Sci* 1992 ; 51 : 2009-18.
55. Kajander KC, Wakisaka S, Bennett GJ. Spontaneous discharge originates in the dorsal root ganglion at the onset of a painful peripheral neuropathy in the rat. *Neurosci Lett* 1992 ; 138 : 225-8.
56. Kajander KC, Bennett GJ. Onset of a painful peripheral neuropathy in rat : a partial and differential deafferentation and spontaneous discharge in Aβ and Aδ primary afferent neurons. *J Neurophysiol* 1992 ; 68(3) : 734-44.
57. Kamei J, Ohhashi Y, Aoki T, Kawasima N, Kasuya Y. Streptozotocin-induced diabetes selectively alters the potency of analgesia produced by μ-opioid agonists, but not by δ- and κ-opioid agonists. *Brain Res* 1992 ; 571 : 199-203.

58. Kappelle AC, Bravenboer B, Van Buren T, Traber J, Erkelens DW, Gispen WH. Amelioration by the Ca^{2+} antagonist, nimodipine of an existing neuropathy in the streptozotocin-induced, diabetic rat. *Br J Pharmacol* 1993 ; 108 : 780-5.
59. Khoury GF, Chen ACN, Garland DE, Stein C. Intra-articular morphine, bupivacaine and morphine/bupivacaine for pain control after knee videoarthroscopy. *Anesthesiology* 1992 ; 77 : 263-6.
60. Khurana G, Bennett MR. Nitric oxide and arachidonic acid modulation of calcium currents in postganglionic neurones of avian cultured ciliary ganglia. *Br J Pharmacol* 1993 ; 109 : 480-5.
61. Kidd BL, Gibson SJ, O'Higgins F, Mapp PI, Polak JM, Buckland-Wright JC, Blake DR. A neurogenic mechanism for symmetrical arthritis. *Lancet* 1989 ; November 11 : 1128-30.
62. Kristensen JD, Svensson B, Gordh T. The NMDA-receptor antagonist CPP abolishes neurogenic "wind-up pain" after intrathecal administration in humans. *Pain* 1992 ; 51 : 249-53.
63. Leah JD, Sandkuhler J, Herdegen T, Murashov A, Zimmermann M. Potentiated expression of fos protein in the rat spinal cord following bilateral noxious cutaneous stimulation. *Neuroscience* 1992 ; 48(3) : 525-32.
64. Leem JW, Willis WD, Chung JM. Cutaneous sensory receptors in the rat foot. *J Neurophysiol* 1993 ; 69(5) : 1684-99.
65. Lembeck F, Donnerer J, Tsushiya M, Nagahisa A. The non-peptide tachykinin antagonist, CP-96,345, is a potent inhibitor of neurogenic inflammation. *Br J Pharmacol* 1992 ; 105 : 527-30.
66. LeVasseur SA, Gibson SJ, Helme RD. The measurement of capsaicin-sensitive sensory nerve fiber function in elderly patients with pain. *Pain* 1990 ; 41 : 19-25.
67. Levine JD, Taiwo YO. Involvement of the mu-opiate receptor in peripheral analgesia. *Neuroscience* 1989 ; 32(3) : 571-5.
68. Levine JD, Coderre TJ, White DM, Finkbeiner WE, Basbaum AI. Denervation-induced inflammation in the rat. *Neurosci Lett* 1990 ; 119 : 37-40.
69. Lewin GR, Ritter AM, Mendell LM. On the role of nerve growth factor in the development of myelinated nociceptors. *J Neurosci* 1992 ; 12(5) : 1896-905.
70. Lindstrom P, Lindblom U. The analgesic effect of tocainide in trigeminal neuralgia. *Pain* 1987 ; 28 : 45-50.
71. Lippe IT, Stabentheiner A, Holzer P. Participation of nitric oxide in the mustard oil-induced neurogenic inflammation of the rat paw skin. *Eur J Pharmacol* 1993 ; 232 : 113-20.
72. Lynn B, Ye W, Cotsell B. The actions of capsaicin applied topically to the skin of the rat on C-fiber afferents, antidromic vasodilatation and substance P levels. *Br J Pharmacol* 1992 ; 107 : 400-6.
73. McLachlan EM, Janig W, Devor M, Michaelis M. Peripheral nerve injury triggers noradrenergic sprouting within dorsal root ganglia. *Nature* 1993 ; 363 : 543-6.
74. Maclean MJ, MacDonald RL. Multiple actions of phenytocin in mouse cord neurones in cell culture. *J Pharmacol Exp Ther* 1984 ; 238 : 727-38.
75. McMahon SB, Koltzenburg M. Novel classes of nociceptors : beyond Sherrington. *TINS* 1990 ; 13(6) : 199-201.
76. Maggi CA. Therapeutic potential of capsaicin-like molecules : studies in animals and humans. *Life Sci* 1992 ; 51 : 1777-81.
77. Malmberg AB, Yaksh TL. Hyperalgesia mediated by spinal glutamate or substance P receptor blocked by spinal cyclooxygenase inhibition. *Science* 1992 ; 257 : 1276-9.
78. Mao J, Price DD, Mayer DJ, Lu J, Hayes RL. Intrathecal MK-801 and local nerve anaesthesia synergistically reduce nociceptive behaviours in rats with experimental peripheral mononeuropathy. *Brain Res* 1992 ; 576 : 254-62.
79. Milner P, Appenzeller O, Qualls C, Burnstock G. Differential vulnerability of neuropeptides in nerves of the vasa nervorum to streptozotocin-induced diabetes. *Brain Res* 1992 ; 574 : 56-62.

80. Moore PK, Babbedge RC, Wallace P, Gaffen ZA, Hart SL. 7-Nitro indazole, an inhibitor of nitric oxide synthase, exhibits anti-nociceptive activity in the mouse without increasing blood pressure. *Br J Pharmacol* 1993 ; 108 : 296-7.
81. Moore UJ, Seymour RA, Rawlins MD. The efficacy of locally applied aspirin and acetaminophen in postoperative pain after third molar surgery. *Clin Pharmacol Ther* 1992 ; 52(3) : 292-6.
82. Morris R, Southam E, Gittins SR, Garthwaite J. NADPH-diaphorase staining in autonomic and somatic cranial ganglia of the rat. *NeuroReport* 1993 ; 4 : 62-4.
83. Moskowitz MA. Neurogenic versus vascular mechanisms of sumatriptan and ergot alkaloids in migraine. *TIPS* 1992 ; 13 : 307-11.
84. Moussaoui SM, Montier F, Carruette A, Blanchard JC, Laduron PM, Garret C. A non-peptide NK_1-receptor antagonist, RP 67580, inhibits neurogenic inflammation postsynaptically. *Br J Pharmacol* 1993 ; 109 : 259-64.
85. Murphy, DF. NSAIDs and postoperative pain. *BMJ* 1993 ; 306 : 1493-4.
86. Nadelhaft I, Vera PL. Reduced urinary bladder afferent conduction velocities in streptozotocin diabetic rats. *Neurosci Lett* 1992 ; 135 : 276-8.
87. Newbold P, Brain SD. The modulation of inflammatory oedema by calcitonin gene-related peptide. *Br J Pharmacol* 1993 ; 108 : 705-10.
88. Nozaki K, Moskowitz MA, Boccalini P. CP-93,129, sumatriptan, dihydroergotamine block c-*fos* expression within rat trigeminal nucleus caudalis caused by chemical stimulation of the meninges. *Br J Pharmacol* 1992 ; 106 : 409-15.
89. Onogi T, Minami M, Kuraishi Y, Satoh M. Capsaicin-like effect of (6)-shogaol on substance P-containing primary afferents of rats : a possible mechanism of its analgesic action. *Neuropharmacol* 1992 ; 31(11) : 1165-9.
90. Parsons CG, Herz A. Peripheral opioid receptors mediating antinociception in inflammation. Evidence for activation by enkephalin-like opioid peptides after cold water swin stress. *J Pharmacol Exp Ther* 1990 ; 255(2) : 795-802.
91. Perkins MN, Campbell EA. Capsazepine reversal of the antinociceptive action of capsaicin *in vivo. Br J Pharmacol* 1992 ; 107 : 329-33.
92. Perkins MN, Campbell E, Dray A. Antinociceptive activity of the bradykinin B_1 and B_2 receptor antagonists, des-Arg^9, [Leu^8]-BK and HOE 140, in two models of persistent hyperalgesia in the rat. *Pain* 1993 ; 53 : 191-7.
93. Piedimonte G, Hoffman JIE, Husseini WK, Bertrand C, Snider RM, Desai MC, Petersson G, Nadel JA. Neurogenic vasodilation in the rat nasal mucosa involves neurokinin$_1$ tachykinin receptors. *J Pharmacol Exp Ther* 1993 ; 265 : 36-40.
94. Poole S, Bristow AF, Lorenzetti BB, Gaines Das RE, Smith TW, Ferreira SH. Peripheral analgesic activities of peptides related to α-melanocyte stimulating hormone and interleukin-1β$^{193-195}$. *Br J Pharmacol* 1992 ; 106 : 489-92.
95. Portnoy RK, Duma C, Foley KM. Acute herpetic and post herpetic neuralgia : clinical review and current management. *Ann Neurol* 1986 ; 20 : 651-64.
96. Prough DS, McLeskey CH, Poehling GG. Efficacy of oral nifedipine in the treatment of reflex sympathetic dystrophy. *Anesthesiology* 1985 ; 62 : 796-9.
97. Przewlocki R, Hassan AHS, Lason W, Epplen C, Herz A, Stein C. Gene expression and localization of opioid peptides in immune cells of inflamed tissue : functional role in antinociception. *Neuroscience* 1992 ; 48(2) : 491-500.
98. Rang HP. The nociceptive afferent neurone as a target for new types of analgesic drug. In : Bond MR, Charlton JE, Woolf CE, eds. Proceedings of the VIth World Congress on Pain. Amsterdam : Elsevier, 1991 : 119-27.
99. Rogers H, Birch PJ, Harrison SM, Palmer E, Manchee GR, Judd DB, Naylor A, Scopes DIC, Hayes AG. GR94839, a κ-opioid agonist with limited access to the central nervous system, has antinociceptive activity. *Br J Pharmacol* 1992 ; 106 : 783-9.

100. Rueff A, Dray A. 5-hydroxytryptamine-induced sensitization and activation of peripheral fibers in the neonatal rat are mediated via different 5-hydroxytryptamine-receptors. *Neuroscience* 1992 ; 50(4) : 899-905.
101. Saito K, Markowitz S, Moskowitz MA. Ergot alkaloids block neurogenic extravasation in dura mater : proposed action in vascular headaches. *Ann Neurol* 1988 ; 24 : 732-7.
102. Salt TE, Hill RG. Neurotransmitter candidates of somatosensory primary afferent fibers. *Neuroscience* 1983 ; 10(4) : 1083-103.
103. Sato J, Perl ER. Adrenergic excitation of cutaneous pain receptors induced by peripheral nerve injury. *Science* 1991 ; 251 : 1608-10.
104. Shepheard SL, Cook DA, Williamson DJ, Hurley CJ, Hill RG, Hargreaves RJ. Inhibition of neurogenic plasma extravasation but not vasodilation in the hindlimb of the rat by the non-peptide NK-1 receptor antagonist (±)RP67580. *Br J Pharmacol* 1992 ; 107 : 150.
105. Shepheard SL, Williamson DJ, Hill RG, Hargreaves RJ. The non-peptide neurokinin$_1$ receptor antagonist, RP 67580, blocks neurogenic plasma extravasation in the dura mater of rats. *Br J Pharmacol* 1993 ; 108 : 11-2.
106. Small JR, Scadding JW, Landon DN. A fluorescence study of changes in noradrenergic sympathetic fibers in experimental peripheral nerve neuromas. *J Neurol Sci* 1990 ; 100 : 98-107.
107. Snutch TP, Reiner PB. Ca^{2+} channels : diversity of form and function. *Curr Opin Neurobiol* 1992 ; 2 : 247-53.
108. Steen KH, Reeh PW, Anton F, Handwerker HO. Protons selectively induce lasting excitation and sensitization to mechanical stimulation of nociceptors in rat skin, *in vitro*. *J Neurosci* 1992 ; 12(1) : 86-95.
109. Stein C, Hassan AHS, Przewlocki R, Gramsch C, Peter K, Herz A. Opioids from immunocytes interact with receptors on sensory nerves to inhibit nociception in inflammation. *Proc Natl Acad Sci* 1990 ; 87 : 5935-9.
110. Stühmer W, Parekh AB. The structure and function of Na^+ channels. *Curr Opin Neurobiol* 1992 ; 2 : 243-6.
111. Swerdlow M. The use of local anaesthetics for chronic pain. *Pain Clin* 1988 ; 2 : 3-6.
112. Szallasi A, Blumberg PM. Resiniferatoxin and its analogs provide novel insights into the pharmacology of the vanilloid (capsaicin) receptor. *Life Sci* 1990 ; 47 : 1399-408.
113. Taiwo YO, Levine JD, Burch RM, Woo JE, Mobley WC. Hyperalgesia induced in the rat by the amino-terminal octapeptide of nerve growth factor. *Proc Natl Acad Sci USA* 1991 ; 88 : 5144-58.
114. Taiwo YO, Levine JD. Serotonin is a directly-acting hyperalgesic agent in the rat. *Neuroscience* 1992 ; 48(2) : 485-90.
115. Tonnaer JADM, Schuijers GJPT, Van Diepen HA, Peeters BWMM. Enhancement of regeneration by Org 2766 after nerve crush depends on the type of neural injury. *Eur J Pharmacol* 1992 ; 214 : 33-7.
116. Verge VMK, Xu Z, Xu XJ, Wiesenfeld-Hallin Z , Hökfelt T. Marked increase in nitric oxide synthase mRNA in rat dorsal root ganglia after peripheral axotomy : *in situ* hybridization and functional studies. *Proc Natl Acad Sci USA* 1992 ; 89 : 11617-21.
117. Verge VMK, Wiesenfeld-Halin Z, Hökfelt T. Cholecystokinin in mammalian primary sensory neurons and spinal cord : *in situ* hybridization studies in rat and monkey. *Eur J Neurosci* 1993 ; 5 : 240-50.
118. Ward SJ, Portenoy RK, Yaksh TL. Nociceptive models : relevance to clinical pain states. In : Basbaum AI, Besson JM, eds. *Towards a new pharmacotherapy of pain*. Chichester : John Wiley & Sons, 1991 : 381-92.
119. Whicher JT, Evans SW. *Biochemistry of inflammation* (Immunology and Medicine series ; 18). Kluwer Academic Publishers, 1992.

120. Wiesenfeld-Hallin Z, Xu XJ, Hao JX, Hokfelt T. The behavioural effects of intrathecal galanin on tests of thermal and mechanical nociception in the rat. *Acta Physiol Scand* 1993 ; 147 : 457-8.
121. Wirth K, Hock FJ, Albus U, Linz W, Alpermann HG, Anagnostopoulos H, Henke St, Breipohl G, König W, Knolle J, Schölkens BA. Hoe 140, a new potent and long acting bradykinin-antagonist : *in vivo* studies. *Br J Pharmacol* 1991 ; 102 : 774-7.
122. Wong E, Mizisin AP, Garrett RS, Miller AL, Powell HC. Changes in aldose reductase after crush injury of normal rat sciatic nerve. *J Neurochem* 1992 ; 58 : 2212-22.

13

Presynaptic control of thin primary afferents : an ultrastructural analysis

S.M. CARLTON

Department of Anatomy and Neuroscience, Marine Biomedical Institute, University of Texas Medical Branch, Galveston, Texas, USA.

Documentation of the relationship between GABAergic and primary afferent axon terminals is of considerable importance since the proposed mechanisms of postsynaptic and presynaptic inhibition are based on interactions involving these neural elements. The following chapter reviews the synaptology of glomerular primary afferent terminals with GABA-containing profiles, documented at the electron microscopic level. The evidence demonstrates that all classes of glomerular primary afferent terminals synapse on GABAergic profiles. Thus, this excitatory input can act as a driving force for an inhibitory system, which in turn can exert inhibitory effects on postsynaptic membranes. On the other hand, not all classes of glomerular primary afferent terminals are subject to GABAergic presynaptic inhibition. There is a paucity of both physiological and anatomical data supporting the direct GABAergic control of a subpopulation of thin primary afferents.

Spinal cord inhibition is brought about by at least 2 different synaptic mechanisms : postsynaptic and presynaptic inhibition [15]. Assumed to be the most commonly occurring mechanism producing inhibition in the spinal cord dorsal horn, postsynaptic inhibition involves synaptic activity at the postsynaptic membrane, counteracting depolarizations produced at other locations by excitatory synapses on the same membrane. In contrast, presynaptic inhibition is believed to involve primary afferent depolarization (PAD), which has the effect of reducing the amount of excitatory transmitter released onto the postsynaptic element, with the consequence being a reduction in the excitatory post-synaptic potential (EPSP). The original work on presynaptic inhibition and PAD was described, and the associated phrases coined, in the late 1950's and early 1960's by Frank and Fuortes [24] and Eccles and coworkers [18, 19]. Presynaptic inhibition was first defined in relation to group Ia primary afferent fibers from muscle spindles and the inhibition of monosynaptic EPSP's produced by Ia afferent volleys in motoneurons [18-20, 24]. The PAD evoked by stimulation of one type of primary afferent fiber was quickly extended to many other types of fibers, including large and medium diameter group Ib muscle afferents, Aβ cutaneous fibers, small diameter, thinly myelinated Aδ fibers, and unmyelinated cutaneous C fibers [18-20, 22]. It was then demonstrated that each of these fiber types were in turn subject to PAD, with the exception of C fibers. In the twenty years since the initial investigations of presynaptic inhibition, physiological findings concerning PAD in unmyelinated C fibers remain equivocal [6, 23, 31, 32, 53, 61].

Pharmacological studies indicate that γ-aminobutyric acid (GABA) plays a major role in PAD [14, 21, 61]. Several years following the physiological and pharmacological descriptions of PAD, anatomical studies documented the presence of GABAergic interactions with central terminals in glomeruli. In this chapter, anatomical evidence will be presented which supports the hypotheses that :
- all classes of glomerular primary afferents are involved in postsynaptic inhibition, feeding their input directly into a GABAergic system which can in turn exert its inhibitory effect on postsynaptic membranes,
- not all classes of glomerular primary afferents are subject to GABAergic presynaptic inhibition.
There is a paucity of physiological and anatomical evidence supporting the direct GABAergic control of a subpopulation of thin primary afferents.

Glomerular primary afferent terminals

Our evidence focuses on the neurocircuitry involving glomerular primary afferents. A glomerulus is a special synaptic arrangement in the dorsal horn consisting of a central primary afferent terminal which is in synaptic contact with several peripheral profiles. The peripheral profiles are mainly dendrites but also include other axon terminals and vesicle-containing dendrites. This complex is "isolated" from the surrounding neuropil by glial processes. Glomeruli have been described by many investigators, in several different species [7, 12, 27, 33-36, 38, 44, 46-49, 54]. Primary afferents participating in glomeruli make up only 5% of the synaptic population in laminae I, II and III ([16, 48, 50, 51]. The majority of primary afferents terminate, however, as simple round or dome-shaped terminals making simple axodendritic synapses. Glomeruli, however, are extremely important dorsal horn structures for they constitute the first site where incoming sensory input can be modified by synaptic events (*i.e.* amplified, inhibited), before the input is relayed to higher centers.

Several lines of evidence indicate that central terminals of glomeruli are primary afferent in origin (*see* [65] for review ; however, *see* [60]). Since much of the anatomical data discussed in this chapter will concern findings in the monkey, a discussion of the glomerular types in this species will be emphasized. Based on morphology, primary afferents that participate in glomeruli in the primate fall into 3 major categories [38]. Similar categories have been described in the rat [45, 57] and cat [41]. One type of central terminal in the glomerulus is a round synaptic vesicle terminal (RSV). It has a light cytoplasm and contains round, clear vesicles of uniform size [38, 49, 57] (Figure 1).

It is believed that RSV terminals arise from large myelinated fibers such as Ia, Ib and large cutaneous afferents [38]. The terminals are found mainly in lamina III-VI. A second type of terminal is a dense sinusoidal axon terminal (DSA) which has a dense axoplasm and contains round clear vesicles of varying sizes [38] (Figure 2). Ralston [49] also observed central terminals with a dark axoplasm, labeling them "Cd" terminals. The third category of terminals contains large dense core vesicles (LDCV). These are very prominent in the monkey [8, 9, 38, 49] (Figure 3). It is believed that

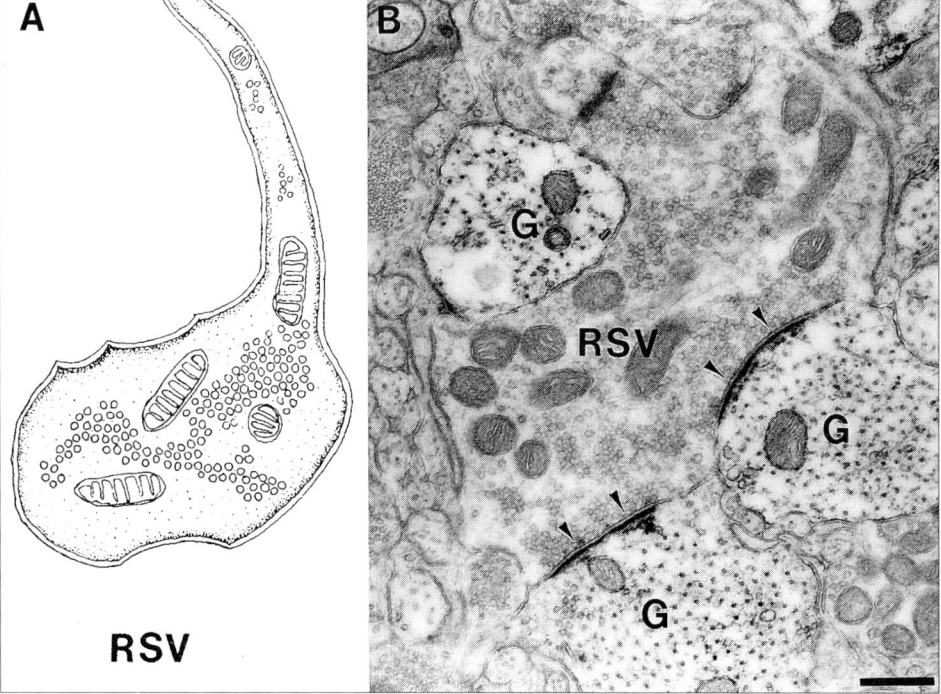

Figure 1. A : Stylized drawing of a "round synaptic vesicle" (RSV) primary afferent terminal, characterized by round clear vesicles of a uniform size and a light axoplasm. B : RSV glomerular terminal from the primate dorsal horn in contact with 3 GABA-immunoreactive (G) dendrites (arrow heads indicate synaptic specializations). (From [7].) Bar = 0.5μm.

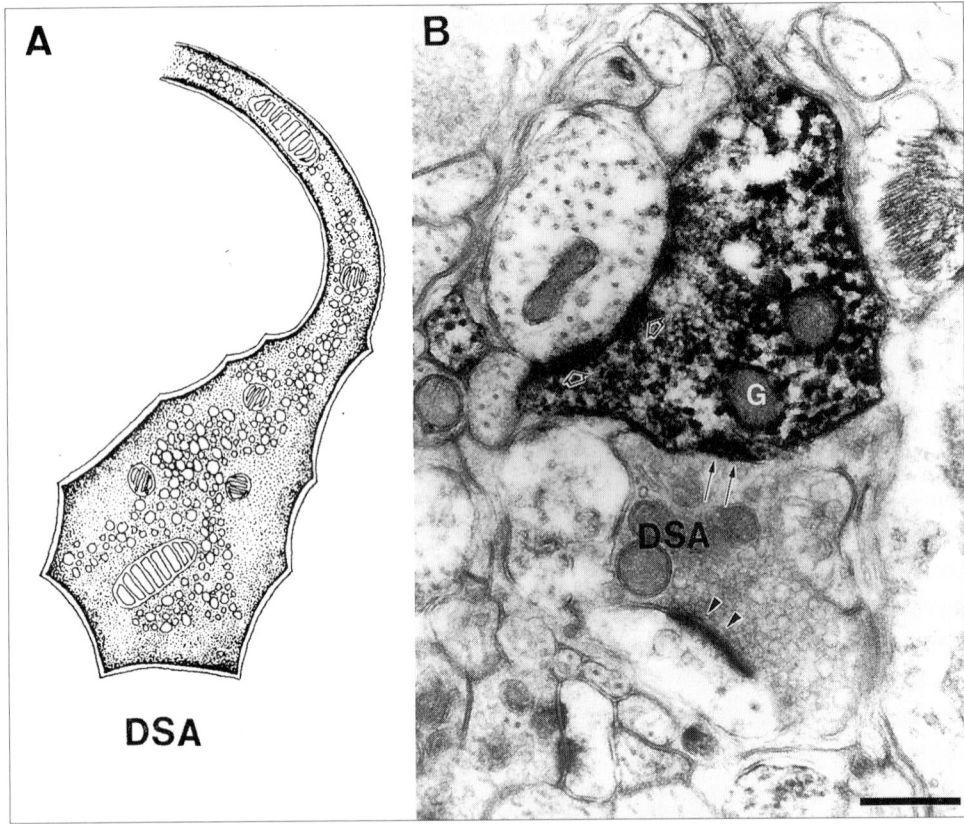

Figure 2. A : Stylized drawing of a "dense sinusoidal axon" (DSA) primary afferent terminal, characterized by round, clear vesicles of varying diameters and a dense axoplasm. B : A DSA terminal synapsing on a GABA-immunoreactive (G) vesicle-containing dendrite (arrows) and an unlabeled dendrite (arrow heads). The GABA-labeled dendrite, in turn, synapses on an unlabeled dendrite (open arrow heads). Bar = 0.5μm.

DSA and LDCV terminals arise from fine myelinated and unmyelinated fibers (Aδ and C fibers) for they are located mainly in laminae I and II and arise from small diameter fibers [37, 38, 45]. LDCV terminal types are relatively uncommon in deeper laminae except for the lateral reticulated region of lamina V [9, 51].

Glomerular involvement in postsynaptic inhibition and PAD

Electron microscopic studies from our laboratory have demonstrated that the 3 major categories of central terminals in the primate synapse on GABA-containing profiles [7]. Through this synaptic arrangement, each class of glomerular primary afferent can

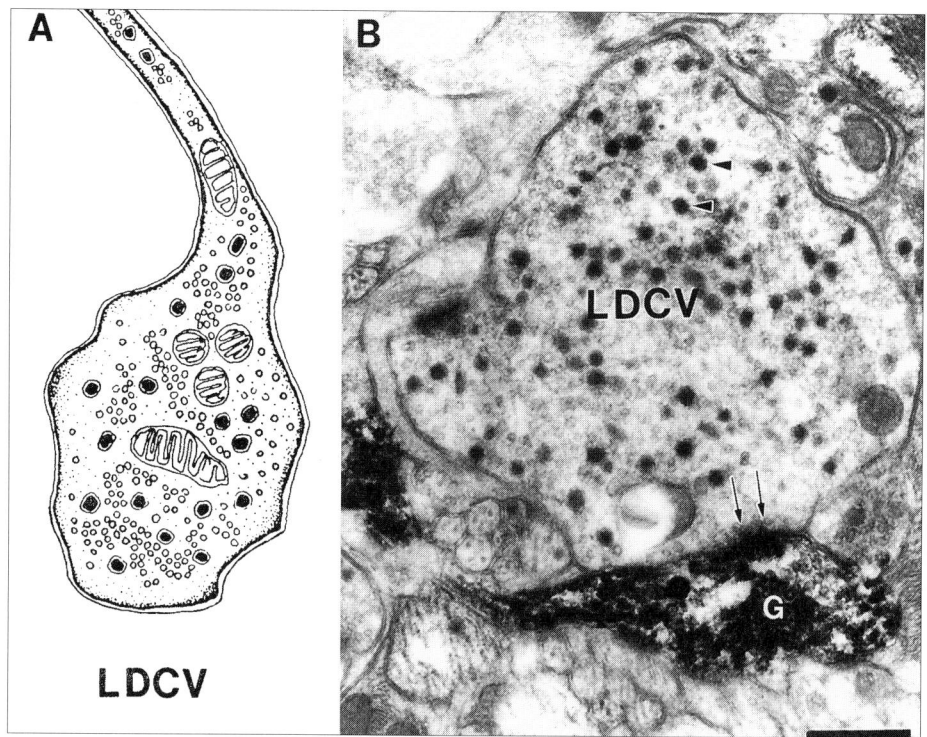

Figure 3. A : Stylized drawing of a "large dense core vesicle" (LDCV) primary afferent terminal, characterized by many dense core vesicles with some clear round vesicles. B : An LDCV terminal synapsing on a GABA-immunoreactive (G) axon (arrows). (From [7].) Bar = 0.5μm.

participate in postsynaptic inhibition. RSV terminals, found in laminae III - VI, where large myelinated fibers predominantly terminate, are most likely modulating innocuous input. Figure 1B demonstrates an RSV glomerular terminal synapsing on several GABA-containing dendrites. DSA glomeruli, concentrated in laminae II, but also found in laminae I, are likely to be modulating noxious input. As shown in Figure 2B, a DSA terminal is observed synapsing on a GABAergic vesicle-containing dendrite which in turn synapses on an unlabeled dendrite. Finally, LDCV terminals, present mainly in laminae I and II, are found presynaptic to GABAergic profiles (Figure 3B). The GABAergic profile in Figure 3B is most likely an axon ; but, GABAergic vesicle-containing dendrites have also been documented postsynaptic to LDCV terminals [30]. Thus, as predicted by the physiological data, our anatomical data indicate that the fiber types represented by the three categories of glomerular primary afferents have the appropriate neurocircuitry for the generation of postsynaptic inhibition : terminals arising from Aβ, Aδ and C fibers synapse on GABAergic profiles and thus can act as a driving force for postsynaptic inhibition. As discussed below, this same neurocircuitry can also serve as the driving force for PAD.

Glomerular involvement in presynaptic inhibition *via* PAD

The anatomical basis for presynaptic inhibition is believed to be axoaxonic interactions [17, 29, 61]. However, dendroaxonic synapses would also be suitable arrangements to provide PAD. Pharmacological studies indicate that γ-aminobutyric acid (GABA) is an important transmitter in the generation of PAD [14, 21]. A decade and a half elapsed before anatomical evidence for these physiologically and pharmacologically based theories was obtained.

Although the chemical content of the presynaptic elements was not known at the time, several laboratories have been successful in the documenting axoaxonic (and dendroaxonic) interactions in which primary afferent terminals were the postsynaptic element [13, 28, 38, 50, 57, 58]. Axoaxonic synapses were demonstrated in experiments in which central terminals arising from rapidly adapting, low threshold mechanoreceptors [40, 52] and hair follicle afferents [39] were specifically identified. Type I and type II slowly adapting afferents were found to be postsynaptic to vesicle-containing profiles [52]. Terminals arising from cutaneous mechanical nociceptors were observed to end in glomeruli and to be postsynaptic to both axon terminals and vesicle-containing dendrites [55]. Axonal profiles were also observed presynaptic to terminals arising from D-hairs [55].

Several different approaches were used to identify the neurochemical content of the vesicle-containing profiles observed presynaptic to glomerular primary afferents. Not surprisingly, studies focussed on the localization of GABA or the enzyme that synthesizes GABA, glutamic acid decarboxylase (GAD). Using autoradiography at the electron microscopic level, Ribeiro-Da Silva and Coimbra [56] demonstrated in rat that some peripheral terminals in synaptic glomeruli sequestered [^{3}H]GABA ; however, in this study unequivocal synaptic interactions and/or the polarity of the interactions were not defined. Following dorsal rhizotomies in rat, degenerating primary afferent terminals were observed postsynaptic to profiles immunostained for GAD [4]. In the cat, Basbaum *et al.* [5] observed GAD-labeled profiles presynaptic to vesicle-containing profiles which resembled scalloped central terminals. In a study of lamina II of the rat dorsal horn, Todd and Lochhead [62] identified GABA-labeled profiles presynaptic to type I synaptic glomeruli. Thus evidence of GABAergic synaptic input onto primary afferent terminals accumulated.

In subsequent experiments employing more advanced techniques, primary afferent fibers were first physiologically identified and then intracellularly injected with horseradish peroxidase (HRP). This tissue was then immunostained for GABA, allowing detailed analysis of primary afferent interactions with GABAergic profiles. Terminals arising from identified hair follicle afferents [43] and arising from Group Ia muscle afferents [42] were observed postsynaptic to GABAergic axon terminals. These afferents terminate in the deeper layers of the dorsal horn and are considered to be RSV type terminals. Although the specific fiber type giving rise to the afferent terminal is unknown, Figure 4 demonstrates a GABAergic vesicle-containing dendrite presynaptic to an RSV terminal [7]. Alvarez et al. [1] demonstrated that terminals arising from identified Aδ high threshold mechanoreceptors participated in GABAergic axoaxonic synapses (Figure 5). Although the density of the axoplasm could not be determined due to the HRP reaction product, the primary afferent terminals demonstrated were very reminiscent of DSA types, containing round clear vesicles of varying sizes and having a very scalloped or sinusoidal appearance. Thus, we conclude that RSV glomerular terminals arising from large myelinated Aβ fibers, and DSA terminals arising from finely myelinated Aδ fibers, are subject to presynaptic inhibition *via* GABAergic mechanisms. What was proposed from physiological and pharmacological studies was confirmed by these anatomical data and there is little disagreement concerning the influence of PAD on myelinated primary afferent fibers.

In contrast, controversy continues to surround the question of presynaptic inhibition of unmyelinated primary afferent fibers. As stated above, there is a lack of compelling physiological data indicating that this group of fibers is subject to PAD [6, 23, 31, 32, 53, 61]. Due to the difficulty in recording from, and subsequent injection of unmyelinated axons, the neural connections made by this fiber type have been derived mainly from studies which identify them by neurochemical content [8, 9, 30, 45, 63, 64], by location in the superficial dorsal horn and/or by morphological criteria [7, 38, 49].

Studies in our laboratory have shown that a subpopulation of finely myelinated and unmyelinated fibers, that terminate as LDCV glomerular terminals, are rarely observed postsynaptic in axoaxonic or dendroaxonic interactions [30]. This subpopulation of LDCV terminals contain calcitonin gene-related peptide (CGRP), which is a well known marker for terminals arising from finely myelinated and unmyelinated primary afferent fibers [11, 25, 45]. In an extensive serial section analysis of 100 CGRP-containing terminals in the primate superficial dorsal horn, only rarely was a vesicle-containing profile observed presynaptic to CGRP-labeled terminals [30]. In fact, only 2 axoaxonic interactions were observed, one in which a GABAergic terminal was presynaptic to the CGRP terminal (Figure 6) and one in which it was postsynaptic to the CGRP terminal (*see* Figure 8 [30]).

Dendroaxonic interactions in which a GABAergic vesicle-containing dendrite was presynaptic to the CGRP terminal was also observed but again these were rare (2/121, *see* Figure 6, [30]). Recently, Alvarez et al. [2] analyzed the synaptic interactions of physiologically identified and intra-axonally injected C fibers in the primate dorsal horn. Both C fibers demonstrated central terminals in glomeruli with many LDCV and were immunoreactive for CGRP. Furthermore, the study confirmed a lack of axoaxonic interactions in relation to these C fiber terminals. Other lines of evidence support the rarity of axoaxonic and dendroaxonic interactions involving LDCV glomerular type terminals : SP-immunoreactive glomeruli in the rat, which contain dense core vesicles and are believed to arise from finely myelinated and unmyelinated fibers, were rarely seen postsynaptic to vesicle-containing profiles [59]. Furthermore, Ralston and Ralston

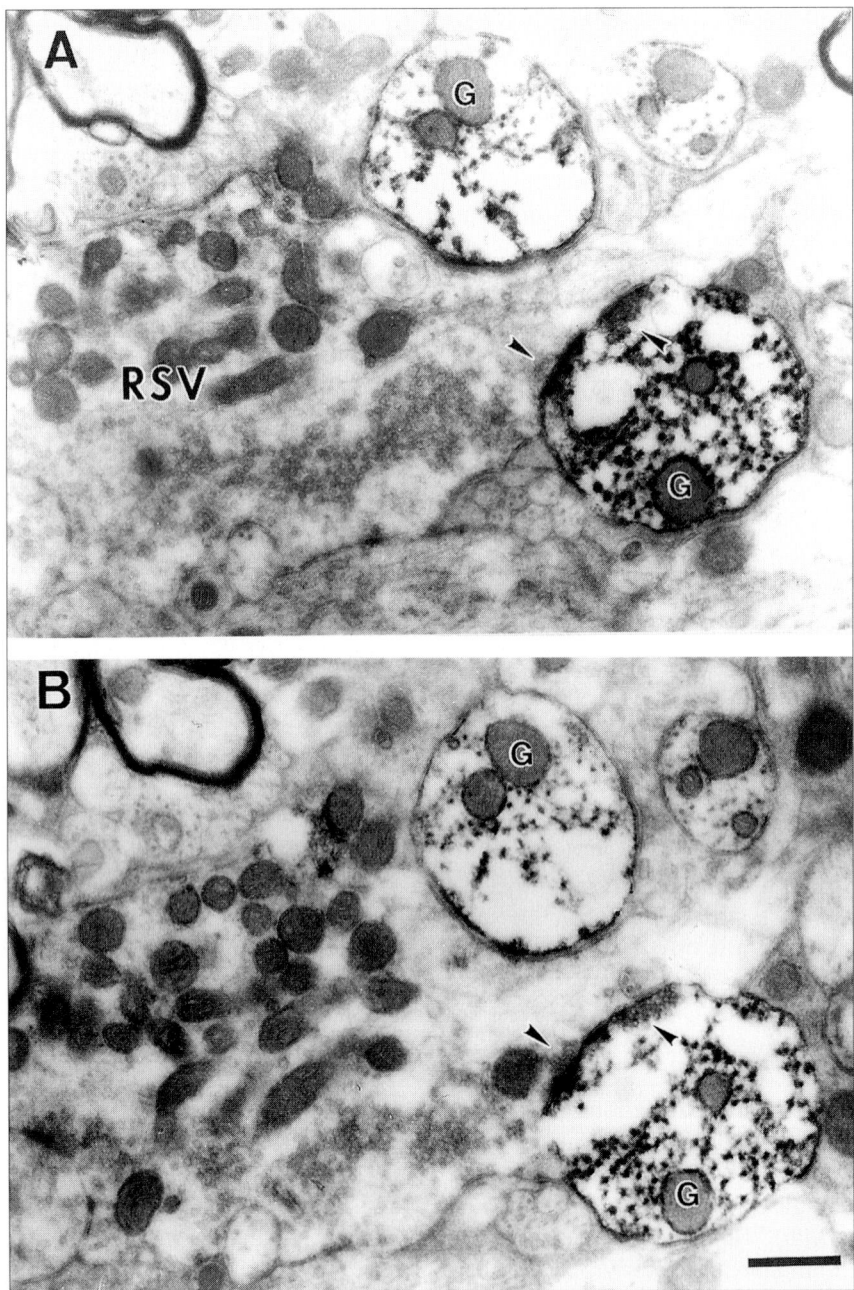

Figure 4. A and B : Serial ultrathin sections demonstrating a reciprocal synapse between an RSV glomerular and a GABA-immunoreactive (G) vesicle-containing dendrite (arrow heads). (From [7]). Bar = 0.5μm.

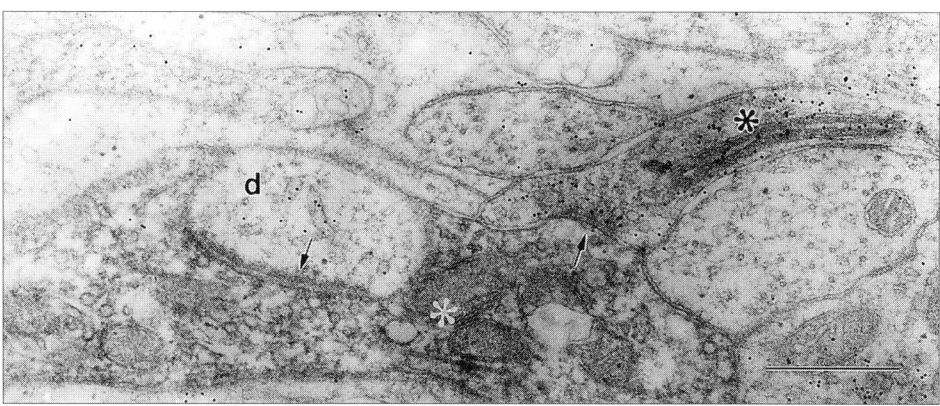

Figure 5. An immunogold-labeled GABA terminal (black asterisk) presynaptic (right arrow) to a terminal arising from a physiologically identified, HRP-filled Aδ fiber (white asterisk). The Aδ terminal is also presynaptic to an unlabeled dendrite (d, left arrow). (From [2].) Bar = 0.5μm.

[50] reported that most of the synapses of primary afferent origin in lamina I were not involved in axoaxonal synapses whereas those terminating in laminae II and III were more often subject to presynaptic inhibition. Thus, anatomical studies demonstrate a lack of a preponderance of axoaxonic interactions for LDCV terminals and this is in agreement with the physiological findings concerning thin primary afferent fibers.

As stated earlier, the central terminal of a glomerulus is not the only arrangement for a primary afferent ending, since the majority of primary afferents terminate as simple round or dome-shaped terminals. Thus, we cannot rule out the occurrence of presynaptic inhibitory endings on non-glomerular primary afferent terminals. In fact, there is evidence that small, round, CGRP-containing terminals are postsynaptic to GABAergic vesicle-containing dendrites (Figure 7). Furthermore, we cannot rule out the possibility that "non-synaptic neurotransmission" may occur. This type of relationship, which is the hypothesized interaction between opiate-containing terminals and primary afferent terminals [26], may also be true of the interaction between GABA profiles and CGRP-containing glomerular afferents.

Conclusion

Evidence that the 3 morphological types of primary afferent glomerular terminals are presynaptic to GABAergic profiles indicates that these afferents can act as a driving force for this inhibitory system. Input being transmitted *via* RSV, DSA and LDCV terminals, arising from Aβ, Aδ, and Aδ or C fibers, respectively, may trigger the activation of a GABAergic inhibitory system. The stimulated GABAergic neurons can, in turn, inhibit cells at the origin of ascending systems such as spinothalamic tract cells [10] through postsynaptic mechanisms. Furthermore, as indicated in the drawing in Figure 8, the primary afferent-activated GABA interneurons can synapse on RSV and

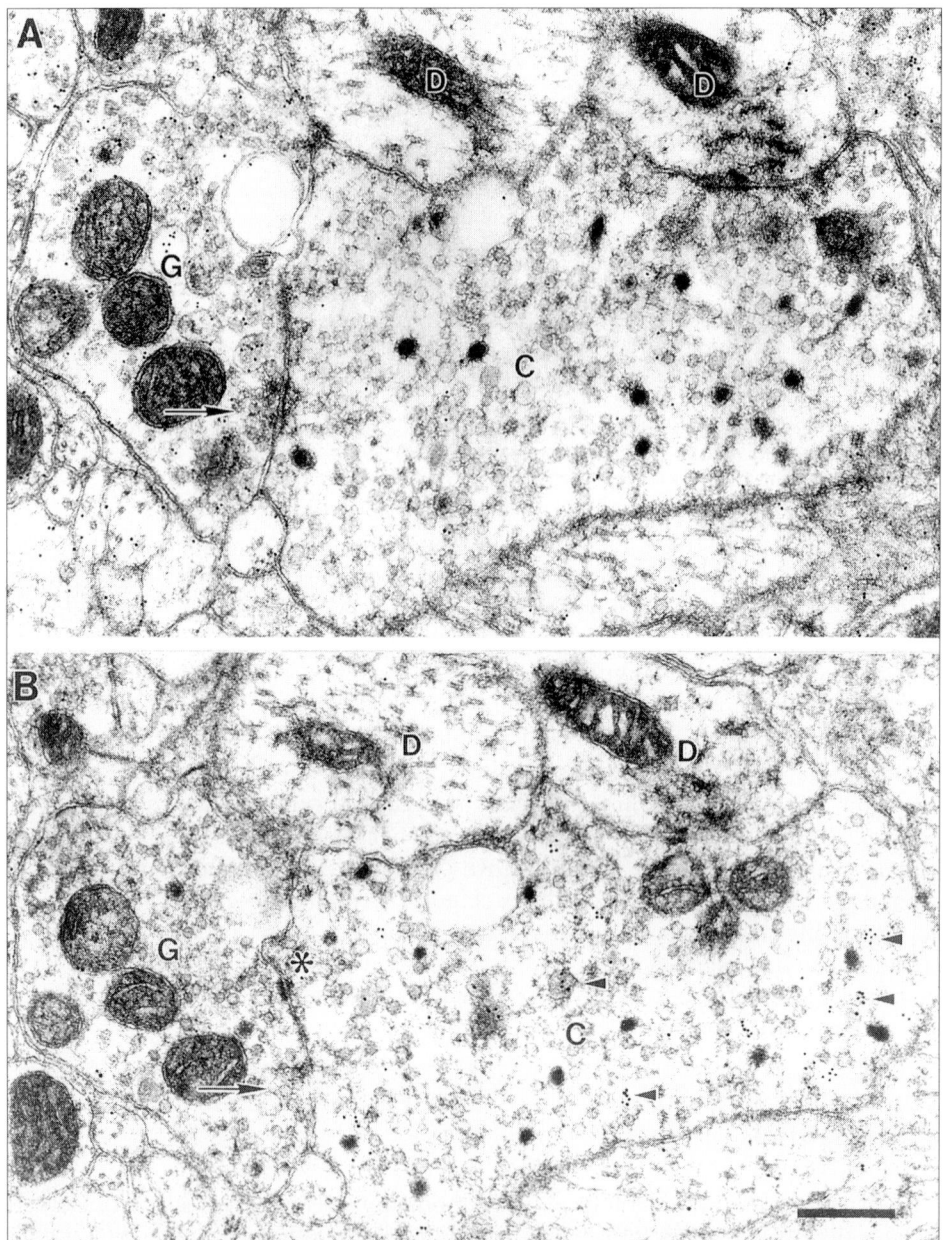

Figure 6. Serial ultrathin sections demonstrating an axoaxonic synapse between a GABA (G) immunogold labeled axon (labeled in A), and a CGRP (C) immunogold labeled terminal (arrow heads indicate CGRP immunogold label in B). (From [30].) Bar = 0.4μm.

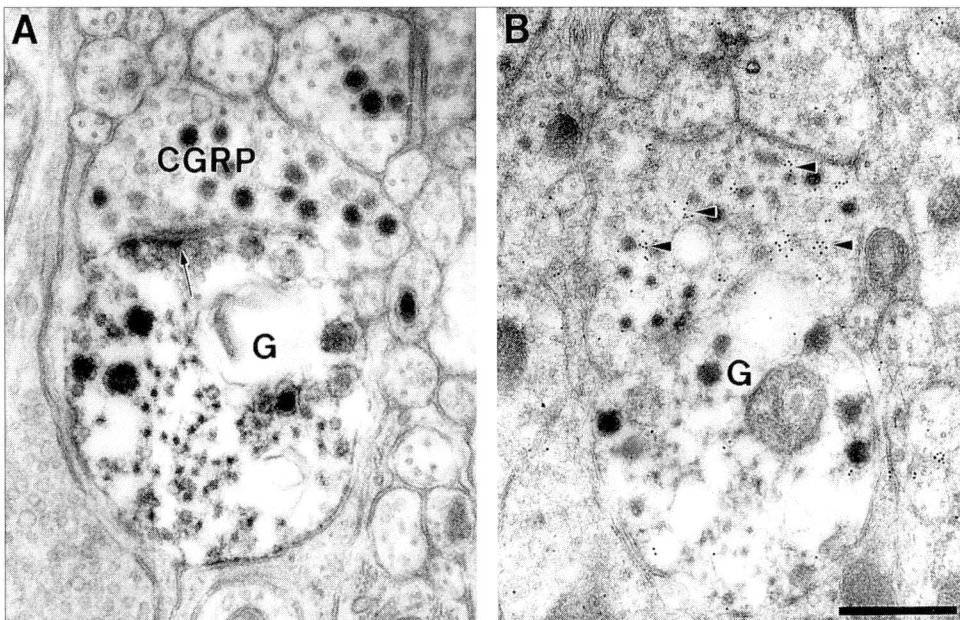

Figure 7. Serial sections demonstrating a dendroaxonic interaction (arrow in A) between a GABAergic vesicle-containing dendrite (labeled with the peroxidase-antiperoxidase method in A) and a simple dome-shaped CGRP terminal (C, labeled with immunogold indicated by arrow heads in B). (From [30].) Bar = 0.5μm.

DSA terminals and effectively inhibit, through presynaptic mechanisms, the EPSP's evoked by primary afferent stimulation. On the other hand, LDCV glomeruli, arising from thin primary afferents, would not be under this inhibitory control. This subpopulation of CGRP-containing terminals may provide the necessary circuitry for tissue-damaging messages to reach consciousness in a timely and unadulterated fashion. This neurocircuitry may also provide for inhibitory surround and contrast enhancement of signals vital to an organism's well-being.

The concept that PAD may be generated through dendroaxonic interactions as well as axoaxonic interactions has minimal impact on the theory. However, the fact that GABAergic neurons can exert their effect through dendritic arbors suggests that widespread inhibition in the dorsal horn could result from minimal primary afferent input. Furthermore, in the case of large muscle and cutaneous afferents, it has been demonstrated that the central latencies for PAD are not shorter that 2.0 ms, which would suggest 2 interneurons in serial order as the simplest pathway for PAD ([3, 19] ; *see* [61] for review). However, anatomical studies would support the possibility that the simplest pathway may involve only one GABAergic interneuron as shown in Figure 8.

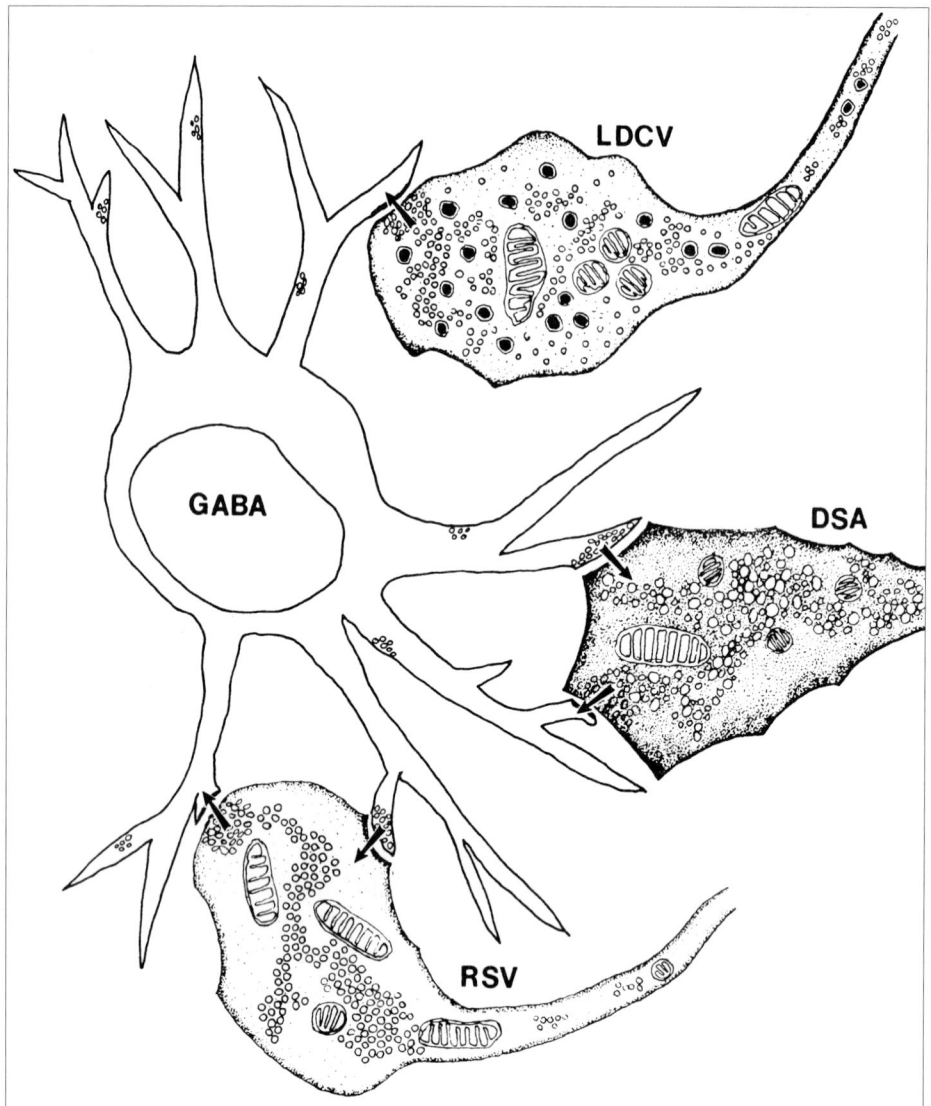

Figure 8. Schematic drawing of the neurocircuitry involving glomerular primary afferents and GABAergic interneurons in the dorsal horn. Glomerular primary afferents synapse on GABAergic dendrites, some of which contain vesicles. GABAergic vesicle-containing dendrites, in turn synapse on DSA and RSV glomerular terminals, providing the basis for presynaptic inhibition. LDCV terminals, however, lack this GABAergic control.

References

1. Alvarez FJ, Kavookjian AM, Light AR. Synaptic interactions between GABA-immunoreactive profiles and the terminals of functionally defined myelinated nociceptors in the monkey and cat spinal cord. *J Neurosci* 1992 ; 12 : 2901-17.
2. Alvarez FJ, Kavookjian AM, Light AR. Ultrastructural morphology, synaptic relationships and CGRP immunoreactivity of physiologically identified C-fiber terminals in the monkey spinal cord. *J Comp Neurol* 1993 ; 329 : 472-90.
3. Andersen P, Eccles JC, Schmidt RF, Yokota T. Depolarization of presynaptic fibers in the cuneate nucleus. *J Neurophysiol* 1964 ; 27 : 92-106.
4. Barber RP, Vaughn JE, Saito K, McLaughlin BJ, Roberts E. GABAergic terminals are presynaptic to primary afferent terminals in the substantia gelatinosa of the rat spinal cord. *Brain Res* 1978 ; 141 : 35-55.
5. Basbaum AI, Glazer EJ, Oertel W. Immunoreactive glutamic acid decarboxylase in the trigeminal nucleus caudalis of the cat : a light- and electron-microscopic analysis. *Somat Res* 1986 ; 4 : 77-94.
6. Calvillo O. Primary afferent depolarization of C fibers in the spinal cord of the cat. *Can J Physiol Pharmacol* 1978 ; 56 : 154-7.
7. Carlton SM, Hayes ES. Light microscopic and ultrastructural analysis of GABA-immunoreactive profiles in the monkey spinal cord. *J Comp Neurol* 1990 ; 300 : 162-82.
8. Carlton SM, McNeill DL, Chung K, Coggeshall RE. A light and electron microscopic level analysis of calcitonin gene-related peptide (CGRP) in the spinal cord of the primate : an immunohistochemical study. *Neurosci Lett* 1987 ; 76 : 145-50.
9. Carlton SM, McNeill DL, Chung K, Coggeshall RE. Organization of calcitonin gene-related peptide-immunoreactive terminals in the primate dorsal horn. *J Comp Neurol* 1988 ; 276 : 527-36.
10. Carlton SM, Westlund KN, Zhang D, Willis WD. GABA-immunoreactive terminals synapse on primate spinothalamic tract cells. *J Comp Neurol* 1992 ; 322 : 528-37.
11. Chung K, Lee WT, Carlton SM. The effects of dorsal rhizotomy and spinal cord isolation on calcitonin gene-related peptide-labeled terminals in the rat lumbar dorsal horn. *Neurosci Lett* 1988 ; 90 : 27-32.
12. Coimbra A, Sodre-Borges BP, Magalhaes MM. The substantia gelatinosa Rolandi of the rat. Fine structure, cytochemistry (acid phosphatase) and changes after dorsal root section. *J Neurocytol* 1974 ; 3 : 199-217.
13. Cruz F, Lima D, Zieglgänsberger, Coimbra A. Fine structure and synaptic architecture of HRP-labelled primary afferent terminations in lamina IIi of the rat dorsal horn. *J Comp Neurol* 1991 ; 305 : 3-16.
14. Curtis DR, Lodge D. The depolarization of feline ventral horn Ia spinal afferent terminations by GABA. *Exp Brain Res* 1982 ; 46 : 215-33.
15. Davidoff RA, Hackman JC. Spinal inhibition. In : Davidoff RA, ed. *Handbook of the spinal cord*. Marcel Dekker Inc, New York 1984 : 385-459.
16. Duncan D, Morales R. Relative numbers of several types of synaptic connections in the substantia gelatinosa of the cat spinal cord. *J Comp Neurol* 1978 ; 182 : 601-10.
17. Eccles JC. The mechanism of synaptic transmission. *Ergebn Physiol* 1961 ; 51 : 299-430.
18. Eccles JC, Eccles RM, Magni F. Central inhibitory action attributable to presynaptic depolarization produced by muscle afferent volleys. *J Physiol Lond* 1961 ; 159 : 147-66.
19. Eccles JC, Kostyuk PG, Schmidt RF. Central pathways responsible for depolarization of primary afferent fibers. *J Physiol* 1962 ; 161 : 237-57.

20. Eccles JC, Magni F, Willis WD. Depolarization of central terminals of group I afferent fibers from muscle. *J Physiol* 1962 ; 160 : 62-93.
21. Eccles JC, Schmidt RF, Willis WD. Pharmacological studies on presynaptic inhibition. *J Physiol (Lond)* 1963 ; 168 : 530-60.
22. Eccles JC, Schmidt RF, Willis WD. Depolarization of the central terminals of cutaneous afferent fibers. *J Neurophysiol* 1963 ; 26 : 646-61.
23. Fitzgerald M, Woolf CJ. Effect of cutaneous nerve and intraspinal conditioning on C-fiber afferent terminal excitability in decerebrate spinal rats. *J Physiol (Lond)* 1981 ; 318 : 25-39.
24. Frank K, Fuortes MGF. Presynaptic and postsynaptic inhibition of monosynaptic reflexes. *Fed Proc* 1957 ; 16 : 39-40.
25. Gibso SJ, Polak JM, Bloom SR, Sabate IM, Mulderry PM, Ghatei MA, McGregor GP, Morrison JF, Kelly JS, Evans RM, Rosenfeld MG. Calcitonin gene-related peptide immunoreactivity in the spinal cord of man and eight other species. *J Neurosci* 1984 ; 4 : 3101-11.
26. Glazer E, Basbaum A. Opioid neurons and pain modulation : an ultrastructural analysis of enkephalin in cat superficial dorsal horn. *Neuroscience* 1983 ; 10 : 357-76.
27. Gobel S. Synaptic organization of the substantia gelatinosa glomeruli in the spinal trigeminal nucleus of the adult cat. *J Neurocytol* 1974 ; 3 : 219-43.
28. Gobel S, Falls WM, Bennett GJ, Hayashi H, Humphrey E. An EM analysis of the synaptic connections of horseradish peroxidase-filled stalked cells and islet cells in the substantia gelatinosa of adult cat spinal cord. *J Comp Neurol* 1980 ; 194 : 781-807.
29. Gray EG. A morphological basis for presynaptic inhibition. *Nature* 1962 ; 193 : 82-3.
30. Hayes ES, Carlton SM. Primary afferent interactions : analysis of calcitonin gene-related peptide-immunoreactive terminals in contact with unlabeled and GABA-immunoreactive profiles in the monkey dorsal horn. *Neuroscience* 1992 ; 47 : 873-96.
31. Hentall ID, Fields HL. Segmental and descending influences on intraspinal thresholds of single C fibers. *J Neurophysiol* 1979 ; 42 : 1527-37.
32. Jänig W, Zimmermann M. Presynaptic depolarization of myelinated afferent fibers evoked by stimulation of cutaneous C fibers. *J Physiol* 1970 ; 214 : 29-50.
33. Kerr FWL. The ultrastructure of the spinal tract of the trigeminal nerve and substantia gelatinosa. *Exp Neurol* 1966 ; 16 : 359-76.
34. Kerr FWL. The fine structure of the subnucleus caudalis of the trigeminal nerve. *Brain Res* 1970 ; 23 : 129-45.
35. Kerr FWL. Pain : a central inhibitory balance theory. *Mayo Clin Proc* 1975 ; 50 : 685-90.
36. Knyihar E, Laszlo I, Tornyos S. Fine structure and fluoride resistant acid phosphatase activity of electron dense sinusoid terminals in the substantia gelatinosa rolandi of the rat after dorsal root transection. *Exp Brain Res* 1974 ; 19 : 529-44.
37. Knyihar-Csillik E, Csillik B. Selective labeling by transsynaptic degeneration of substantia gelatinosal cells : an attempt to decipher intrinsic wiring in the Rolando substance of primates. *Neurosci Lett* 1981 ; 23 : 131-6.
38. Knyihar-Csillik E, Csillik B, Rakic P. Periterminal synaptology of dorsal root glomerular terminals in the substantia gelatinosa of the spinal cord in the Rhesus monkey. *J Comp Neurol* 1982 ; 210 : 376-99.
39. Maxwell DJ, Bannatyne BA, Fyffe REW, Brown AG. Ultrastructure of hair-follicle afferent fiber terminations in the spinal cord of the cat. *J Neurocytol* 1982 ; 11 : 571-82.
40. Maxwell DJ, Bannatyne BA, Fyffe REW, Brown AG. Fine structure of primary afferent axon terminals projecting from rapidly adapting mechanoreceptors of the toe and foot pads of the cat. *Q J Exp Physiol* 1984 ; 69 : 381-92.
41. Maxwell DJ, Christie WM, Short AD, Storm-Mathisen J, Ottersen OP. Central boutons of glomeruli in the spinal cord of the cat are enriched with L-glutamate-like immunoreactivity. *Neuroscience* 1990 ; 36 : 83-104.

42. Maxwell DJ, Christie WM, Short AD, Brown AG. Direct observations of synapses between GABA-immunoreactive boutons and muscle afferent terminals in lamina VI of the cat's spinal cord. *Brain Res* 1990 ; 530 : 215-22.
43. Maxwell DJ, Noble R. Relationships between hair-follicle afferent terminations and glutamic acid decarboxylase-containing boutons in the cat's spinal cord. *Brain Res* 1987 ; 408 : 308-12.
44. Maxwell DJ, Rethelyi M. Ultrastructure and synaptic connections of cutaneous afferent fibers in the spinal cord. *TINS* 1987 ; 10 : 117-22.
45. McNeill DL, Coggeshall RE, Carlton SM. A light and electron microscopic study of calcitonin gene-related peptide in the spinal cord of the rat. *Exp Neurol* 1988 ; 99 : 699-708.
46. Ralston HJ. The organization of the substantia gelatinosa Rolandi in the cat lumbosacral cord. *Z Zellforsch* 1965 ; 67 : 1-23.
47. Ralston HJ. The fine structure of neurons in the dorsal horn of the cat spinal cord. *J Comp Neurol* 1968 ; 132 : 275-302.
48. Ralston HJ. The synaptic organization in the dorsal horn of the spinal cord and in the ventrobasal thalamus in the cat. In : Dubner R, Kawamura Y, eds. *Oral-facial sensory and motor mechanisms.* Appleton-Century-Crofts, New York 1971 : 229-50.
49. Ralston HJ. The fine structure of laminae I, II, and III of the macaque spinal cord. *J Comp Neurol* 1979 ; 184 : 619-42.
50. Ralston HJ, Ralston DD. The distribution of dorsal root axons in laminae I, II and III of the macaque spinal cord : a quantitative electron microscope study. *J Comp Neurol* 1979 ; 184 : 643-84.
51. Ralston HJ, Ralston DD.The distribution of dorsal root axons to laminae IV, V, and VI of the macaque spinal cord : a quantitative electron microscopic study. *J Comp Neurol* 1982 ; 212 : 435-48.
52. Ralston HJ III, Light AR, Ralston DD, Perl ER. Morphology and synaptic relationships of physiologically identified low-threshold dorsal root axons stained with intra-axonal horseradish peroxidase in the cat and monkey. *J Neurophysiol* 1984 ; 59 : 777-92.
53. Randic M. Presynaptic effects of γ-aminobutyric acid and substance P on intraspinal single cutaneous C- and A-fibers. In : Brown AG, Rethelyi M, eds. *Spinal cord sensation.* Edinburgh : Scottish Academic Press, 1981 : 285-94.
54. Rethelyi M, Szentágothai J. The large synaptic complexes of the substantia gelatinosa. *Exp Brain Res* 1969 ; 7 : 258-74.
55. Rethelyi M, Light AR, Perl ER. Synaptic complexes formed by functionally defined primary afferent units with fine myelinated fibers. *J Comp Neurol* 1982 ; 207 : 381-93.
56. Ribeiro-Da Silva A, Coimbra A. Neuronal uptake of [^{3}H] glycine in laminae I-III (substantia gelatinosa Rolandi) of the rat spinal cord. An autoradiographic study. *Brain Res* 1980 ; 188 : 449-64.
57. Ribeiro-Da Silva A, Coimbra A. Two types of synaptic glomeruli and their distribution in laminae I-III of the rat spinal cord. *J Comp Neurol* 1982 ; 209 : 176-86.
58. Ribeiro-Da Silva A, Pignatelli D, Coimbra A. Synaptic architecture of glomeruli in superficial dorsal horn of rat spinal cord, as shown in serial reconstructions. *J Neurocytol* 1985 ; 14 : 203-20.
59. Ribeiro-Da Silva A, Tagari P, Cuello AC. Morphological characterization of substance P-like immunoreactive glomeruli in the superficial dorsal horn of the rat spinal cord and trigeminal subnucleus caudalis : a quantitative study. *J Comp Neurol* 1989 ; 281 : 497-515.
60. Ruda MA, Gobel S. Ultrastructural characterization of axonal endings in the substantia gelatinosa which take up [^{3}H]serotonin. *Brain Res* 1980 ; 184 : 57-83.
61. Schmidt RF. Presynaptic inhibition in the vertebrate central nervous system. *Ergeb Physiol* 1971 ; 63 : 20-101.

62. Todd AJ, Lochhead V. GABA-like immunoreactivity in type I glomeruli of rat substantia gelatinosa. *Brain Res* 1990 ; 514 : 171-4.
63. Traub RJ, Solodkin A, Ruda MA. Calcitonin gene-related peptide immunoreactivity in the cat lumbosacral spinal cord and the effects of multiple dorsal rhizotomies. *J Comp Neurol* 1989 ; 287 : 225-37.
64. Traub RJ, Allen B, Humphrey E, Ruda MA. Analysis of calcitonin gene-related peptide-like immunoreactivity in the cat dorsal spinal cord and dorsal root ganglia provide evidence for a multisegmental projection of nociceptive C-fiber primary afferents. *J Comp Neurol* 1990 ; 302 : 562-74.
65. Willis WD Jr, Coggeshall RE. *Sensory mechanisms of the spinal cord,* 2nd ed. New York : Plenum Press, 1991 : 1-575.

14

A possible relation between neuropathic pain and central sensory sprouting following peripheral nerve lesions

R.E. COGGESHALL

Anatomy and Neuroscience, Physiology and Biophysics, and Marine Biomedical Institute, University of Texas Medical Branch, Galveston, Texas, USA.

The present paper is concerned with the central primary afferent sprouting that follows peripheral nerve transection in adult mammals. The main finding is that central primary afferent fibers expand to end in different spinal laminae following peripheral nerve transection. In particular, large primary afferent fibers, which are normally confined to laminae III and below, enter laminae I and II after nerve transection, and there make synaptic connections with post-synaptic cells. Since large primary afferent fibers normally carry discriminative information such as fine touch, and since the cells in laminae I and II normally process nociceptive information, the hypothesis is that mild stimuli are now exciting cells that would normally transmit nociceptive information to higher centers. If so, this could provide at least part of the explanation as to why peripheral nerve injuries sometimes lead to intractable neuropathic pain.

The present paper concerns the reorganization of central sensory fibers that follows peripheral nerve lesions. Two relatively recent developments make this a particularly interesting topic at present. First, there is the discovery that the growth associated protein, GAP-43 [20], is expressed in the dorsal horn following peripheral nerve lesions [24]. Second, there are the transganglionic tracing techniques that allow one to trace the central connections of different types of primary afferent fibers in relative isolation

[16]. The discussion will be restricted to spinal changes of primary afferents following peripheral nerve or dorsal root lesions, and it is assumed that the reader understands the general organization of the dorsal root ganglion cell (a pseudo-unipolar cell with at least one peripheral process that receives information from the periphery and at least one central process that transmits this information into the spinal cord and brain stem). The particular goal of this paper is to provide some suggestions as to how such changes might bear on pain, particularly the severe deafferentation pain that sometimes follows peripheral nerve lesions.

Central changes that follow peripheral nerve lesions are both degenerative and regenerative in nature. The regenerative changes are often referred to as sprouting (*e.g.* [7]). For heuristic reasons, the central regenerative changes will be subdivided into 3 broad areas and the discussion is restricted to data from adult animals :
- collateral spouting (central processes of undamaged or unconditioned dorsal root ganglion cells sprout into a neighboring denervated region of spinal cord, as in Figure 1),
- reactive collateral sprouting (central processes of only conditioned dorsal root ganglion cells sprout into a neighboring denervated region of spinal cord, as in Figure 2),
- reactive sprouting (central processes of conditioned dorsal root ganglion cells sprout into different laminae of the cord as in Figures 3 and 4). In 2 and 3 above, conditioning is achieved by cutting the distal processes of those dorsal root ganglion cells whose peripheral axons travel in a peripheral nerve. We will concentrate on simple reactive sprouting because the lesion, simple nerve transection, is what happens commonly in humans.

Collateral sprouting

Early ideas were that central sensory axons had no regenerative or restorative responses following peripheral nerve lesions in adult mammals. Any changes that could be assumed to represent sprouting or other regenerative processes were described as "abortive" [14]. Then Liu and Chambers [10] demonstrated an increased area of silver staining following transection of a dorsal root whose axons project into denervated cord as contrasted to transection of the same segmental root whose axons project into normal undenervated cord. This type of sprouting is usually referred to as "collateral" sprouting, and the term implies that the central processes of undamaged cells are sprouting or growing into a neighboring area where synaptic vacancies have occurred (Figure 1). The subject is controversial, however, in that some studies report collateral sprouting after denervation alone [7, 9], but others do not [11-13, 17, 18]. The conclusion would seem to be that central collateral sprouting of adult mammalian primary afferent fibers from otherwise normal cells occurs following denervation alone under some conditions, such as destroying the peripheral nerve with pronase [9], but not in others. If this is so, the conditions that allow such sprouting as well as those that

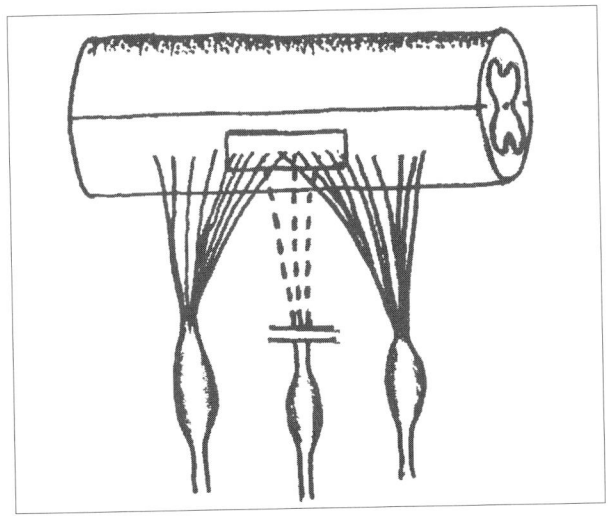

Figure 1. A sketch showing classical collateral sprouting. Note that cutting the central dorsal root (double line) results in denervation of an area of spinal cord (box) into which the axons from neighboring roots grow.

prevent it are of obvious interest. It would also be desirable to see how such sprouting, when it occurs, could provide a substrate for the pain that sometimes follows peripheral nerve lesions.

Reactive collateral sprouting

In recent years, several investigators noted that if sensory cells are "primed" or "conditioned" by cutting their peripheral processes, their central processes sprout vigorously into denervated areas [11,12] (Figure 2).

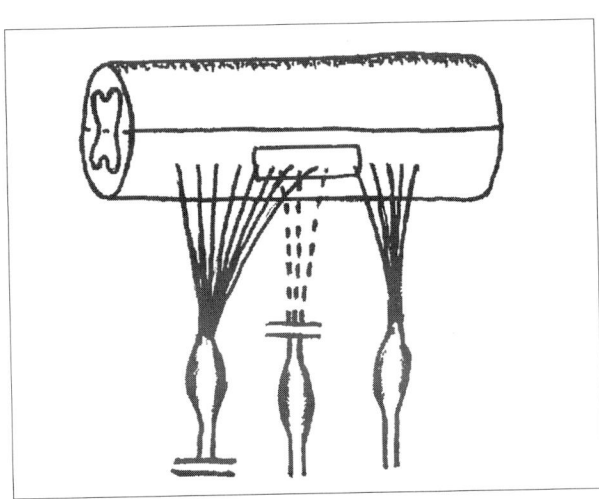

Figure 2. A sketch showing reactive collateral sprouting. Section of a dorsal root, the middle root in this picture, results in a denervation of an area of spinal cord (box). Axons from the neighboring lower root, which arise from undamaged (unconditioned) sensory cells do not sprout into the denervated region. By contrast, axons from the neighboring upper root, which arise from sensory cells whose peripheral prosses are transected, do sprout into the denervated region.

The hypothesis is that the central sprouting is the result of a combination of cell conditioning and an area of central denervation into which the central axons can sprout. Certainly the data presented in these papers are convincing, and the hypothesis seems to have considerable merit. But, as with collateral sprouting after simple denervation, it is not immediately clear how such findings bear on pain. One suggestion, however, is that recovery of function or mitigation of deafferentation pain could be enhanced by a reversible injury to neighboring intact nerves. The idea is that the peripheral lesion would allow or enhance the sprouting of sensory axons from neighboring nerves into the denervated region, and the assumption is that this would be beneficial [11]. The advantage of this suggestion is that it is susceptible to experimental verification.

Reactive sprouting

The above studies provide important information as to the responses of primary afferent axons to injury. But the lesions are more complicated than simple nerve crush or transection, which are the commonest clinical lesions, and the experimental paradigms are concerned with axons from "other" nerves projecting into a region denervated by some experimental manipulation. Thus, we felt it would be desirable to see what happens to the axons from cells whose peripheral processes are cut by a simple crush or transection within the normal central territory of that particular nerve. That reactive or regenerative activity occurs in the central processes of dorsal root ganglion cells after nerve crush has long been suggested, but the first convincing indication, in my opinion, is the demonstration that the growth associated protein, GAP-43, is immunohistochemically demonstrable following sciatic nerve crush or transection within the territory where the central axons from the sciatic nerve normally distribute [24]. GAP-43 is a growth associated protein [2, 3, 19, 20] that is expressed in growing neurons and axons, and whose expression stops once the target is innervated [6, 8, 15]. GAP-43 is rapidly reexpressed in adult dorsal root ganglion cells and in the growing tips of peripheral regenerating sensory axons following nerve lesions [21]. GAP-43 is not expressed in the cord if root sections are done [25] indicating that the GAP-43 in the cord is in primary afferent axons. In addition, electron microscopic observation shows that this material is found in axons, synaptic terminals and growth cones [5]. Thus, it is reasonable to conclude that GAP-43 is a good general marker of axonal regenerative events, and for primary afferent fibers in particular, its occurrence in the dorsal horn following peripheral nerve transection strongly suggests that there is regenerative activity in central afferent fibers whose cell bodies have had their peripheral processes transected by a nerve injury.

Finding that central processes of primary afferent axons from conditioned cells express GAP-43 in the spinal cord provides strong support for the hypothesis that there is some sort of regenerative central reorganization of primary afferents following peripheral simple nerve lesions. It might be asked, however, whether this reorganization occurs in axons from cells whose peripheral processes have been transected, or whether it represents sprouting from central processes of undamaged primary afferent neurons in nearby areas. That it is primarily the former is indicated by several findings. First, the labelling is restricted to but extends throughout the known territory of the sciatic nerve distribution [22]. It is true that there is some overlap of central primary afferent axons whose associated peripheral processes travel in different nerves, but most of the primary afferent input into the sciatic nerve territory is from cells whose peripheral axons project in that nerve. Second, transganglionic markers applied to the central stump of the transected sciatic nerve show sprouting of large fibers from lamina III to laminae I and II ([25], *see* below). Third, individually labelled large fibers in the sciatic nerve that normally end only in lamina III travel into laminae I and II following nerve section [25]. Accordingly, although it is not certain that the sprouting is only from fibers that arise from cells whose peripheral processes are cut, it seems certain that the large majority are.

Given that there is sprouting of central fibers from cells whose peripheral processes are transected within the sciatic nerve, the two obvious questions are what is the mechanism that underlies this sprouting and what are the implications of this finding in considerations of deafferentation pain ? Any discussion as to mechanisms for the phenomenon of central primary afferent sprouting following simple peripheral nerve lesions must remain speculative at present. Nevertheless, it seems reasonable to suggest that the sprouting occurs because of a combination of conditioning the cells (by cutting their peripheral processes) and a central denervated field. The conditioning of the cells is easy to understand, but one might well ask why central denervation occurs when a peripheral nerve is transected. One reason is that some dorsal root ganglion cells die when a peripheral nerve is transected [1]. This finding rests on nerve cell counts, which admittedly need to be repeated by modern methods, and also on the demonstration of dying dorsal root ganglion cells and central primary afferent axons. In addition recent work suggests that there is a loss of glomerular terminals in lamina II following peripheral nerve section, and one of the explanations of this finding is that there is an uncoupling of central pre- and postsynaptic processes following peripheral nerve section [4]. Much work remains to be done on both of these phenomena, but the bottom line is that a peripheral nerve lesion seems to do two seemingly contradictory things :
- prime the sensory cells so they are better able to sprout centrally,
- partially denervate that area of the cord into which the central axons of the cut nerve normally project. The result seems to be central sprouting following simple peripheral nerve lesions.

The next point concerns the possible relation of the above findings to neuropathic pain. One characteristic of studies of collateral sprouting, from axons of either normal or conditioned cells, is that the data are primarily of the areal extent of labelled fibers. Another type of topography is found in the spinal cord, however, namely the laminae which are dorso-ventral subdivisions of the grey matter that have considerable functional meaning [5]. In particular, different types of primary afferent fibers enter specific laminae of the dorsal horn. For the case of reactive sprouting following simple nerve transection, the sprouting was manifest, not by a greater areal extent over which the sprouted fibers spread, but by the demonstration that large primary afferents, which are normally restricted to laminae III and below (Figure 3), now extend into laminae I and II [25] (Figure 4).

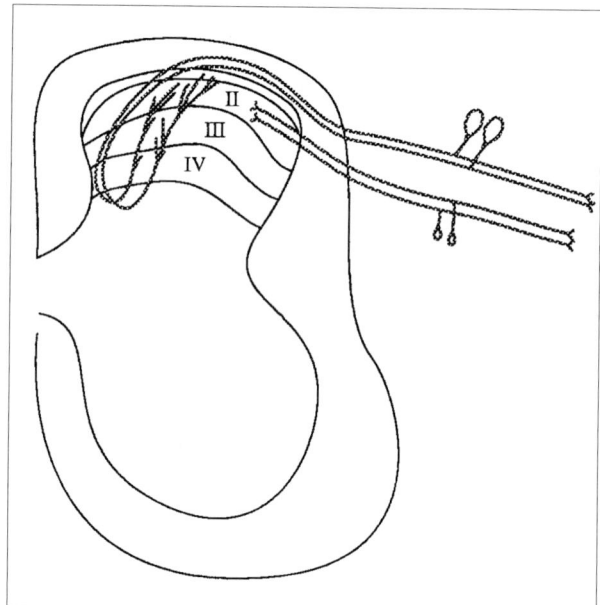

Figure 3. A sketch showing the normal arrangement of large primary afferent fibers which are normally distributed to lamina III and below and fine primary afferent fibers which are distributed to the superficial dorsal horn, particularly lamina II.

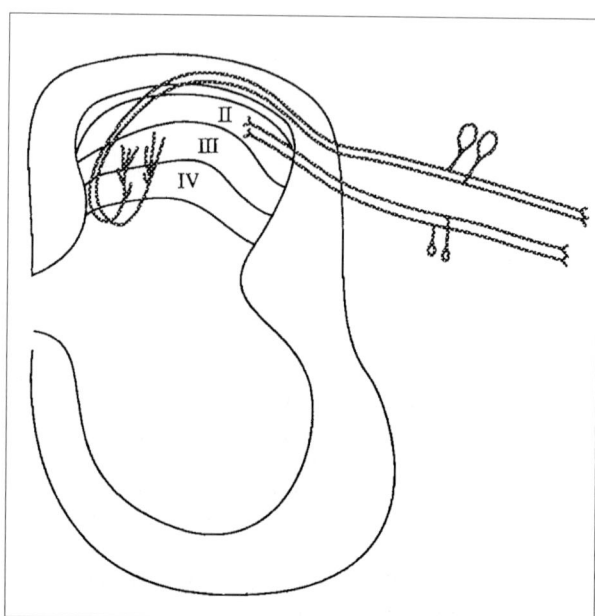

Figure 4. A sketch showing the redistribution of large primary afferent fibers following peripheral nerve section. Note that the large primary afferent fibers now enter laminae I and II.

Thus, large fiber input is now entering an area of the cord normally concerned only with fine fiber input. This is shown not only by the transganglionic transport of choleragenoid-labelled horseperoxidase (B-HRP), which labels the large primary afferent fibers [16], but also by single fiber fills of large sensory fibers [25]. The upshot is that simple nerve transection results in large afferent fibers that normally are concerned with light touch and fine discrimination [23] entering more superficial areas that are usually concerned with nociceptive information processing [23]. Furthermore, we have obtained preliminary evidence that these sprouting fibers are actually making synaptic contacts with dendrites or cell bodies in superficial laminae. Thus, it is reasonable to hypothesize that spinal cells that normally only respond to nociceptive input are now receiving light touch or similar discriminative information. Presumably this implies that stimuli normally interpreted as mild touch or vibration are now exciting long tract cells that normally transmit nociceptive information centrally. This would presumably contribute to the intractable touch-evoked pain that can sometimes follow nerve injury. Further work to prove this hypothesis is underway.

Acknowledgements

My work is supported by NIH grants NS11255 and NS10161. I thank Drs Susan Carlton and Helena Lekan for their critical reading of the manuscript.

References

1. Aldskogius H, Arvidsson J, Grant G. The reaction of primary sensory neurons to peripheral nerve injury with particular emphasis on transganglionic changes. *Brain Res Rev* 1985 ; 10 : 27-46.
2. Benowitz LI, Apostolides PJ, Perrone-Bizzozzero N, Finkelstein SP, Zwiers H. Anatomical distribution of the growth-associated protein GAP43/B-50 in the adult rat brain. *J Neurosci* 1988 ; 8 : 339-52.
3. Benowitz LI, Routenberg AA. Membrane phosphoprotein associated with neural development, axonal regeneration, phospholipid metabolism, and synaptic plasticity. *TINS* 1987 ; 10 : 527-31.
4. Castro-Lopes JM, Coimbra A, Grant A, Arvidsson J. Ultrastructural changes of the central scalloped (C1) primary afferent ending of synaptic glomeruli in the substania gelantinosa Rolandi of the rat after peripheral neurotomy. *J Neurocytol* 1990 ; 19 : 329-37.
5. Coggeshall RE, Reynolds ML, Woolf CJ. Distribution of the growth association protein GAP-43 in the central processes of axotomized primary afferents in the adult rat spinal cord ; presence of growth cone-like structures. *Neurosci Lett* 1991 ; 131 : 37-41.
6. Fitzgerald M, Reynolds ML, Benowitz LI. GAP-43 expression in the developing rat lumbar spinal cord. *Neuroscience* 1991 ; 41 : 187-99.
7. Goldberger ME, Murray M. Patterns of sprouting and implications for recovery of function. *Adv Neurol* 1988 ; 47 : 361-83.
8. Jacobson RD, Virag I, Skene JHP. A protein associated with growth, GAP 43, is widely distributed and developmentally regulated in rat CNS. *J Neurosci* 1986 ; 6 : 2570-663.
9. LaMotte CC, Kapadia SE, Kocol CM. Deafferentation-induced expansion of saphenous terminal field labelling in the adult rat dorsal horn following pronase injection of the sciatic nerve. *J Comp Neurol* 1989 ; 288 : 311-25.

10. Liu CN, Chambers WW. Intraspinal sprouting of dorsal root axons. *Arch Neurol* 1958 ; 79 : 46-61.
11. McMahon SB, Kett-White R. Sprouting of peripherally regenerating primary sensory neurones in the adult central nervous system. *J Comp Neurol* 1991 ; 304 : 307-15.
12. Molander C, Kinnman E, Aldskogius H. Expansion of spinal cord primary sensory afferent projection following combined sciatic nerve resection and saphenous nerve crush : a horseradish peroxidase study in the adult rat. *J Comp Neurol* 1988 ; 276 : 436-41.
13. Pubols LM, Bowen DC. Lack of central sprouting of primary afferent fibers after ricin deafferentation. *J Comp Neurol* 1988 ; 275 : 282-7.
14. Ramon y Cajal S. *Degeneration and regeneration of the nervous system.* New York : Hafner Publishing Company, 1959.
15. Reynolds ML, Fitzgerald M, Benowitz LI. GAP-43 expression in developing cutaneous and muscle nerves in the rat hindlimb. *Neuroscience* 1991 ; 41 : 201-11.
16. Robertson B, Grant GA. Comparison between wheat germ agglutinin- and choleragenoid-horseradish peroxidase as anterogradely transported markers in central branches of primary sensory neurones in the rat with some observations in the cat. *Neuroscience* 1985 ; 14 : 895-905.
17. Rodin BE, Kruger L. Absence of intraspinal spouting in dorsal root axons caudal to a partial spinal hemisection : a horseradish peroxidase transport study. *Somatosen Res* 1984 ; 2 : 171-92.
18. Rodin BE, Sampogna SL, Kruger L. An examination of intraspinal sprouting in dorsal root axons with the tracer horseradish peroxidase. *J Comp Neurol* 1983 ; 215 : 187-98.
19. Skene HJP, Willard M. Axonally transported proteins associated with growth in rabbit central and peripheral nervous system. *J Cell Biol* 1981 ; 89 : 96-103.
20. Skene HJP. Axonal growth-associated proteins. *Annu Rev Neurosci* 1989 ; 12 : 127-56.
21. Sommervaille T, Reynolds ML, Woolf CJ. Time-dependent differences in the increase in GAP-43 expression in dorsal root ganglion cells after peripheral axotomy. *Neuroscience* 1991 ; 45 : 213-20.
22. Swett JE, Woolf CJ. Somatotopic organization of primary afferent terminals in the superficial dorsal horn of the rat spinal cord. *J Comp Neurol* 1985 ; 231 : 66-71.
23. Willis WD, Coggeshall RE. *Sensory mechanisms of the spinal cord.* 2nd ed. New York : Plenum Press, 1991.
24. Woolf CJ, Reynolds ML, Molander C, O'Brien C, Lindsay RM, Benowitz LI. The growth-associated protein GAP-43 appears in dorsal root ganglion cells and in the dorsal horn of the rat spinal cord following peripheral nerve injury. *Neuroscience* 1990 ; 34 : 465-78.
25. Woolf CJ, Shortland P, Coggeshall RE. Peripheral nerve injury triggers central sprouting of myelinated afferents. *Nature* 1992 ; 355 : 75-8.

15

Deafferentation-induced alterations in the adult rat dorsal horn

C.C. LAMOTTE

Section of Neurosurgery, Yale University School of Medicine, New Haven, USA.

We have developed a spinal cord model of plasticity evoked by primary deafferentation to study the effects of making a very selective lesion of just one system that contributes to spinal circuitry. The model is based on selective destruction of sciatic dorsal root ganglion cells by injecting the nerve with proteolytic enzymes (pronase). One week after injection, the synaptic terminals of these nerve fibers in the spinal dorsal horn die, indicating that an effective lesion has been made. Four months after the pronase injection, there is sprouting of noninjured saphenous afferents into the deafferented territory demonstrated by injecting tracers (WGA-HRP and BHRP) into the saphenous nerve. We have determined several aspects of this phenomenon :
  - the different classes of primary sensory afferents sprout into appropriate laminar regions of the spinal dorsal horn,
  - the profiles of synaptic terminals sprouted by the saphenous nerve are larger and make more synaptic contacts than normal saphenous terminals ; this is particularly evident for the terminals which arise from small diameter afferents. In most cases the sprouted terminals resemble sciatic terminals more than the control saphenous terminals do,
  - synaptic terminals which contain substance P (SP) and calcitonin gene related peptide (CGRP) are initially eliminated in the sciatic territory in the dorsal horn, but substantially replenished after 4 months. This correlates well with the sprouting of the saphenous afferents, and indicates that they not only sprout but also have the peptide identity of the original terminals,
  - current studies of receptor changes in the dorsal horn indicate that there is an increase of SP receptors associated with the early loss of SP terminals and that after 4

months, the receptor level is returned to normal, correlating with the return of SP terminals,

- in a recent time course study, the expression of a guidance factor (NCAM) and a growth associated protein (GAP43) increased in the superficial dorsal horn by 10 days after pronase injection. By 20-30 days, NCAM and GAP43 spread into the deep dorsal horn. By 30-45 days, NCAM returned to normal, but GAP43 persisted throughout the dorsal horn until 60-90 days.

In summary, we have observed that the sprouted terminals are distributed to appropriate dorsal horn laminae by class ; this may be directed by guidance factors. The terminals have at least some of the normal array of peptides ; the initial loss and later recovery of these peptides are accompanied by receptor changes. In addition, although the terminals formed are also of the correct type for the laminae, there is proliferation, hypertrophy, and increased synapse formation, particularly for small diameter afferents.

Sprouting of afferents following spinal lesions or nerve injury

For many years anatomical investigations of possible sprouting of non-injured central processes of dorsal root afferents following a spinal or primary afferent lesion yielded quite conflicting results. Interpretation was complicated by significant variables, including labeling techniques, type of lesion, species and age of subjects, and type of afferents studied (*see* [26] for review). Nevertheless, a growing number of models which examine the central effects of damage to primary afferents have been developed, and certain consistent features have become evident. The models include damage to either the peripheral or the central processes, or to the ganglion itself. Each of these approaches has merit in that they represent forms of naturally occurring injury which may occur, or they are designed to selectively injure a known group of afferents in order to clarify interpretation of the results.

Rhizotomy of several consecutive dorsal roots eliminates all primary afferents over a defined area and results in sprouting of descending and interneuronal elements [18, 31, 51]. A quantitative electron microscopic study of sprouting [31] revealed the replacement of synaptic terminals following dorsal rhizotomy of several lumbar segments in the adult cat. In the dorsal horn, large glomerular terminals were replaced by small round terminals, presumably arising from either local or central neurons, whereas at least some of the synaptic replacement in Clarke's nucleus resembled primary afferents and may have been from other dorsal root afferents.

In a spared root rhizotomy the surviving primary afferents show evidence of sprouting, although it may be limited to the normal root projection area, with no greater rostral or caudal extent [17, 57]. More recently, in rats with a unilateral spared L5 root preparation, sciatic injection of BHRP, which preferentially labels myelinated afferents, resulted in increased density of labeling in the deep dorsal horn and the nucleus of Clarke on the lesioned side [35].

Crush, transection, and loose ligature of a peripheral nerve produce various degrees of degeneration of the central terminals of the afferents. However, the resulting reorganization includes at least partial regeneration of terminals from the injured nerve ; these terminal patterns may be altered, including extension of myelinated afferents into lamina II [56]. In contrast, there appears to be little or no sprouting by neighboring, non-injured afferents, although there may be a rearrangement of terminal fields within normal boundaries of the afferents' distribution [22, 36, 46]. Nevertheless, there are some exceptions when the experimental conditions are modified. For example, the territory of the adult rat saphenous nerve did not increase following either sciatic section or saphenous crush alone, but did increase approximately 10% following combination of the two lesions [29]. Additional studies using HRP methods have shown sprouting of non-injured dorsal root afferents after peripheral nerve lesions in the neonate [39], but a failure to sprout in the older animal [13]. Sprouting in the neonate has also been demonstrated following treatment with capsaicin, which destroys a majority of nonmyelinated (C) dorsal root afferents ; this results in sprouting of large diameter primary afferents into areas of the adult rat superficial dorsal horn normally occupied by C fibers [32, 38].

In summary, injury to a peripheral nerve in the adult results in regeneration of the injured nerve's central processes ; elimination of the primary afferents by rhizotomy results in sprouting by other spinal systems ; and elimination of a selected group of afferents by spared root results in central sprouting of normal, neighboring afferents.

A model of deafferentation using pronase injection

At the beginning of our studies, we hypothesized that the reason for failure of sprouting by non-injured afferents after peripheral nerve section in adult animals, in contrast to neonates, could be due to an alteration of the stimulus to sprout, rather than to an inability to generate collateral sprouts in the adult animal. That is, peripheral nerve section may induce severe ganglion cell death and central terminal atrophy in the neonate [1], but since many ganglion cells survive in the older animal after nerve section [12, 19, 58], fewer primary afferent terminals are eliminated. In that case, sprouting would be less likely or less abundant.

We sought to determine if injection of a mixture of proteolytic enzymes (pronase) into the sciatic nerve could be used as an effective method of lesioning its ganglion cells, based on a report by Parnas and Bowling [33] in which pronase was used to lesion single neurons in the leech. This technique was chosen as one which would be safer for laboratory use than injection of ricin, and because of some question that suicide transport of ricin may or may not result in spread in the dorsal root ganglia [53]. Pronase produced death of the majority of myelinated and nonmyelinated sciatic axons, along with nerve scarring and mast cell invasion [26] ; within the dorsal root ganglion many cells also were destroyed [25]. Leakage to adjacent nonsciatic ganglion cells, or to adjacent axons in the root entry zone or dorsal columns did not appear to occur, since neighboring ganglion cells and the adjacent dorsal column areas were normal in appearance. Further, degenerating terminals in the dorsal horn were restricted to the normal sciatic terminal field when compared to mapping of the sciatic with HRP and WGA-HRP. Thus, pronase produced many more degenerated terminals than nerve section, and the degenerated area was well localized to the sciatic territory, in contrast to the widespread degeneration produced by rhizotomy [21, 25].

There were also significant deafferentation responses of the dendrites of dorsal horn cells and of the spinal glia which were similar after either rhizotomy, nerve section, or pronase injection [21, 25]. Postsynaptic dendritic cavitation, darkening, and accumulation of osmiophilic floccular material resulted within 2-3 weeks from all three types of dorsal horn deafferentation ; further, glial reactivity was clearly evident, including glial expansions and wrapping of thin sheaths around degenerating terminals and dendrites (Figure 1). Loss of terminals from dendritic and somatic spines was common, with replacement by glial sheaths. Although similar changes have been described following nerve section [16, 48] and in the nuclei of other deafferented systems [2, 7, 8, 14, 15, 30, 34, 45, 52], such changes had not been previously reported in the dorsal horn following rhizotomy. More recently, immunostaining for MAP 2 (microtubule-associated protein 2), a cytoskeletal protein present specifically in dendrites, has confirmed the reduction of dendritic mass in the dorsal horn after dorsal rhizotomy [20] ; we have seen a similar, but temporary reduction after pronase injection (Figure 2). These findings suggest that the degree of reorganization that occurs within the dorsal horn following injury to dorsal root afferents is substantial. Particularly, the dendritic atrophy and glial engulfment of dendrites as well as terminals result in loss not only of primary afferent synapses but also of other systems impinging on that region of the dendrite. Such changes would drastically alter the influence of remaining inputs on the soma and surviving dendrites. Furthermore, possible restructuring by sprouting and reestablishment of synapses is likely to be even more complex than previously thought, considering that postsynaptic structures and other terminals are partially eliminated and possibly restored.

Central sprouting of saphenous afferents after sciatic pronase injection

After finding that injection of the sciatic nerve with pronase would allow selective destruction of sciatic ganglion cells and their central terminals, we injected pronase into the sciatic nerve of adult rats in order to determine if a profound loss of sciatic afferents would produce afferent collateral sprouting in the adult rat. Four months later, saphenous terminal fields were labeled bilaterally by injecting the saphenous nerves

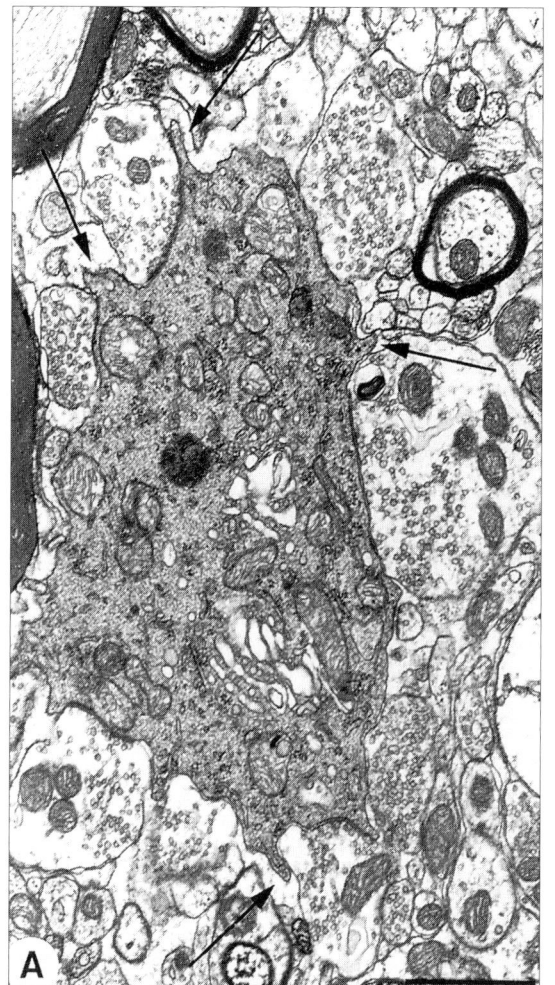

Figure 1. A dendrite from lamina IV dorsal horn at L4, 20 days after pronase injection of the ipsilateral sciatic nerve. Ultrastructural changes include darkening, loss of terminals on dendritic spines, and replacement by glial extensions (arrows). Note several degenerating terminals in contact with the dendrite. Bar = 1 μm [25].

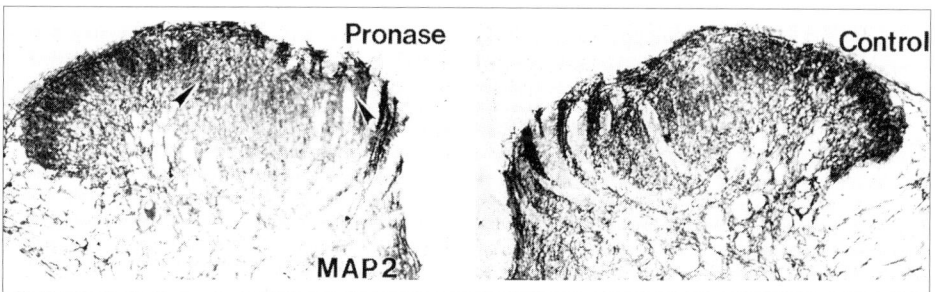

Figure 2. Photomicrograph of MAP 2 immunostaining in the left and right dorsal horn from a section at the L4 level of the spinal cord, from a rat in which the left sciatic nerve was injected with pronase 3 weeks prior to sacrifice. The immunostaining is reduced in a medial and central area of the superficial dorsal horn, corresponding to the sciatic territory. The reduction suggests loss of dendrites, which normally stain well for MAP 2.

with WGA-HRP ; on the lesioned side, the terminal field of the saphenous nerve was expanded in the medial, lateral and caudal directions (Figure 3). The expansion resulted in a total saphenous area 26% larger than the control side [26].

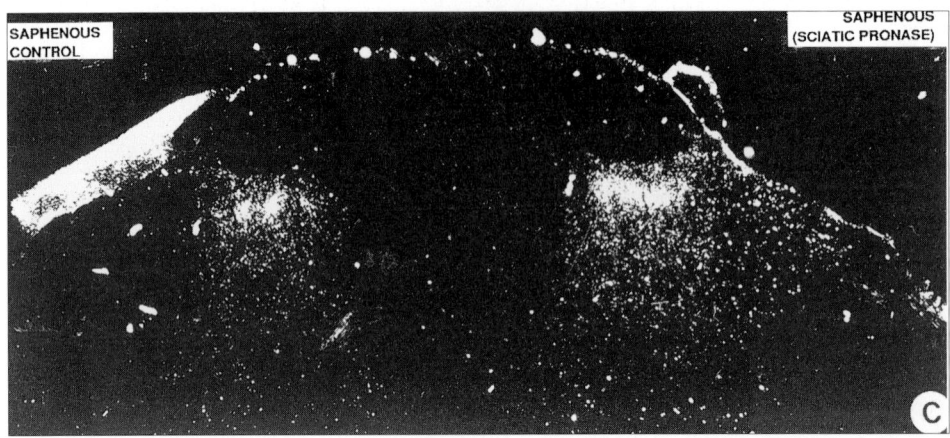

Figure 3. Darkfield photomicrograph of a section at the L3/4 level of the rat cord from a rat in which the right sciatic nerve was injected with pronase 4 months prior to labeling both the left and right saphenous nerves with WGA-HRP and HRP. These tracers primarily labeled nonmyelinated and finely myelinated afferents. The terminal field of the right saphenous nerve is expanded medially and lateraly and increased in density. Note that the laminar distribution of these afferents is restricted to the superficial dorsal horn and not altered on the pronase side. [26].

Thus, the pronase model appears to most closely parallel the spared root rhizotomy preparation ; that is, it eliminates a group of selected primary afferents and promotes sprouting of neighboring, normal afferents [18, 35, 57]. However, the pronase model may have certain advantages. It is simpler and less invasive, with less potential damage to the spinal cord, and it produces a small, discrete region of central deafferentation.

There is a similar expansion of the saphenous territory in laminae III and IV, demonstrated by using the tracer BHRP (B subunit of cholera toxin conjugated to HRP) to label myelinated afferents [28] (Figure 4). BHRP was chosen because several studies have demonstrated that it selectively labels myelinated axons of all sizes that distribute to laminae I, III, IV and V of the dorsal horn, as well as to the ventral horn and other targets of myelinated axons [27, 41, 43, 44].

The use of differential labeling of large and small diameter saphenous afferents, using BHRP or WGA-HRP, respectively, also showed that although both afferent types have expanded territories into the sciatic region, there is no crossover of laminar fields by either fiber group ; that is, the small diameter afferents remain in the superficial dorsal horn, and the large afferents in the deep dorsal horn. This finding is of particular interest to us. BHRP labeled afferents are not normally found in lamina II and there is no crossing of the lamina II border by sprouting BHRP labeled afferents from laminae

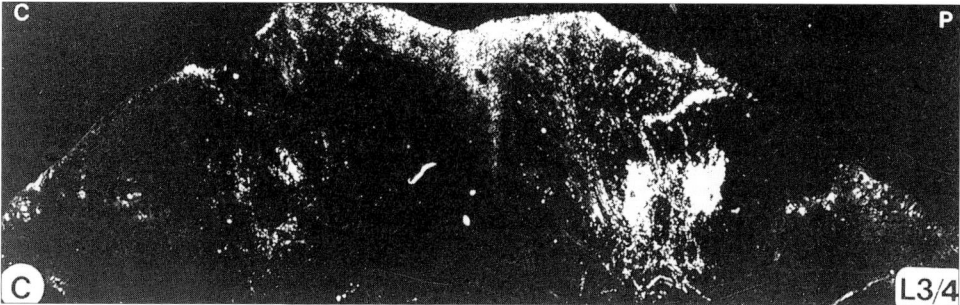

Figure 4. Darkfield photomicrograph of a section at the L3/4 level of the spinal cord from a rat in which the right sciatic nerve was injected with pronase 4 months prior to labeling both the left and right saphenous nerves with BHRP. This tracer labels only myelinated axons of all sizes. The terminal field of the right saphenous nerve is expanded medially and laterally and increased in density. Note that the laminar distribution of these afferents is restricted to lamina I and to the deeper dorsal horn and not altered on the pronase side. [28].

III-V. Thus, the integrity of the substantia gelatinosa is preserved, such that types of intact primary afferents which are not normally found in the area cannot penetrate there in the adult under the experimental conditions described in the pronase model. This result contrasts, however, with the effects of other experimental conditions which have been reported to alter projections of primary afferents to lamina II. Diffuse lesions of the monkey spinal cord increased the density of dorsal root terminals in laminae I and II, when measured 14-18 months later [3] ; however, it was not determined if these terminals arose from small or large diameter afferents. Two other studies have indicated that the specific removal of nonmyelinated (C) afferents in the neonate induces a laminar shift of the larger diameter afferents. HRP labeling was used by Nagy and Hunt [32] to demonstrate that neonatal capsaicin treatment, which destroys a majority of nonmyelinated (C) dorsal root afferents, results in sprouting of large diameter primary afferents into areas of the rat superficial dorsal horn normally occupied by C fibers. Rethelyi *et al.* [38] also observed neonatal administration of capsaicin in the rat to produce a spread of thick primary afferents from laminae III and IV into lamina II, with a differential distribution of hairy skin and non hairy skin afferent fiber types in the lateral and medial areas, respectively. Laminar boundaries can also be trespassed by collaterals of injured axons, as shown recently by Woolf *et al.* [56] ; they used BHRP labeling to demonstrate that axotomized sciatic and sural myelinated afferents sprout into lamina II after 1 to 15 weeks. In our study, the absence of sprouting into the substantia gelatinosa by BHRP labeled afferents may reflect competition by the sprouting C and A delta fibers observed in the substantia gelatinosa ; as long as these fibers are available to sprout they appear to maintain dominance in the area and exclude invasion of the superficial dorsal horn by larger afferents.

Sprouting of saphenous afferents is not limited to the dorsal horn. The saphenous afferents within the nucleus gracilis also expand their territory when the sciatic is injected with pronase [27] (Figure 5).

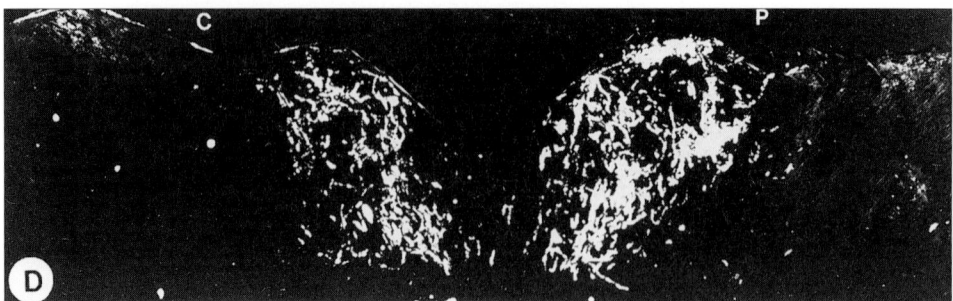

Figure 5. Darkfield photmicrograph of the nucleus gracilis from a section near the obex of a rat in which the right sciatic nerve was injected with pronase 4 months prior to labeling both the left and right saphenous nerves with BHRP. The labeled terminals are concentrated in the gracile nucleii the density and territory is increased on the pronase treated side [28].

Ultrastructure and differentiation of sprouted terminals

The WGA-HRP and BHRP label in both the normal and expanded territories of the saphenous nerve is primarily contained in axons and terminals, with minor transneuronal labeling [26]. Labeled terminals in the expanded areas are both simple terminals with round, clear vesicles, and glomerular terminals with multiple synaptic contacts ; these terminal types resemble those previously described for primary afferents in the superficial dorsal horn [5, 40].

The changes in sprouted terminals are also interesting when one compares profiles of control and pronase side saphenous terminals to normal sciatic terminals (Table I). There are two main types of glomerular terminals in the rat laminae II and III. These are Type I terminals, found predominantly in lamina II and thought to arise from fine diameter axons ; and Type II terminals, found more commonly in lamina III and thought to arise from myelinated axons [5, 40]. The mean number of synaptic contacts found on profiles of normal Type I saphenous terminals was significantly less than on normal sciatic terminals. However, the mean number of synaptic contacts of the saphenous terminal profiles on the experimental side, selected from the area of expanded terminal field, was equal to mean of sciatic profiles. This was also true for the population of Type II terminal profiles labeled by WGA-HRP. The number of synaptic contacts of Type II profiles labeled by BHRP were the same for control, experimental, and sciatic. In summary, in each case, the experimental saphenous profiles matched the sciatic profiles, but the control saphenous profiles were different from the sciatic in three out of four populations. The perimeter of the Type I terminals also increased with the increase in number of synapses, to the point that the sprouted saphenous terminal profiles were larger than either the control saphenous or the sciatic. The Type II terminal profiles showed less change in size, and the experimental terminals either increased in size (WGA-HRP terminals), matching the sciatic terminals, or did not change (BHRP

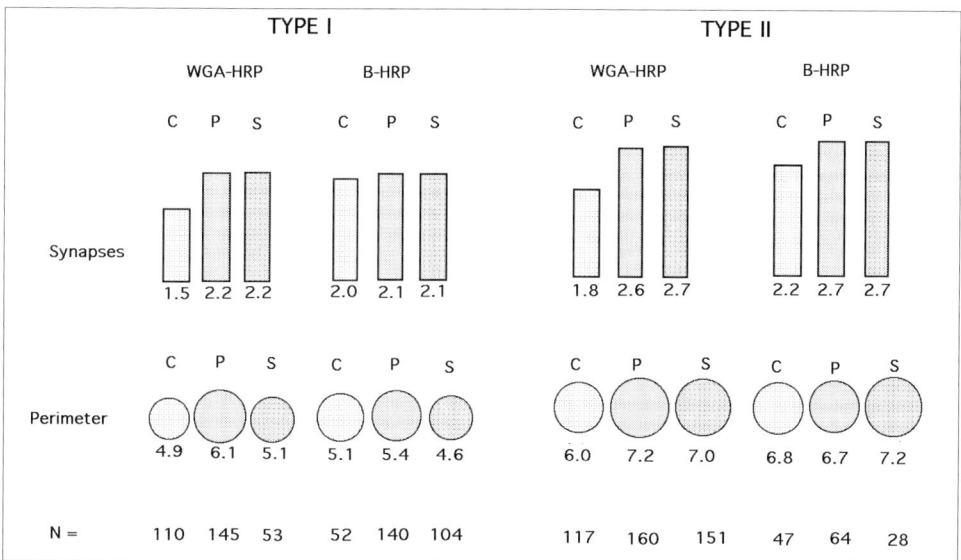

Table I. Summary of analysis of labelled synaptic terminals in pronase and control material. Type I and Type II indicate types of synaptic glomeruli. WGA-HRP and B-HRP indicate the type of tracer injected into a nerve. C and P indicate data for labelled saphenous terminals from the control and pronase treated side of rats surviving 4 months after pronase injection of the sciatic nerve. S indicates data for labelled normal sciatic terminals. Bars indicate the average number of synaptic specializations observed on single cross-sections of Type I or II terminals in the superficial dorsal horn ; value of the bars is given in the numbers below each bar. Circles indicate the average perimeter of the same terminals ; numbers below indicate perimeter in microns. N indicates the number of terminals analyzed in each case.

terminals) in size when the control saphenous matched the sciatic. (It should be noted that these results are based on the measurement of profiles of terminals, and do not give information on the three dimensional properties of the terminals and their synaptic contacts ; therefore there may be sampling bias in the actual counts and measurements, but the direction of the changes would not be likely affected).

The overall increase in terminal size and synaptic contacts, which was especially prominent for WGA terminals, when considered by label, and for Type I terminals, when considered by type, strongly implicates the C and A delta afferents as being more active in modifying their typical morphology when creating new terminals (El-Bohy and LaMotte in preparation).

Peptide and receptor changes

In order to assess changes in peptidergic structures in the dorsal horn in the pronase model, we have studied 20 experimental rats immunostained for SP, CGRP, CCK, SS,

NPY, galanin and VIP. Using a computerized densitometry analysis system, segments L2-3 and L4-5 were studied, using paired data in which a pair represents the control and the pronase values of a single section. Although there was little change in NPY or galanins, four peptides, *i.e.* CGRP, SP, CCK and SS, were significantly decreased in staining density in the superficial dorsal horn on the pronase side in both the short (10 days) and long (4 months) survival groups [10] (Figure 6). In each case, the decrease was greater in the L4-5 region than in the L1-3 region, matching the distribution pattern of sciatic afferents to these segments. The greatest effect was shown by CGRP and SP ; after an initial depletion, there was a 70-80% recovery by four months. CGRP terminals in the dorsal horn are presumed to arise only from primary afferents ; no other sources have been found to project to this area [4, 49]. The recovery seen in the long term animals may be due to sprouting of afferents from other nerves, such as the saphenous. The saphenous sprouting occurs mainly in L3 and at the L3/4 border, and this is where the recovery of CGRP was greatest. A similar, but slightly less effect, was obtained for SP. Most SP in the dorsal horn arises from primary afferents, but there are also local neurons and descending sources ; these multiple contributors likely dilute the effect of the primary afferent loss. The data for CCK and SS, which are also derived from multiple sources, showed only a slight recovery with time. In summary, these results may indicate that primary afferents which sprout following deafferentation may not only establish synaptic connections which morphologically resemble those which were removed, but also may neurochemically resemble the replaced synapses. We have found little change in either short term or long term animals for immunostaining of VIP, NPY, enkephalin, GABA and 5-HT immunoreactivity, using the same paradigm. However, galanin increased in the short term animals and returned to normal by four months [11].

We have recently begun a quantitative receptor autoradiography study to determine the distribution and density of peptidergic (SP, CGRP, mu, delta, and kappa opiates),

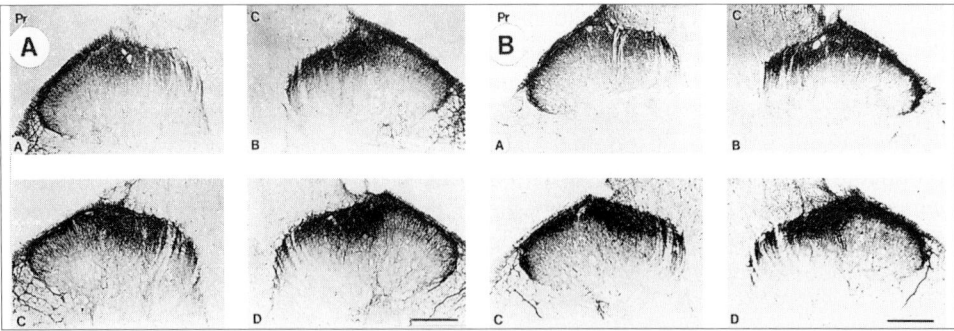

Figure 6. Photomicrographs of CGRP (left pairs) and SP (right pairs) immunostaining at the L4 level of the dorsal horn from a short-term (A,B) and long-term (C,D) animal. The CGRP and SP immunoreactivity is reduced in the central and medial area of the short-term dorsal horn on the pronase treated side and partially recovered in the long-term animals. Bar = 200 µm [10].

inhibitory neurotransmitter (GABA, 5-HT) and excitatory amino acid (glutamate) binding sites in the dorsal horn of short and long term pronase injected animals. Our preliminary results indicate an increase in SP binding by 10 days, correlating with the loss of SP immunostaining, and a return to normal levels of binding by 4 months, correlating with the partial restoration of SP observed by this time (Figure 7).

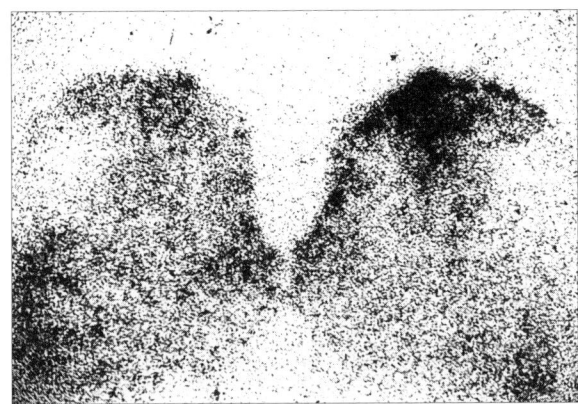

Figure 7. Photomicrograph of autoradiograph of SP binding at the L4 level of the dorsal horn from a short term animal, illustrating increased binding (arrow) in the dorsal horn on the pronase treated (right) side.

Terminal guidance and growth

One approach to understanding the process by which sprouted processes establish their distinct locations on their target neurons and differentiate into synaptic terminals is to examine the growth of these terminals at different stages in their development and to determine changes in their environment and the extracellular matrix. Some of these events can be detected by immunohistochemical demonstration of several substances, including GAP 43 and NCAM.

GAP 43 (growth-associated protein) is found in growth cones and is thought to influence neurite elongation and synaptic formation [55]. GAP 43 increases within 4 days in the superficial dorsal horn after sciatic cut or crush, reaches a maximum at 21 days, and drops to normal by 9 weeks after crush and by 36 weeks after sciatic cut [23, 47, 55]. GAP 43 increases in the superficial dorsal horn by 10 days after injection of the sciatic nerve with pronase. By 20 days it spreads into the deep dorsal horn, and surrounds many neurons (Figure 8) ; after one month the immunostaining returns to normal.

NCAM (neural cell adhesion molecule) is thought to mediate adhesion of neurons to neurons and to other types of cells (glia, muscle) and may affect formation and distribution of new synaptic contacts. It is highly concentrated in developing structures, but much reduced in most areas in the adult [6, 9, 50]. NCAM immunostaining shows a similiar pattern to GAP 43 in the pronase model ; NCAM increases in the superficial

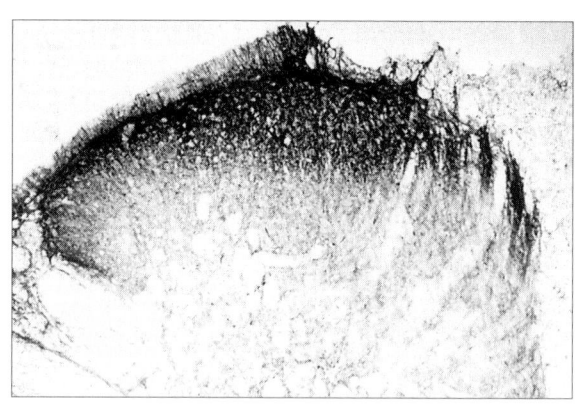

Figure 8. Photomicrograph of GAP 43 immunostaining in the left dorsal horn from a section at the L4 level of the spinal cord, from a rat in which the left sciatic nerve was injected with pronase 3 weeks prior to sacrifice. Although GAP 43 immunoreactivity is normally low, the density of GAP 43 is greatly increased in the dorsal horn on the pronase treated side, as shown.

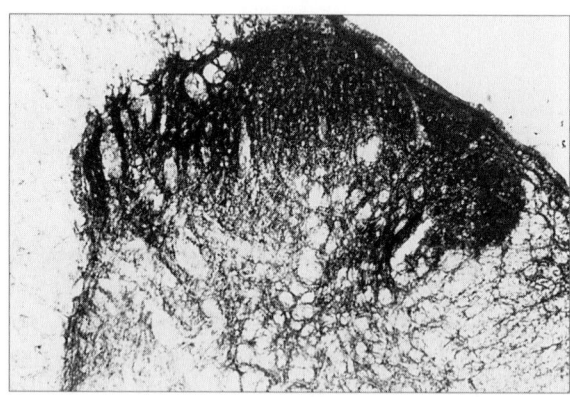

Figure 9. Photomicrograph of NCAM immunostaining in the left dorsal horn from a section at the L4 level of the spinal cord, from a rat in which the left sciatic nerve was injected with pronase 3 weeks prior to sacrifice. Although NCAM immunoreactivity is normally low, the density of NCAM is greatly increased in the dorsal horn on the pronase treated side, as shown.

dorsal horn by 10 days after pronase injection, and it spreads into the dorsal horn by 20 days (Figure 9); after one month staining returns to normal.

We interpret the data from this time series as indicating that different classes of axons may begin the process of sprouting at different times, and that sprouting may be correlated both with the timecourse of degeneration of the lesioned afferents and with the expression of guidance factors. The very early appearance of NCAM, and GAP 43 in laminae I and II may imply that the small diameter afferents begin the process of sprouting earlier than the larger diameter afferents that sprout in the deep dorsal horn. The delayed appearance of NCAM and GAP 43 in the deep dorsal horn supports this idea. The sprouting of terminals in laminae I and II before sprouting in the deeper dorsal horn may be related to the observation that primary afferents which terminate in the superficial dorsal horn degenerate and are removed within the first few days after rhizotomy, while degeneration of terminals in the deeper dorsal horn persists for more than a week [24, 37]. Thus early degeneration and clearance may precipitate early sprouting.

The persistence of GAP 43 for 1-2 months beyond the expression of NCAM may indicate that the first few weeks after injury are devoted to the guidance of sprouting axons to their targets, and that there is then a longer period of growth and maturation of the terminals and establishment of functional synapses.

Acknowledgement

Supported by NIH grants NS10174, NS 13335, NS 28876, and grants from the Spinal Cord Research Foundation of the Paralyzed Veterans Association and the Eastern Paralyzed Veterans Association.

References

1. Aldskogius H, Risling M. Effect of sciatic neurectomy on neuronal number and size distribution in the L7 ganglion of kittens. *Exp Neurol* 1981 ; 74 : 597-604.
2. Benes FM, Parks TN, Rubel EW. Rapid dendritic atrophy following deafferentation : an EM morphometric analysis. *Brain Res* 1977 ; 205 : 289-98.
3. Bullitt EW, Stofer D, Vierck CJ, Perl ER. Reorganization of primary afferent nerve terminals in the spinal dorsal horn of the primate caudal to anterolateral chordotomy. *J Comp Neurol* 1988 ; 270 : 549-58 ; 272 : 383-408.
4. Carlton SM, McNeill DL, Chung K, Coggeshall RE. A light and electron microscopic level analysis of calcitonin gene-related peptide (CGRP) in the spinal cord of the primate : an immunohistochemical study. *Neurosci Lett* 1987 ; 82 : 145-50.
5. Cruz F, Lima D, Zieglgansberger W, Coimbra A. Fine structure and synaptic architecture of HRP-labelled primary afferent terminations in lamina IIi of the rat dorsal horn. *J Comp Neurol* 1991 ; 305 : 3-16.
6. Daniloff J, Levi G, Grumet M, Rieger F, Edelman GM. Altered expression of neuronal cell adhesion molecules induced by nerve injury and repair *J Cell Biol* 1986 ; 103 : 929-45.
7. Deitch JS, Rubel EW. Rapid changes in ultrastructure during deafferentation-induced dendritic atrophy. *J Comp Neurol* 1989 ; 281 : 234-58.
8. Deitch JS, Rubel EW. Changes in neuronal cell bodies in N laminaris during deafferentation-induced dendritic atrophy. *J Comp Neurol* 1989 ; 281 : 259-68.
9. DiFiglia M, Marshall P, Covault J, Yamamoto M. Ultrastructural localization of molecular subtypes of immunoreactive neural cell adhesion molecule (NCAM) in the adult rodent striatum. *J Neurosci* 1989 ; 9 : 4158-69.
10. El-Bohy A, LaMotte CC. Deafferentation-induced changes in neuropeptides of the adult rat dorsal horn following pronase injection of the sciatic nerve. *J Comp Neurol* 1993 ; 336 : 1-10.
11. El-Bohy A, Arsenault KE, LaMotte CC. Deafferentation induced increase of galanin in the rat dorsal horn. *Soc Neurosci* 1992 ; 18 : 133 (Abstract).
12. Faull RL, Villiger JW. Opiate receptors in the human spinal cord : a detailed anatomical study comparing the autoradiographic localization of 3Hdiprenorphine binding sites with the laminar pattern of substance P myelin and nissl staining. *Neuroscience* 1987 ; 20(2) : 395-407.
13. Fitzgerald M. The sprouting of saphenous nerve terminals in the spinal cord following early postnatal sciatic nerve section in the rat. *J Comp Neurol* 1985 ; 240 : 407.
14. Gentschev T, Sotelo C. Degenerative patterns in the ventral cochlear nucleus of the rat after primary deafferentation : an ultrastructural study. *Brain Res* 1973 ; 62 : 37-60.

15. Ghetti B, Hovoupian DS, Wisniewski HM. Transynaptic response of the lateral geniculate nucleus and the pattern of degeneration of the nerve terminals in the rhesus monkey after eye enucleation. *Brain Res* 1972 ; 45 : 31-48.
16. Gobel S. An electron microscopic analysis of the transsynaptic effects of peripheral nerve injury subsequent to tooth pulp extirpations on neurons in laminae I and II of the medullary dorsal horn. *J Neurosci* 1984 ; 4 : 2281-90.
17. Goldberger ME, Murray M. Lack of sprouting and its presence after lesions of the cat spinal cord. *Brain Res* 1982 ; 241 : 227-39.
18. Goldberger ME, Murray M. Recovery of function and anatomical plasticity after damage to the adult and neonatal spinal cord. In : Cotman C, ed. *Synaptic plasticity*. New York : Guilford, 1985 : 77-110.
19. Himes BT, TesslerA. Death of some dorsal root ganglion neurons and plasticity of others following sciatic nerve section in adult and neonatal rats. *J Comp Neurol* 1989 ; 284 : 215-30.
20. Hirakawa M, Kawata M. Changes of chemoarchitectural organization of the rat spinal cord following ventral and dorsal root transection. *J Comp Neurol* 1992 ; 320 : 339-52.
21. Kapadia SE, LaMotte CC. Deafferentation-induced alterations in the rat dorsal horn : I. Comparison of peripheral nerve injury vs rhizotomy effects on presynaptic postsynaptic and glial processes. *J Comp Neurol* 1987 ; 266 : 183-97.
22. Kerr FWL. The potential of cervical primary afferents to sprout in the spinal nucleus of V following long term trigeminal denervation. *Brain Res* 1972 ; 43 : 547-60.
23. Knyihar-Csillik E, Csillik B, Oestreicher AB. Light and electron microscopic localization of B-50 (GAP 43) in the rat spinal cord during transganglionic degenerative atrophy and regeneration. 1992 ; 32(1) : 93-109.
24. LaMotte CC. Distribution of the tract of Lissauer and dorsal root fibers in the primate spinal cord. *J Comp Neurol* 1977 ; 172 : 529-61.
25. LaMotte CC, Kapadia SE. Deafferentation-induced alterations in the rat dorsal horn : II. Effects of selective poisioning by pronase of the central processes of a peripheral nerve. *J Comp Neurol* 1987 ; 266 : 198-208.
26. LaMotte CC, Kapadia SE, Kocol CM. Deafferentation-induced expansion of saphenous terminal field labelling in the adult rat dorsal horn following pronase injection of the sciatic nerve. *J Comp Neurol* 1989 ; 288 : 311-25.
27. LaMotte CC, Kapadia SE, Shapiro CM. Central projections of the sciatic saphenous median and ulnar nerves of the rat demonstrated by transganglionic transport of choleragenoid-HRP (B-HRP) and wheat germ agglutinin-HRP(WGA-HRP). *J Comp Neurol* 1991 ; 311 : 546-62.
28. LaMotte CC, Kapadia SE. Deafferentation-induced terminal field expansion of myelinated saphenous afferents in the adult rat dorsal horn and the nucleus gracilis following pronase injection of the sciatic nerve. *J Comp Neurol* 1993 ; 330 : 83-94.
29. Molander C, Kinnman E, Aldskogius H. Expansion of spinal cord primary sensory afferent projection following combined sciatic nerve resection and saphenous nerve crush : a horseradish peroxidase study in the adult rat. *J Comp Neurol* 1988 ; 276 : 436-.41
30. Mouren-Mathieu A, Colonnier M. The molecular layer of the adult cat cerebellar cortex after lesion of the parallel fibers : an optic and electron microscope study. *Brain Res* 1969 ; 16 : 307-23.
31. Murray M, Goldberger ME. Replacement of synaptic terminals in lamina II and Clarke's nucleus after unilateral lumbosacral dorsal rhizotomy in adult cats. *J Neurosci* 1986 ; 6 : 3205-17.
32. Nagy JI, Hunt SP. The termination of primary afferents within the rat dorsal horn : evidence for rearrangement following capsaicin treatment. *J Comp Neurol* 1983 ; 218 : 145-58.
33. Parnas I, Bowling D. Killing of single neurones by intracellular injection of proteolytic enzymes. *Nature* 1977 ; 270 : 626-8.

34. Pinching AJ, Powell TPS. Ultrastructural features of transneuronal cell degeneration in the olfactory system. *J Cell Sci* 1971 ; 8 : 253-87.
35. Polistina D, Murray M, Goldberger ME. Myelinated fibers contribute to dorsal root sprouting after partial deafferentation in rats ? *Soc Neurosci* 1987 ; 13 : 4710 (Abstract).
36. Pubols LM, Bowen DC. Lack of central sprouting of primary afferent fibers after ricin deafferentation. *J Comp Neurol* 1988 ; 275 : 282-7.
37. Ralston HJ, Ralston DD. The distribution of dorsal root axons in laminae I II and III of the macaque spinal cord : a quantitative electron microscopic study. *J Comp Neurol* 1979 ; 184 : 643-84.
38. Rethelyi M, Salim MZ, Jansco G. Altered distribution of dorsal root fibers in the rat following neonatal capsaicin treatment. *Neuroscience* 1986 ; 18 : 749-61.
39. Rhoades RW, Mooney RD, Chiaia NL, Bennett-Clarke CA. Development and plasticity of the serotoninergic projection to the Hamster's superior colliculus. *J Comp Neurol* 1990 ; 299 : 151-66.
40. Ribeiro-da-Silva A, Coimbra A. Two types of synaptic glomeruli and their distribution in laminae I-III of the rat spinal cord in the cat. *J Comp Neurol* 1982 ; 209 : 176-86.
40. Rivero-Melian C, Grant G. Somatotopic organization of hindlimb muscle afferent projections to the column of Clarke of the rat studied with choleragenoid horseradish peroxidase conjugate. *Soc Neurosci* 1988 ; 14(1) : 693 (Abstract).
42. Rivero-Melian C, Grant G. Distribution of lumbar dorsal root fibers in the lower thoracic and lumbosacral spinal cord of the rat studied with choleragenoid horseradish peroxidase conjugate. *J Comp Neurol* 1990 ; 299 : 470-81.
43. Robertson B, Arvidsson J. Transganglionic transport of wheat germ agglutinin-HRP and choleragenoid-HRP in rat trigeminal primary sensory neurons. *Brain Res* 1985 ; 348 : 44-51.
44. Robertson B, Grant G. A comparison between wheat germ agglutinin and choleragenoid-horseradish peroxidase as anterogradely transported markers in central branches of primary sensory neurones in the rat with some observations in the cat. *Neuroscience* 1985 ; 14 : 895-905.
45. Rustioni A, Sotelo C. Some effects of chronic deafferentation on the ultrastructure of the nucleus gracilis of the cat. *Brain Res* 1974 ; 73 : 527-33.
46. Seltzer Z, Devor M. Effect of nerve section on the spinal distribution of neighboring nerves. *Brain Res* 1984 ; 306 : 31-7.
47. Sommervaille T, Reynolds ML, Woolf CJ. Time-dependent differences in the increase in GAP-43 expression in dorsal root ganglion cells after peripheral axotomy. *Neuroscience* 1991 ; 45 : 213-20.
48. Sugimoto T, Gobel S. Dendritic changes in the spinal dorsal horn following transection of a peripheral nerve. *Brain Res* 1984 ; 321 : 199-208.
49. Traub R, Solodkin JA, Ruda MA. Calcitonin gene-related peptide immunoreactivity in the cat lumbosacral spinal cord and the effects of multiple dorsal rhizotomies. *J Comp Neurol* 1989 ; 287 : 225-37.
50. Van den Pol AN, Kim WT. NILE/L1 and NCAM-polysialic acid expression on growing axons of isolated neurons. *J Comp Neurol* 1993 ; 332 : 237-57.
51. Wang S, Goldberger E, Murray M. Plasticity of spinal systems after unilateral lumbosacral dorsal rhizotomy in the adult rat. *J Comp Neurol* 1991 ; 304 : 555-68.
52. Wells J, Tripp LN. Time course of the reaction of glial fibers in the somatosensory thalamus after lesions in the dorsal column nuclei. *J Comp Neurol* 1987 ; 255 : 476-82.
53. Wiley RG, Neural lesioning with ribosome-inactivating proteins : suicide transport and immunolesioning. *TINS* 1992 ; 15 : 285-90.
54. Wiesenfeld-Hallen Z. Substance P and somatostatin modulated spinal cord excitability via physiologically different sensory pathways. *Neurosci Lett* 1986 ; 372 : 172-5.

55. Woolf CJ, Reynolds ML, Molander C, O'Brien C, Lindsay RM, Benowitz LI. The growth-associated protein GAP-43 appears in dorsal root ganglion cells and in the dorsal horn of the rat spinal cord following peripheral nerve injury. *Neuroscience* 1990 ; 34 : 465-78.
56. Woolf CJ, Shortland P, Coggeshall RE. Peripheral nerve injury triggers central sprouting of myelinated afferents. *Nature* 1992 ; 355 : 75-8.
57. Wu LF, Petry-Battisti W, Goldberger ME, Murray M. Spared root deafferentation of cat spinal cord : anatomical recovery. *Soc Neurosci* 1986 ; 12 : 114 (Abstract).
58. Yip HK, Rich KM, Lampe PA, Johnson EM. The effects of nerve growth factor and its antiserum on the postnatal development and survival after injury of sensory neurons in rat dorsal root ganglia. *J Neurosci* 1984 ; 12 : 2986-92.

16

Plasticity of sensory transmission and modulation following peripheral nerve lesion with special emphasis on peptidergic, nitric oxidergic, α_2 adrenergic and opioidergic systems

X.J. XU, Z. WIESENFELD-HALLIN

Department of Clinical Physiology, Section of Clinical Neurophysiology, Karolinska Institute, Huddinge University Hospital, Huddinge, Sweden.

The chemical composition of primary sensory neurons is dramatically altered after injury to their peripheral axons. There are complex changes in the levels of peptides, as well as other chemical mediators, such as nitric oxide synthase (NOS), in the somata of sensory neurons and their terminals. In addition, the receptor systems in the spinal cord which normally exert a role in modulating sensory input can be also altered after peripheral nerve lesion. The present article reviews results from experimental studies conducted in our laboratory in recent years concerning the functional significance of some of these plastic changes in sensory neurons and spinal cord involved in sensory transmission and modulation, as well as the occurrence of experimental neuropathic pain.

Peptides of the tachykinin family found in primary afferents, such as substance P (SP) and neurokinin A (NKA), normally participate in the generation of spinal cord hyperexcitability in rats after repetitive conditioning stimulation (CS) of unmyelinated afferents. After nerve section, vasoactive intestinal peptide (VIP), which is upregulated in primary sensory afferents after axotomy, takes over the role of SP in mediating spinal hyperexcitability after C-fiber CS of cutaneous nerves. Another upregulated peptide, galanin, however, apparently has an endogenous inhibitory role in sensory transmission in axotomized rats. Nitric oxide (NO), whose synthetic enzyme is also upregulated in sensory neurons, is involved in both the induction of spinal hyperexcitability after C-fiber CS, as well as in the generation of spontaneous activity in A-fibers by dorsal root ganglia.

The sensitivity of the spinal cord flexor reflex to the depressive effect of morphine and clonidine was also changed after peripheral nerve lesion. In rats which autotomized following axotomy, a possible indication of the presence of neuropathic pain, the efficacy of the reflex depressive effect of morphine was decreased. In contrast, the effect of clonidine was enhanced in axotomized rats. The changes in the sensitivity of the spinal cord to these two drugs after nerve injury was reflected by their differential effectiveness with chronic intrathecal (i.t.) application on autotomy behavior. The ineffectiveness of morphine was reversed by the cholecystokinin (CCK)-B receptor antagonist CI988, indicating that morphine insensitivity was related to the upregulation of CCK in primary afferents after axotomy.

The present series of studies demonstrated that complex functional plasticity in the transmission and modulation of sensory signals occurs as a result of peripheral nerve injury. Some of the changes may be involved in the induction and maintenance of sensory abnormalities associated with nerve injury. Based on these plasticities, drugs that affect peptidergic, NO-ergic and α_2-adrenergic systems may be useful in treating neuropathic pain.

Effects of peripheral nerve injury on the expression and functions of neuropeptides in primary sensory afferents

Peripheral nerve injury causes complex physiological and biochemical changes in sensory neurons and the spinal cord, including dramatic alteration in peptide synthesis. Thus, a few days after axotomy of the peripheral branch of sensory nerves, there is a significant decrease in the number of SP and somatostatin (SOM) containing dorsal root ganglion (DRG) cells and SP and SOM content in afferent terminals in the spinal cord [4, 21, 37], which was recently demonstrated to be due to decreased synthesis in sensory neurons [30]. Similar, but less profound and slower reduction of the level of calcitonin gene-related peptide (CGRP) level has also been reported [47]. In contrast, the levels of VIP, galanin (GAL), neuropeptide Y (NPY) and cholecystokinin (CCK) are dramatically increased in sensory neurons [17, 26, 37, 44, 49], which is due to upregulated peptide synthesis [30, 44, 46].

The functional significance of these changes in peptide levels after peripheral axotomy has been unclear, although it has been proposed that peptides like VIP may have trophic functions to promote neuronal regeneration [24]. In recent years, our laboratory has been engaged in examining the involvement of peptidergic systems in studies of plasticity in primary afferent and spinal cord functions after peripheral nerve injury and some of the results have been reviewed [59, 61, 66, 69]. We have employed an electrophysiological preparation in which the spinal nociceptive flexor reflex was recorded in decerebrate, spinalized, unanesthetized rats with intact peripheral nerves or after unilateral section of the sciatic nerve. The reflex is exquisitely sensitive to either i.t. or systemically applied drugs, with increased excitability following the application of hyperalgesic and decreased reflex magnitude after analgesic substances. In behavioral studies, we have used the autotomy model [52] to examine the involvement of some peptides in altering this behavioral sign of neuropathic pain.

A transient CS train of 20 shocks at 1 Hz applied to unmyelinated afferents elicits a pronounced increase in spinal cord excitability, lasting from a few minutes following cutaneous nerve stimulation to about one hour after activation of muscle afferents, as indicated by a prolonged facilitation of the flexor reflex [53]. This phenomenon, known as central sensitization, may reflect the hyperalgesia that occurs after tissue injury and can be blocked by peptide and non-peptide SP antagonists [60, 72], indicating that central sensitization may be mediated by the release of SP from C-afferents in rats with intact sciatic nerves. This conclusion seems, however, to be contradictory to the fact that there is severe depletion of SP from primary sensory afferents after nerve transection [4, 21] and yet the brief central sensitization remained in axotomized rats [54]. I.t. VIP, which is upregulated in DRG after nerve section [26, 37], is also capable of inducing spinal hyperexcitability [56]. We tested whether the ability of C-fibers to induce central sensitization may reflect the substitution of SP´s function by VIP. We compared the effect of the tachykinin antagonist spantide II [60] and the VIP-antagonist, (Ac-Tyr^1, D-Phe^2)-GRF (1-29) [48], on the facilitation of the flexor reflex induced by cutaneous C-fiber CS in rats with intact and sectioned sciatic nerves. In rats with intact sciatic nerves, pretreatment with spantide II effectively blocked reflex facilitation by the sural afferent CS with similar potency and duration to its blocking effect of i.t. SP [60] whereas no effect was found with the VIP-antagonist [70]. Ten to 14 days post axotomy, i.t. spantide II and the VIP-antagonist maintained their ability to block the reflex facilitation caused by i.t. SP and VIP respectively, just as in rats with intact sciatic nerves [61]. Furthermore, the sural CS caused comparable facilitation of the flexor reflex in rats with intact and sectioned sciatic nerves. However, the VIP-antagonist, but not spantide II, blocked the sural CS-induced reflex facilitation at 10-14 days post-axotomy [61]. Experiments performed at various times after nerve section revealed a linear decrease in the effectiveness of spantide II to block sural CS-induced reflex facilitation, which had the same time course as the decrease of SP synthesis in DRG after axotomy [30]. These results suggested that the normal role of tachykinins in inducing spinal hyperexcitability was taken over by VIP after peripheral nerve section. This was later confirmed morphologically, as a coexpression of VIP and SP mRNA was observed in some DRG neurons a few days after axotomy, indicating that VIP is produced in the same neurons after axotomy that previously produced SP [19].

GAL, a neuropeptide consisting of 29 amino acids, has been shown to occur in a relatively small population of DRG cells, primarily with small somata (*see* [65] for review). Previous studies in this and other laboratories have indicated that GAL may have inhibitory actions upon nociceptive transmission at the spinal level [33, 58, 59, 69, 79] ; *see* [65] for review). An increase in GAL synthesis and levels in primary sensory neurons and afferent terminals was demonstrated after peripheral nerve axotomy [17, 46]. Correspondingly, there was increased out-transport of newly synthesized GAL in both central and peripheral branches of primary sensory neurons [47]. These findings suggested that GAL may have a particularly important role in modulating sensory input in axotomized rats. Coadministration of GAL with the sural CS does-dependently suppressed reflex facilitation induced by the sural CS in animals with intact, as well as sectioned, nerves [58, 59, 69]. There was no significant difference in the ability of GAL to antagonize the facilitatory effect of sural CS before and after nerve section [69]. The antagonistic effect of GAL on sural CS induced spinal hyperexcitability in nerve intact rats was attributed, at least partly, to a post-synaptic antagonism of the facilitatory effect of i.t. SP and CGRP, peptides that coexist with GAL normally [69]. After nerve section, GAL blocked the reflex facilitation induced by VIP and CGRP, but not by SP. Meanwhile, a strong coexistence between GAL and VIP emerged in deafferented DRG cells [69].

With the help of a series of chimeric peptides that are high affinity GAL antagonists [5], we have examined the role of endogenous GAL in the mediation of spinal cord hyperexcitability and autotomy behavior. The GAL antagonist M35 [GAL (1-12)-Pro-bradykinin (2-9)-amide] potentiated the facilitation of the flexor reflex induced by sural nerve CS, an effect that was significantly enhanced in rats with sectioned sciatic nerves and after up-regulation of GAL in sensory neurons [66]. Similarly, chronic i.t. infusion of M35 through an osmotic minipump significantly exaggerated autotomy behavior in rats after unilateral sciatic nerve transection compared to saline treatment, without noticeably influencing the level of GAL mRNA in corresponding DRG and the dorsal horn [45]. Thus, GAL may play an endogenous inhibitory role in somatosensory transmission and along with an increase in GAL level in sensory neurons, this role may be enhanced after peripheral nerve injury. Therefore, GAL may possess an inhibitory control upon the expression of neuropathic pain related symptoms.

Effect of peripheral nerve injury on the expression and function of nitric oxide in primary sensory afferents

NO is a recently identified messenger in the nervous system and may have a variety of functions [8]. NO may mediate mechanical, chemical and thermal nociceptive input in the somatosensory system at the spinal level [16, 28]. NO is synthesized from L-arginine by the enzyme NO synthase (NOS). Due to its high lipophilicity, NO can diffuse through cell membranes and influence adjacent cells. NO has been suggested to function as a signalling system in rat dorsal root ganglia between sensory and satellite cells [29]. There was a marked increase in NOS mRNA in rat DRG within two days after peripheral nerve section, which was maintained for at least two months [43], and was paralleled by increase in NOS protein [80]. The increase in NOS mRNA in axotomized ganglion cells was similar to the increased levels of several neuropeptides and NOS mRNA was found to partially co-exist with the mRNA for these neuropeptides after axotomy [43]. We have conducted functional studies to examine the possible role of NO in somatosensory transmission in rats after peripheral nerve injury.

In the first series of experiments, we have examined the involvement of NO in the spinal cord and DRG in the mediation of spinal cord hyperexcitability after CS of cutaneous C-afferents [43]. The NOS inhibitor nitro-L-arginine methyl ester (L-NAME) applied i.t. blocked with similar efficacy the facilitation of the flexor reflex induced by C-afferent CS in rats with intact and sectioned sciatic nerves, indicating that NO may have a role in some aspect of nociceptive transmission at the spinal level which was not influenced by peripheral nerve section, which is in agreement with the finding that the level of NOS mRNA in the dorsal horn interneurons was unchanged after axotomy (Zhang et al., unpublished observation). In contrast, L-NAME applied intravenously was much more effective in blocking C-fiber CS-induced reflex facilitation in axotomized than in normal rats, suggesting that L-NAME may have a peripheral action involving C-fiber activation which was enhanced by axotomy and may be related to the upregulation of NOS in DRG.

Peripheral nerve injury can promote the development of ongoing discharges in both myelinated and unmyelinated afferents originating in the neuroma at the proximal stump of the axotomized nerve [50, 51], as well as in the DRG of associated segments [50]. We have examined whether NO was involved in such abnormal neural activity in axotomized rats. Ongoing discharges which were influenced by electrical stimulation of the proximal end of the sectioned sciatic nerves were recorded in dorsal rootlets L4-5. The latency of the evoked response nerves indicated that the activity originated from afferents with myelinated axons. In order to identify the site of the effect of L-NAME on ongoing discharges, *i.e.* the DRG and/or the neuroma, the sciatic nerve was sectioned in some rats proximal to the neuroma, thus the sciatic origin of the ongoing activity in the rootlets was established by electrical stimulation. The nerve section induced a brief, intense discharge, followed by stable ongoing discharge in all cases, which was not appreciably different from that recorded prior to cutting the nerve, suggesting that the ongoing activity recorded from the dorsal rootlets arose mainly, if not exclusively, from DRG. In rootlets activated by sciatic nerve stimulation, 100 mmol/kg i.v. L-NAME totally abolished the ongoing activity. L-arginine, the precursor of NO synthesis, briefly reversed the effect of L-NAME.

Ongoing activity was also recorded from more caudal or rostral rootlets in axotomized rats which were not influenced by sciatic stimulation, as well as from dorsal rootlets in normal rats that could be influenced by flexion or extension of the hindlimb, presumably reflecting activity in proprioceptor afferents. Ongoing activity in rootlets that were not responsive to stimulation of the sciatic nerve or in rats with intact sciatic nerves was not influenced by 200 or 400 μmol/kg L-NAME. The lack of effect of L-NAME in normal rootlets may be correlated to the low level of NOS enzyme and NOS mRNA in normal DRG [43] and indicated that the depressive effect of L-NAME on activity originating in axotomized DRG was not due to unspecific effects, such as changes in vasomotor tone.

Results from our physiological studies indicated that NO may act as an intra- and intercellular messenger within DRG cells after axotomy. A transmitter-like function has been assigned to NO. Activation of the N-methyl-D-aspartate (NMDA) receptor subtype for glutamate triggers NO formation, which activates soluble guanylate cyclase, leading to the formation of intracellular cGMP [14]. A role for NO in synaptic transmission involving the NMDA receptor at spinal cord has also been suggested [28]. NMDA receptor mRNA has been observed in rat sensory ganglion cells [38]. It is possible that after peripheral nerve section activation of these receptors may lead to the production of NO. However, at the present time there is little evidence that receptors on DRG cell bodies are activated synaptically. Moreover, DRG neurons are not sensitive to NMDA [1] and DRG exposed to NMDA *in vitro* exhibit no change in basal cGMP levels [29]. Thus, it is unclear if this mechanism is involved in the generation of ongoing discharges in axotomized DRG cells. Ongoing activity in DRG has been associated with the accumulation of K^+ in the extracellular space. NO, acting as an intracellular second messenger [8], may be involved in generation of ongoing activity. Another possible mechanism for initiating ongoing discharges is the presence of cross-excitation among injured nerve fibers [11]. It has been suggested that the cross-excitation among DRG neurons may be mediated by non-synaptic release of neuroactive compounds [11]. Due to the unusual features of NO, such as its ability to diffuse between neurons and to increase cellular cGMP, it may represent a good candidate for a neuroactive compound involving the interaction between DRG neurons.

Plasticity of the role of spinal α_2 adrenergic and opioidergic antinociceptive mechanisms following peripheral nerve injury

Spinal application of opioid and α_2 adrenoceptor agonists produces antinociception mediated by both pre- and postsynaptic receptors located in the dorsal spinal cord (*see* [76, 77] for review). The spinal opioidergic and noradrenergic systems and their receptors are subjected to complex changes after peripheral nerve injury. Axotomy induces a small, but significant, decrease of μ and δ opioid binding sites in superficial dorsal horn [7] whereas more dramatic loss of opioid receptor are observed after multiple dorsal rhizotomy [7]. Peripheral nerve constriction injury also caused a decrease in δ binding sites [39]. However, the effect of this type of nerve injury on μ-binding sites is unclear [7, 39]. Nerve constriction, but not axotomy, also caused a dramatic increase in dynorphin synthesis and content in the spinal cord [12]. In contrast to the changes in opioid system, nerve constriction caused an increase in the biosynthesis of α_2 adrenoceptors [68]. Moreover, dorsal rhizotomy decreased the content of monoamines in the spinal cord [9]. We have compared the effect of the opioid agonist morphine and α_2 agonist clonidine, both clinically used spinal analgesics, on the flexor reflex in normal and axotomized rats in order to assess the sensitivity of the spinal cord to the antinociceptive effect of morphine and clonidine after peripheral nerve injury [71, 73]. Furthermore, we have examined the effect of chronically administered morphine and α_2 agonists on autotomy behavior in order to establish the clinical relevance of using these drugs for treating neuropathic pain [34, 35, 75].

As expected, i.t. morphine and clonidine dose-dependently depressed the flexor reflex in rats with intact sciatic nerves. Both drugs caused an initial facilitation of the reflex at low doses, which may be related to the intraspinal release of tachykinins [23, 64]. In animals which did not develop autotomy after nerve section or in which autotomy had ceased for several days prior to the acute experiments, i.t. morphine had a similar depressive effect on the flexor reflex as in animal with intact nerves. However, in rats which were autotomizing at the time of the acute experiment, the threshold dose of the depressive effect of morphine was increased 3-5 fold, indicating a decrease in the sensitivity of the spinal cord to the antinociceptive effect of morphine [71]. The potency of the effect of morphine was unchanged as higher doses of morphine elicited a similar effect in all groups. In contrast to the changes that occurred with morphine, the sensitivity of the spinal cord to the depressive effect of clonidine was enhanced in axotomized rats irrespective of the level of autotomy [73]. The opposite changes in the sensitivity of the flexor reflex to morphine and clonidine were further reinforced by the behavioral observation that chronic i.t. clonidine and dexmedetomidine, another α_2 agonist, but not morphine, effectively suppressed autotomy in rats after sciatic nerve section. Moreover, after nerve constriction injury, the effect of clonidine on the response to noxious thermal stimuli of the engaged hindpaw was enhanced compared to normals, whereas the effect of morphine was decreased [10]. Our results agree in general with findings of receptor binding studies and support the clinical observation that morphine and other opioids may be relatively ineffective for treating neuropathic pain [3]. Furthermore, our data suggest that spinal application of α_2 adrenoceptor agonists may be useful in such conditions.

Up-regulation of cholecystokinin in sensory neurons and its role in morphine insensitivity of neuropathic pain-related behavior in rats

Ever since the publication of the clinical study by Arnér and Meyerson [3] indicating that neuropathic pain is not relieved by morphine, the subject of morphine as a therapeutic agent for neuropathic pain has been fiercely debated [32]. As described above, our experimental data of the lack of effect of morphine on autotomy [75] and the reduced sensitivity of the spinal cord to the reflex depressive effect of morphine [74] tended to support the notion that opiates have a poor effect on neuropathic pain.

The mechanism(s) for a lack (or reduced) effect of morphine on neuropathic pain is unclear, but this phenomenon is similar to the appearance of morphine tolerance, *i.e.*

under both circumstances morphine fails to elicit the expected analgesic effect. CCK, being an endogenous peptide and well documented physiological opioid antagonist [13, 62], has been convincingly implicated in the development of morphine tolerance [55, 74, 81]. CCK normally exists in spinal cord interneurons, but not primary sensory neurons, in rat [18]. We recently demonstrated that peripheral nerve injury caused a marked increase in CCK synthesis in rat DRG cells primarily with small somata [44]. We examined whether endogenous CCK is involved in controlling the development of autotomy, as well as morphine insensitivity, after peripheral nerve section with CI988, a highly selective and potent antagonist of the CCK-B receptor [20, 62]. Autotomy behavior was not influenced by chronic i.t. injection of saline or morphine, nor by subcutaneous (s.c.) saline or CI988 alone. However, the combination of s.c. CI988 plus i.t. morphine significantly suppressed autotomy behavior [75]. This finding suggested that increased release of CCK from the terminals of primary sensory afferents may antagonize the actions of opioid analgesics released either endogenously or applied exogenously, resulting in the development of neuropathic pain-related behavior in rats and the ineffectiveness of opioids. Another source of CCK in the spinal cord is from the terminals of descending tracts and spinal interneurons, but there was no evidence for increased CCK synthesis in these areas after peripheral nerve injury (Verge *et al.*, unpublished observation). Thus, the clinical use of CCK receptor antagonists alone or in combination with opioid analgesics may provide a promising alternative in the pharmacological management of chronic neuropathic pain.

Differential interaction between morphine and clonidine with neuropeptides in the spinal cord

The differential changes of the sensitivity of the spinal cord to the depressive effect of morphine and clonidine raised a further question concerning the mechanisms by which these drugs possess their antinociceptive effect. While some data suggested the involvement of the spinal opioid system in α_2 agonist-induced analgesia, most studies indicated that opioids and α_2 adrenoceptor agonists produce analgesia through independent receptor systems (see [77] for review). However, there is considerable evidence that i.t. co-administration of opioid and α_2 agonists produce synergistic antinociception [40, 67, 78]. Two mechanisms have been proposed to explain the synergism between opioids and α_2 agonists. On the one hand, opioid and α_2 receptors may coexist in single dorsal horn neurons and primary afferent terminals and there may be a convergence of each receptor type on Gi-protein mediated common second messenger systems which are able to regulate K^+ and/or Ca^{2+} channels, resulting in synergism between these two classes of compounds [42]. On the other hand, it has also been suggested that the interaction between opioids and α_2 receptor agonists could be *via* separate neuronal pathways. Thus, α_2 agonists may inhibit nociceptive response of dorsal horn neurons that are relatively insensitive to opioids and *vice versa*, resulting in a supra-additive inhibition of the final common pathway when both opioids and α_2 agonist are applied [67].

The spinal antinociceptive effect of opioids is differentially modulated by peptides. Cholecystokinin (CCK) and FLFQPQRF-amide (F8A) behave as opioid antagonists as they block morphine-induced analgesia [13, 25, 57]. As summarized above, this property, at least for CCK, is physiologically important as morphine-induced analgesia is potentiated by selective CCK receptor antagonists [62]. On the other hand, morphine's analgesic effect can be potentiated by i.t. galanin (GAL) [63]. The mechanism by which these peptides influence opioid-induced analgesia is unknown, but may be related to the actions of these peptides on second messenger systems and ionic channels. For example, F8A is known to produce a prolonged membrane depolarization *via* the closure of the K^+ channel [15] in contrast to the hyperpolarization involving the opening of K^+ channels by opioids [31]. Similarly, GAL hyperpolarizes neurons and is able to activate pertussis toxin sensitive Gi-protein to exert an inhibitory action in a number of neuronal systems [6].

If a convergence of opioid receptors and α_2 receptors on Gi protein-mediated second messenger system regulating ionic channels is responsible for the interaction between opioids and α_2 agonists, one would expect that peptides which influence opioid-induced analgesia by acting on common second messenger systems and ionic channels would also be able to modulate the antinociceptive effect of α_2 adrenoceptor agonists. This hypothesis is supported by a recent report where spinally applied F8A attenuated the inhibition of dorsal horn neurons by the α_2 agonist dexmedetomidine [41], which was similar to the blocking effect of F8A on opioid-induced inhibition of dorsal horn neurons [25]. We recently addressed this question by examining the effects of i.t. CCK and GAL on the depression of the spinal nociceptive flexor reflex by the α_2 agonist clonidine and compared it with results from studies where the interaction between i.t. CCK, GAL and morphine was examined [57, 62, 63].

GAL and CCK, at doses that modulated the spinal antinociceptive effect of morphine [57, 62, 63], did not influence the depressive effect of i.t. clonidine on the flexor reflex. This morphine-selective modulating effect by GAL and CCK was not due to receptor selectivity as there is no evidence that either peptide binds to opioid receptors. Thus, there are important differences in the mechanism of action of morphine and clonidine, as they are differentially modulated by GAL and CCK. The convergence of opioid receptors and α_2 receptors on common second messenger systems in single dorsal horn neurons or primary afferent terminals probably does not play a significant role in mediating the depressive effect of these drugs. It is likely that morphine and clonidine exert their antinociceptive effect by acting on different populations of dorsal horn neurons or by acting on the same neuronal pathway, but through different mechanisms with morphine's effect being more susceptible to modulation by GAL and CCK. The lack of interaction between CCK and clonidine may partly explain the increased sensitivity of the spinal cord to the reflex depressive effect of clonidine in contrast to a decreased effect of morphine.

Conclusions

Our physiological and behavioral studies, together with morphological data, have established a complex plasticity of the role of peptides, NO, opioidergic and α_2 adrenergic systems in somatosensory transmission and modulation at spinal level after peripheral axotomy, including a substitution of VIP in some of the functions of tachykinins, an enhanced role for GAL as an endogenous inhibition, a role for CCK as an endogenous antagonist of opioids and a role for NO. Some of these functional changes may reflect abnormal sensory processing in the spinal cord after peripheral nerve injury. It is possible that drugs which can manipulate the function of peptidergic and NO systems, such as VIP and CCK antagonist, GAL agonists and NOS inhibitors may be useful in treating neuropathic pain.

The diverse changes in sensitivity to the spinal depressive effect of morphine and clonidine after axotomy, as well as the differential interaction between morphine, clonidine and peptides may also have clinical significance. The findings that peripheral axotomy caused up-regulation of CCK synthesis in DRG cells and that a CCK-B receptor antagonist reversed the ineffectiveness of i.t. morphine in suppressing autotomy behavior in axotomized rats may indicate that upregulation of the CCK system after nerve injury may in part be associated with the lack of effect of opioid analgesics in neuropathic pain. The increased sensitivity to the depressive effect of clonidine, the effectiveness of clonidine on autotomy behavior and the lack of interaction between clonidine and CCK may suggest that α_2 adrenoceptor agonists may be useful in treating neuropathic pain after peripheral nerve injury.

Acknowledgements

These studies have been supported by the Swedish MRC (project. 07913), the Bank of Sweden Tercentenary Foundation, Astra Pain Control AB, Marcus and Amalia Wallenbergs Minnesfond, Lars Hiertas Minnes Stiftelsen and research funds of the Karolinska Institute. We thank Mrs. U. Petersson for her secretarial assistance.

References

1. Agrawal SG, Evans RH. The primary afferent depolarizing action of kainate in the rat. *Br J Pharmacol* 1986 ; 87 : 345-55.
2. Amir R, Devor M. Axonal cross-excitation in nerve- and neuromas : comparison of A- and C-fibers. *J Neurophysiol* 1992 ; 68 : 1160-6.
3. Arnér S, Meyerson B. Lack of analgesic effect of opioids on neuropathic and idiopathic forms of pain. *Pain* 1988 ; 33 : 11-23.
4. Barbut D, Polak JM, Wall PD. Substance P in spinal cord dorsal horn decreases following peripheral nerve injury. *Brain Res* 1981 ; 205 : 289-98.
5. Bartfai T, Fisone G, Langel Ü. Galanin and galanin antagonists : molecular and biochemical perspectives. *Trends Pharmacol Sci* 1992 ; 13 : 312-7.

6. Bedecs K, Langel Ü, Bartfai T, Wiesenfeld-Hallin Z. Galanin receptors and their second messengers in the lumbar spinal cord ; the effect of GTP and sciatic nerve transection. *Acta Physiol Scand* 1992 ; 144 : 213-20.
7. Besse D, Lombard MC, Perrot S, Besson JM. Regulation of opioid binding sites in the superficial dorsal horn of the rat spinal cord following loose ligation of the sciatic nerve : comparison with sciatic nerve section and lumbar dorsal rhizotomy. *Neuroscience* 1992 ; 50 : 921-33.
8. Bredt DS, Snyder SH. Nitric oxide, a novel neuronal messenger. *Neuron* 1992 ; 8 : 3-11.
9. Colado MI, Arnedo A, Peralta E, Del-Rio J. Unilateral dorsal rhizotomy decrease monoamine levels in the rat spinal cord. *Neurosci Lett* 1988 ; 87 : 302-6.
10. Desmeules J, Kayser V, Attal N, Guilbaud G. Distinctive antinociceptive effects elicited by morphine and clonidine in rats with unilateral mononeuropathy. *Eur J Neurosci* 1991 ; (Suppl) 4 : 37.
11. Devor M, Wall PD. Cross-excitation in dorsal root ganglia of nerve-injured and intact rats. *Neurophysiology* 1990 ; 64 : 1733-46 .
12. Draisci G, Kajander KC, Dubner R, Bennett GJ, Iadarola MJ . Up-regulation of opioid gene expression in spinal cord evoked by experimental nerve injuries and inflammation. *Brain Res* 1991 ; 560 : 186-92.
13. Faris PL, Komisaruk BR, Watkins LR, Mayer DJ. Evidence for the neuropeptide cholecystokinin as an antagonist of opiate analgesia. *Science* 1983 ; 219 : 310-2.
14. Garthwaite J, Charles SL, Chess-Williams R. Endothelium-derived relaxing factor release on activation of NMDA receptors suggest a role as intracellular messenger in the brain. *Nature* 1988 ; 326 : 385-7.
15. Guzman A, Legendre P, Allard M, Geoffre S, Vincent JD, Simonnet G. Electrophysiological effects of FLFQPQRFamide, an endogenous brain morphine modulating peptide, on cultured mouse spinal-cord neurons. *Neuropeptides* 1989 ; 14 : 253-61.
16. Haley JE, Dickenson AH, Schachter M. Electrophysiological evidence for a role of nitric oxide in prolonged chemical nociception in the rat. *Neuroscience* 1992 ; 31 : 251-8.
17. Hökfelt T, Wiesenfeld-Hallin Z, Villar MJ, Melander T. Increase of galanin-like immunoreactivity in rat dorsal root ganglion cells after peripheral axotomy. *Neurosci Lett* 1987 ; 83 : 217-20.
18. Hökfelt T, Herrera-Marschitz M, Seroogy K, Ju G, Staines WA, Holets V, Schalling M, Ungerstedt U, Post C, Rehfeld JF, Frey P, Fischer J, Dockray G, Hamaoka T, Walsh JH, Goldstein M. Immunohistochemical studies on cholecystokinin (CCK) immunoreactive neurons in the rat using sequence specific antisera and with specific reference to the caudate nucleus and primary sensory neurons. *J Chem Neuroanat* 1988 ; 1 : 11-52.
19. Hökfelt T, Verge VMK, Wiesenfeld-Hallin Z, Eriksson M. Upregulation of vasoactive intestinal peptide in substance P expressing primary sensory neurons after injury. *Soc Neurosci* 1991 ; 17 : 439 (Abstract).
20. Hughes J, Boden P, Costall B, Domeney A, Kelly E, Horwell DC, Hunter JC, Pinnock RD, Woodruff GN. Development of class of selective cholecystokinin type B receptor antagonists having potent anxiolytic activity. *Proc Natl Acad Sci USA* 1990 ; 87 : 6728-32.
21. Jessell T, Tsunoo A, Kanazawa I, Otsuka M. Substance P : depletion in the dorsal horn of rat spinal cord after section of the peripheral processes of primary sensory neurons. *Brain Res* 1979 ; 168 : 247-59.
22. Lee JH, Wilcox GL, Beitz AJ. Nitric oxide mediates Fos expression in the spinal cord induced by mechanical noxious stimulation. *Neuroreport* 1992 ; 3 : 841-4.
23. Luo L, Wiesenfeld-Hallin Z. Intrathecal clonidine release tachykinins in rat spinal cord. *Eur J Pharmacol* 1993 ; 235 : 157-9.
24. Magistretti PJ, Morrison JH, Shoemaker WJ, Sapin V, Bloom FE. Vasoactive intestinal

polypeptide induced glycogenolysis in mouse cortical slices : a possible regulatory mechanism for the local control of energy metabolism. *Proc Natl Acad Sci USA* 1981 ; 78 : 6535-9.
25. Magnusson DSK, Sullivan AF, Simonnet G, Roques BP, Dickenson AH. Differential interaction of cholecystokinin and FLFQPQRF-NH2 with μ and δ opioid antinociception in the rat spinal cord. *Neuropeptides* 1990 ; 16 : 213-318.
26. McGregor GP, Gibson SJ, Sabate IM, Blank MA, Christofides ND, Wall PD, Polak JM, Bloom SR. Effect of peripheral nerve section and nerve crush on spinal cord neuropeptides in the rat : increased VIP and PHI in the dorsal horn. *Neuroscience* 1984 ; 13 : 207-16.
27. Meller ST, Dykstra C, Gebhart GF. Production of endogenous nitric oxide and activation of soluble guanylate cyclase are required for N-methyl-D-aspartate-produced facilitation of the nociceptive tail-flick reflex. *Eur J Pharmacol* 1992 ; 214 : 93-6.
28. Meller ST, Pechman PS, Gebhart GF, Maves TJ . Nitric oxide mediates the thermal hyperalgesia produced in a model of neuropathic pain in the rat. *Neuroscience* 1992 ; 50 : 7-10.
29. Morris R, Southam E, Braid DJ, Garthwaite J. Nitric oxide may act as a messenger between dorsal root ganglion neurones and their satellite cells. *Neurosci Lett* 1992 ; 137 : 29-32.
30. Nielsch U, Keen P. Reciprocal regulation of tachykinin- and vasoactive intestinal peptide-gene expression in rat sensory neurones following cut and crush injury. *Brain Res* 1989 ; 481 : 25-30.
31. North RA, Yoshimura M. The actions of noradrenaline on neurones of the rat substantia gelatinosa *in vitro*. *J Physiol* 1984 ; 349 : 43-55.
32. Portenoy RK, Foley KM, Inturrisi CE. The nature of opioid responsiveness and its implications for neuropathic pain : new hypothesis derived from studies of opioid infusions. *Pain* 1991 ; 43 : 273-86.
33. Post C, Alari L, Hökfelt T. Intrathecal galanin increases the latency in the tail flick and hot plate tests in mouse. *Acta Physiol Scand* 1988 ; 132 : 583-4.
34. Puke MJC, Xu XJ, Wiesenfeld-Hallin Z. Intrathecal administration of clonidine suppress autotomy, a behavioral sign of chronic pain in rats after sciatic nerve section. *Neurosci Lett* 1991 ; 133 : 199-202.
35. Puke MJC, Wiesenfeld-Hallin Z. The differential effects of morphine and the α_2 adrenoceptor agonists clonidine and dexmedetomidine on the prevention and treatment of experimental neuropathic pain. *Anesth Analg* 1993 ;77 : 104-9.
36. Randic M, Gerber G, Ryu PD, Kangrga I. Inhibitory actions of galanin and somatostatin 28 on rat spinal dorsal horn neurons. *Soc Neurosci* 1987 ; 13 : 1308 (Abstract).
37. Shehab SAS, Atkinson ME. Vasoactive intestinal polypeptide (VIP) increases in the spinal cord after peripheral axotomy of the sciatic nerve originates from primary afferent neurons. *Brain Res* 1986 ; 372 : 37-44.
38. Shigemoto R, Ohishi H, Nakanishi S, Mizuno N. Expression of the mRNA for the rat NMDA receptor (NMDAR1) in the sensory and autonomic ganglion neurons. *Neurosci Lett* 1992 ; 144 : 229-32.
39. Stevens CW, Kajander KC, Bennett GJ, Seybold VS. Bilateral and differential changes in spinal mu, delta and kappa opioid binding sites in rat with a painful unilateral neuropathy. *Pain* 1991 ; 46 : 315-26.
40. Sullivan AF, Dashwood MR, Dickenson AH. α_2 adrenoceptor modulation of nociception in rat spinal cord : location, effects and interaction with morphine. *Eur J Pharmacol* 1987 ; 138 : 169-77.
41. Sullivan AF, Kalso EA, McQuay HJ, Dickenson AH. FLFQPQRF-amide modulates α_2 adrenergic antinociception in the rat dorsal horn *in vivo*. *Brain Res* 1991 ; 562 : 327-8.
42. Sullivan AF, Kalso EA, McQuay HJ, Dickenson AH. Evidence for the involvement of the μ but not δ opioid receptor subtype in the synergistic interaction between opioid and α_2 adrenergic antinociception in the rat spinal cord. *Neurosci Lett* 1992 ; 139 : 65-8.

43. Verge VMK, Xu Z, Xu XJ, Wiesenfeld-Hallin Z, Hökfelt T. Marked increase in nitric oxide synthase mRNA in rat dorsal root ganglia after peripheral axotomy : *in situ* hybridization and functional studies. *Proc Natl Acad Sci USA* 1992 ; 89 : 11617-21.
44. Verge VMK, Wiesenfeld-Hallin Z, Hökfelt T. Cholecystokinin in mammalian primary sensory neurons and spinal cord : *in situ* hybridization studies on rat and monkey spinal ganglia. *Eur J Neurosci* 1993 ; 5 : 240-50.
45. Verge VMK, Xu XJ, Langel Ü, Hökfelt T, Wiesenfeld-Hallin Z, Bartfai T. Evidence for endogenous inhibition of autotomy by galanin in the rat after sciatic nerve section : demonstrated by chronic intrathecal infusion of a high affinity galanin receptor antagonist. *Neurosci Lett* 1993 ; 149 : 193-7.
46. Villar MJ, Cortés R, Theodorsson E, Wiesenfeld-Hallin Z, Schalling M, Fahrenkrug J, Emson PC, Hökfelt T. Neuropeptide expression in rat dorsal root ganglion cells and spinal cord after peripheral nerve injury with special reference to galanin. *Neuroscience* 1989 ; 33 : 587-604.
47. Villar MJ, Wiesenfeld-Hallin Z, Xu XJ, Theodorsson E, Emson P, Hökfelt T. Further studies on galanin-, substance P-, and CGRP-like immunoreactivities in primary sensory neurons and spinal cord : effects of dorsal rhizotomies and sciatic nerve lesions. *Exp Neurol* 1991 ; 112 : 29-39.
48. Waelbroeck M, Robberecht P, Coy DH, Camus JC, De Neef P, Christopher J. Interaction of growth hormone-releasing factor (GRF) and 14 GRF analogs with vasoactive intestinal peptide (VIP) receptors of rat pancreas Discovery of (N-Ac-Tyr^1, D-Phe^2)-GRF-(1-29)-NH$_2$ as a VIP antagonist. *Endocrinology* 1985 ; 116 : 2643-9.
49. Wakisaka S, Kajander KC, Bennett GJ. Increased neuropeptide Y (NPY)-like immunoreactivity in rat sensory neurons following peripheral axotomy. *Neurosci Lett* 1991 ; 124 : 200-3.
50. Wall PD, Devor M. Sensory afferent impulse originate from dorsal root ganglia as well as from the periphery in normal and nerve injured rats. *Pain* 1983 ; 17 : 321-39.
51. Wall PD, Gutnick K. Ongoing activity in peripheral nerves : the physiology and pharmacology of impulses originating from a neuroma. *Exp Neurol* 1974 ; 43 : 580-93.
52. Wall PD, Devor M, Inbal R, Scadding JW, Schonfield D, Seltzer Z, Tomkiewicz MM. Autotomy following peripheral nerve lesions : experimental anaesthesia dolorosa. *Pain* 1979 ; 7 : 103-13.
53. Wall PD, Woolf CJ. Muscle but not cutaneous C-afferent input produces prolonged increases in the excitability of the flexion reflex in the rat. *J Physiol* 1984 ; 356 : 443-58.
54. Wall PD, Woolf CJ. The brief and prolonged facilitatory effects of unmyelinated afferent input on the rat spinal cord are independently influenced by peripheral nerve section. *Neuroscience* 1986 ; 17 : 1199-205.
55. Watkins LR, Kinscheck IB, Mayer DJ. Potentiation of opiate analgesia and apparent reversal of morphine tolerance by proglumide. *Science* 1984 ; 224 : 395-6.
56. Wiesenfeld-Hallin Z. Nerve section alters the interaction between C-fiber activity and intrathecal neuropeptides on the flexor reflex in rat. *Brain Res* 1989 ; 489 : 129-36.
57. Wiesenfeld-Hallin Z, Duranti R. Intrathecal cholecystokinin interacts with morphine, but not substance P in modulating the nociceptive flexion reflex in the rat. *Peptides* 1987 ; 8 : 153-8.
58. Wiesenfeld-Hallin Z, Villar MJ, Hökfelt T. The effect of intrathecal galanin and C-fiber stimulation on the flexor reflex in the rat. *Brain Res* 1989 ; 486 : 205-13.
59. Wiesenfeld-Hallin Z, Xu XJ, Villar MJ, Hökfelt T. The effect of intrathecal galanin on the flexor reflex in rat : increased depression after sciatic nerve section. *Neurosci Lett* 1989 ; 105 : 149-54.
60. Wiesenfeld-Hallin Z, Xu XJ, Håkansson R, Feng DM, Folkers K. The specific antagonistic effect of intrathecally injected spantide II on substance P- and C-fiber conditioning stimulation-induced facilitation of the nociceptive flexor reflex in rat. *Brain Res* 1990 ; 526 : 284-90.
61. Wiesenfeld-Hallin Z, Xu XJ, Håkansson R, Feng DM, Folkers K. Plasticity of the peptidergic mediation of spinal reflex facilitation. *Neurosci Lett* 1990 ; 116 : 293-8.
62. Wiesenfeld-Hallin Z, Xu XJ, Hughes HJ, Horwell DC, Hökfelt T. PD 134308, a selective antagonist of cholecystokinin type-B receptor, enhances the analgesic effect of morphine and

synergistically interacts with intrathecal galanin to depress spinal nociceptive reflexes. *Proc Natl Acad Sci USA* 1990 ; 87 : 7105-9.
63. Wiesenfeld-Hallin Z, Xu XJ, Villar MJ, Hökfelt T. Intrathecal galanin potentiates the spinal analgesic effect of morphine : electrophysiological and behavioral studies. *Neurosci Lett* 1990 ; 109 : 217-21.
64. Wiesenfeld-Hallin Z, Xu XJ, Håkansson R, Feng DM, Folkers K. Low-dose intrathecal morphine facilitates the spinal flexor reflex by releasing different neuropeptides in rats with intact and sectioned peripheral nerves. *Brain Res* 1991 ; 551 : 157-62.
65. Wiesenfeld-Hallin Z, Bartfai T, Hökfelt T. Galanin in sensory neurons in the spinal cord. *Front Neuroendocrinol* 1992 ; 13 : 319-43.
66. Wiesenfeld-Hallin Z, Xu XJ, Langel Ü, Bedecs K, Hökfelt T, Bartfai T. Galanin mediated control of pain : enhanced role after nerve injury. *Proc Natl Acad Sci USA* 1992 ; 89 : 3334-7.
67. Wilcox GL, Carlsson KH, Jochim A, Jurna I. Mutual potentiation of antinociceptive effects of morphine and clonidine on motor and sensory responses in rat spinal cord. *Brain Res* 1987 ; 405 : 84-93.
68. Williams F, Birnbaum A, Wilcox GL, Beitz A. Hybridization histochemical analysis of spinal neurons that express the α_2 adrenergic receptors in a rat model of peripheral mononeuropathy. *Soc Neurosci* 1991 ; 17 : 1370 (Abstract).
69. Xu XJ, Wiesenfeld-Hallin Z, Villar MJ, Fahrenkrug J, Hökfelt T. On the role of galanin, substance P and other neuropeptides in primary sensory neurons of rat : studies on spinal reflex excitability and peripheral axotomy. *Eur J Neurosci* 1990 ; 2 : 733-43.
70. Xu XJ, Wiesenfeld-Hallin Z. An analogue of growth hormone releasing factor (GRF), (Ac-Tyr^1, D-Phe^2)-GRF-(1-29), specifically antagonizes the facilitation of the flexor reflex induced by intrathecal vasoactive intestinal peptide in rat spinal cord. *Neuropeptides* 1991 ; 18 : 129-35.
71. Xu XJ, Wiesenfeld-Hallin Z. The threshold for the depressive effect of intrathecal morphine on the spinal nociceptive flexor reflex is increased during autotomy after sciatic nerve section in rats. *Pain* 1991 ; 46 : 223-9.
72. Xu XJ, Dalsgaard CJ, Wiesenfeld-Hallin Z. Intrathecal CP-96, 345 blocks reflex facilitation induced in rats by substance P and C-fiber-conditioning stimulation. *Eur J Pharmacol* 1992 ; 216 : 337-44.
73. Xu XJ, Puke MJC, Wiesenfeld-Hallin Z. The depressive effect of intrathecal clonidine on the spinal flexor reflex in enhanced after sciatic nerve section in rats. *Pain* 1992 ; 51 : 145-51.
74. Xu XJ, Wiesenfeld-Hallin Z, Hughes J, Horwell DC, Hökfelt T. CI988, a selective antagonist of cholecystokinin B receptors, prevents morphine tolerance in the rat. *Br J Pharmacol* 1992 ; 105 : 591-6.
75. Xu XJ, Puke MJC, Verge VMK, Wiesenfeld-Hallin Z, Hughes J, Hökfelt T. Up-regulation of cholecystokinin in primary sensory neurons is associated with morphine insensitivity in experimental neuropathic pain. *Neurosci Lett* 1993 ; 152 : 129-32.
76. Yaksh TL. Pharmacology of spinal adrenergic systems which modulate spinal nociceptive processing. *Pharmacol Biochem Behav* 1985 ; 22 : 845-58.
77. Yaksh TL, Noueihed R. The physiology and pharmacology of spinal opiates. *Annu Rev Pharmacol Toxicol* 1985 ; 25 : 433-62.
78. Yaksh TL, Reddy SV. Studies in the primate on the analgesic effects associated with intrathecal actions of opioids, a-adrenergic agonists and baclofen. *Anesthesiology* 1981 ; 34 : 451-67.
79. Yanagisawa M, Yagi N, Otsuka M, Yanaihara C, Yanaihara N. Inhibitory effects of galanin on the isolated spinal cord of the newborn rat. *Neurosci Lett* 1986 ; 70 : 278-82.
80. Zhang X, Verge V, Wiesenfeld-Hallin Z, Ju G, Bredt D, Snyder SH, Hökfelt T. Nitric oxide synthase-like immunoreactivity in lumbar dorsal root ganglia and spinal cord of rat and monkey and effect of peripheral axotomy. *J Comp Neurol* 1993 ; 335 : 563-75.

81. Zhou Y, Sun YH, Zhang ZW, Han JS. Accelerated expression of cholecystokinin gene in the brain of rats rendered tolerant to morphine. *Neuroreport* 1992 ; 3 : 1121-3.

17

The release of neuropeptides in the spinal cord following peripheral stimuli : *in vivo* studies

A.W. DUGGAN

Department of Preclinical Veterinary Sciences, University of Edinburgh, Summerhall, Edinburgh, UK.

A vast amount of data is available on the peptides contained within dorsal root ganglion neurones [7, 16, 21, 26, 34, 38]. In nearly all cases it is only small diameter neurones which contain a particular neuropeptide and within this population, indirect evidence suggests that a proportion of these neurones do not contain any neuropeptides. Although it seems an attractive experiment to determine the neuropeptide content of dorsal root ganglion cells characterized functionally under *in vivo* conditions, only one such study has appeared [32] and the limited results illustrate the difficulty of this approach.

A decade ago it was hoped that it would be possible to link a particular neuropeptide to a particular functional type of primary afferent fiber and thus that a given neuropeptide served as the neurotransmitter of the information conveyed by that fiber. If this were true, it contains the inherent problem as to why there is a need to effect excitatory transmission in such a multiplicity of ways. Indeed, there are good reasons to believe that neuropeptides do not function as simple neurotransmitters of information within primary afferent fibers. The first of these is the description of coexistence of more than one neuroactive compound within single afferent fibers. The combinations are multiple and varied and include coexistent neuropeptides [3, 15, 26] and peptides coexistent with an excitant amino acid [1]. It is the latter combination in particular which makes it improbable that a particular neuropeptide is signalling accurately the onset, offset and intensity of a peripheral noxious stimulus. The latter probably requires a short latency, rapidly inactivated compound, and what is known of neuropeptides in the periphery does not favour such an action, but does not exclude it. Considerable evidence suggests that neuropeptides released from primary afferent fibers act to alter the efficacy of transmission of impulses by rapidly degraded compounds and such alterations can last for relatively prolonged periods.

From a functional view point it is important to determine what compounds are released centrally from the central terminals of primary afferent fibers when these are invaded from the periphery. Provided that the peripheral stimuli can be graded, and are distinct physiological entities, then such studies of release can form a baseline to investigate the functional roles of differing compounds released from primary afferent fibers.

Release studies have an important caveat which requires early consideration. The transmission of information arriving in primary afferent fibers results in activation of many spinal neurones both excitatory and inhibitory. Thus there can be difficulties in relating the release of a compound within the spinal cord to a particular structure. This difficulty is at its worst when examining a likely widely used transmitter such as L-glutamate and if the technology used collects the compound diffusely from the whole spinal cord such as with surface perfusion *in vivo* or perfusion of a spinal cord slice *in vitro*.

Anatomy can sometimes help. For example, calcitonin gene-related peptide is contained within a proportion of primary afferent fibers of the cat and rat and also within motoneurones but virtually no other spinal neural structure [6]. Thus release into the spinal cord following a peripheral stimulus almost certainly results from release from the central terminals of primary afferents. If release can be localised anatomically with some precision, then the probability of release from a known structure is increased. Thus although substance P containing neurones occur in various areas of the spinal cord and within descending fibers (particularly in the ventral horn), the detection by antibody microprobes of release in the region of the substantia gelatinosa of spinal cats following a peripheral noxious stimulus almost certainly represents release predominantly from the central terminals of nociceptors since these are concentrated in this area [8, 22, 34].

Release of tachykinins

The tachykinins have been intensively investigated in the spinal cord mainly in relation to the function of nociceptors. Such a role was inferred from the association of substance P with small diameter dorsal root ganglion cells [21]. Of the tachykinin family of peptides, substance P, neurokinin A, neurokinin B, neuropeptide K and neuropeptide gamma occur in vertebrates. Although neuropeptide K has been identified in human cerebrospinal fluid [47], release studies in the spinal cord *in vivo* have only dealt with substance P and neurokinin A. The methodologies used under *in vivo* conditions have included perfusion of the spinal cord surface, invasive collection tubes and antibody microprobes.

Spinal cord perfusion

Perfusion of the surface of the spinal cord of the anaesthetized cat has shown a release of immunoreactive (ir) substance P following electrical stimulation of high threshold primary afferents [49]. In subsequent experiments [19] intense heat (metal places at 75°C applied to the hind limbs intermittently for 30 minutes) produced small increases in ir substance P in the spinal perfusate. Although there is difficulty in knowing the source of substance P in these experiments, the finding that intense, probably damaging thermal stimuli caused this neuropeptide to appear in the perfusate is in accord with results subsequently obtained with antibody microprobes.

Push pull cannulae and microdialysis

The most extensive studies using push pull cannulae to measure ir substance P release have come from Kuraishi and his colleagues. They found in rabbits that noxious mechanical, but not thermal stimuli, produced a 10-fold increase in ir SP in a perfusate of the dorsal horn [30]. The thermal stimulus used was a focused light bulb and the temperatures attained were measured with a subcutaneous thermocouple. The maximum temperature attained was 48.5°C and it was stated that subdermal temperatures of 44°C were exceeded for more than 11 minutes of the 20 minute stimulus period. In a subsequent study [29] this group found that severe thermal stimuli did result in a spinal release of substance P and they suggested an association with peripheral tissue damage since subcutaneous formalin also increased release. Rather puzzling are the observations of McCarson and Goldstein [36] who found that noxious mechanical cutaneous stimulation increased spinal release of substance P but that injection of formalin subcutaneously decreased release.

Antibody microprobes

Substance P

Antibody microprobes are glass micropipettes having antibodies to a peptide of interest immobilized to their outer surfaces. They cause minimal disturbance when introduced and can localise sites of release to fine structures [10].

Studies with antibody microprobes have shown that, in the anaesthetized spinal cat, electrical stimulation of large diameter primary afferents of the tibial nerve does not produce release of ir substance P within the spinal cord but that increasing the stimulus strength to include unmyelinated (C) fibers resulted in release of this peptide in the region of the substantia gelatinosa of the ipsilateral dorsal horn [9] (Figure 1).

When using noxious peripheral stimuli a release of ir substance P was produced both in the region of the substantia gelatinosa but also at the cord surface by noxious thermal, mechanical and chemical stimuli [11]. With noxious heat the hind paw was immersed

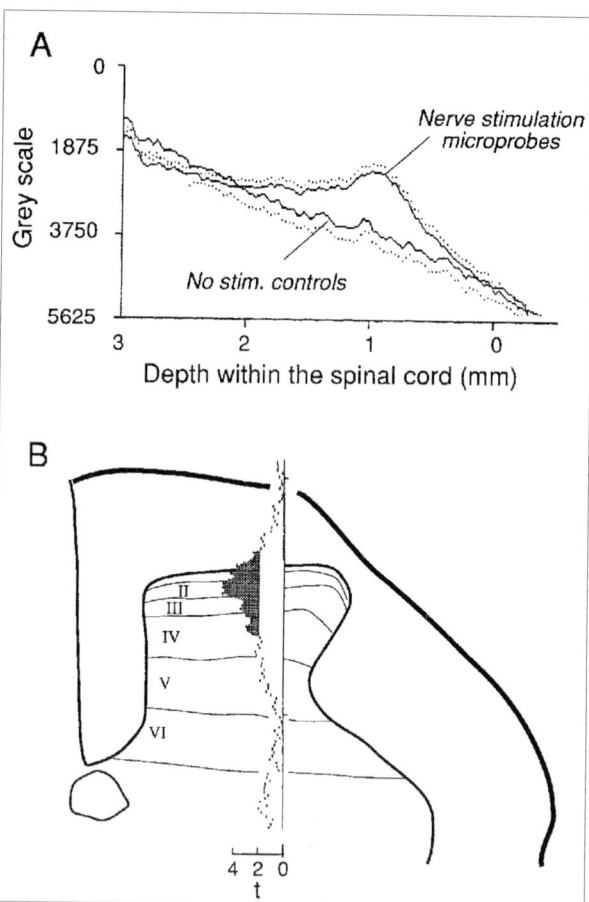

Figure 1. The sites of release of ir-substance P in the dorsal horn following electrical stimulation of the ipsilateral tibial nerve of the anaesthetised cat. A : The image analyses of two groups of antibody microprobes are shown. Those present in the spinal cord for 15 minutes and in the absence of any stimulation and a comparable group present during electrical stimulation of myelinated and unmyelinated fibers of the ipsilateral tibial nerve. The analysis was performed in 30 μm intervals but the means have been joined as a line. The standard errors of the means are plotted at each analysis point. B : The t-statistics derived from the differences of the means shown in A are plotted in relation to the laminae of the spinal cord. The hatched area outlines where the differences are significant at the $P<0.5$ level.

in a water bath and, although temperatures of 45°- 48°C are generally regarded as painful, both in man and cat [50], a bath temperature of 50°C was needed to produce release of irSP in the dorsal horn. The noxious mechanical stimulus was pinching of the skin of digital pads with small alligator clips. Non noxious mechanical stimulation did not result in ir substance P release. The noxious chemical stimulus was painting the skin of digital pads with methylene chloride and produced considerable swelling of the hind paws. Although these early experiments required stimulus times of 15 to 30 minutes, later microprobe experiments [20, 44] have shown release of ir substance P with 10 minutes of noxious pinch.

Because of the need to use relatively severe stimuli to produce release of ir substance P into the substantia gelatinosa, it was suggested that tissue damage was the more effective stimulus. This is known to produce sensitization of peripheral nociceptors and to produce firing in the so-called "silent nociceptor" group [46]. Support for this proposal came from experiments using antibody microprobes to measure spinal release of ir substance P in the cat before and after induction of inflammation in a knee joint by injection of kaolin and carrageenan [45]. Both before and from 3 to 8 hours after joint injection, joint movement failed to produce a central release of substance P. Beyond that period, joint flexion produced a massive release of substance P both in the superficial dorsal horn and deep in spinal laminae VI and VII. Compression of an inflamed joint resulted in a similarly large release of substance P. When compression of an inflamed joint was resulting in a wide spread presence of ir substance P in the dorsal horn, noxious pinch to the uninflamed digital pads of these animals resulted in a discrete zone of release restricted to the region of the substantia gelatinosa. The significance of these contrasting patterns, which are illustrated in Figure 2, will be discussed subsequently when considered degradation, and protection from degradation, of released tachykinins.

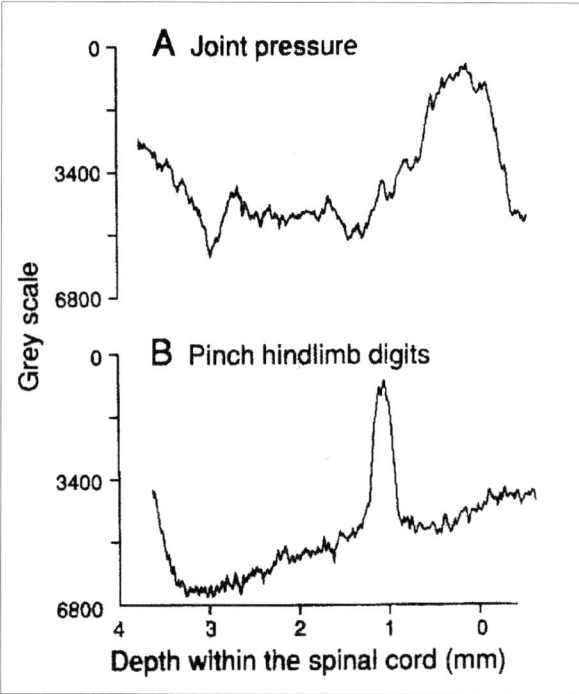

Figure 2. Contrasting effects of pressure to an inflamed joint and of pinching normal skin on the release of ir substance P in the spinal cord. Both records are single microprobe analyses. Both bore monoclonal antibodies to the c-terminus of substance P and were inserted 4 mm into the spinal cord. A : The joint was squeezed 5 times within the 15 minutes the microprobe was present in the spinal cord. B : Alligator clips were applied with a sequence of 2 minutes on one minute off to the digital pads of the ipsilateral hind paw. (Reproduced with permission from [45].)

Neurokinin A

Neurokinin A is a tachykinin which extensively coexists with substance P in dorsal root fibers of the rat [7]. Studies of the release of this compound, however, have shown important differences from substance P. In the anaesthetized cat, peripheral cutaneous thermal and mechanical stimuli produced a spinal release of ir neurokinin A [12]. Unlike the relatively focal release of ir substance P in the substantia gelatinosa, ir neurokinin A was detected widely in the dorsal horn. Because of the relative resistance of neurokinin A to enzyme degradation [41], it was suggested that this neuropeptide diffused widely from sites of release and was likely to affect neurones within relatively large areas of the spinal cord. Further support for this proposal came from experiments in which ir neurokinin A was found to require 60 to 90 minutes to return to basal levels following 30 minutes of peripheral nerve stimulation [24].

Spinal release of ir neurokinin A was also studied following the induction of peripheral arthritis [23]. Unlike substance P, spinal release of ir neurokinin A occurred immediately after joint injection and widespread presence in the spinal cord was observed. As with peripheral nerve stimulation, these elevated levels of ir neurokinin A persisted. It is important to emphasize the differences between the two tackykinins in these experiments. ir neurokinin A appeared with joint injection and persisted in the spinal cord irrespective of any peripheral stimulus whereas ir substance P release did not occur till some hours after joint injection and required an active stimulus. These results have an interesting peripheral counterpart where arthroscopy of joints in humans was associated with detectable levels of neurokinin A in synovial fluid but not of substance P.

If the widespread presence of ir neurokinin A following release is due to resistance to degradation, then a similar pattern should be observed for ir substance P if this compound could be protected from degradation. Such an effect was shown by Duggan *et al.* [13] following microinjection of the mixed peptidase inhibitor kelatorphan into the superficial dorsal horn of the cat. Under these conditions, released ir substance P not only diffused widely in the spinal cord but also persisted for prolonged periods following release. The same type of response was produced by microinjecting calcitonin gene-related peptide into the superficial dorsal horn [44]. Figure 3 compares the distribution of ir substance P produced by nerve stimulation in normal animals with that following inhibition of peptidases. Calcitonin gene-related peptide has been shown to inhibit an endopeptidase degrading substance P [33] and this raises interesting possibilities on controls of the sites accessed by co-released tachykinins.

It may be that the persistence and spread of or neurokinin A results from its greater susceptibility to inhibition of degradation through coreleased calcitonin gene-related peptide. The functional significance of this wide diffusion is presently obscure but it may act to produce widespread increases in excitability of spinal neurones. This action would be reinforced by substance P if the release of calcitonin gene-related peptides were to be enhanced, since this would result in substance P reaching sites not normally accessed. Levels of calcitonin gene-related peptide have been shown to be increased in the spinal cords of arthritic rats [35] and the release of calcitonin gene-related peptide was shown to be enhanced from slices of the spinal cord of such animals [2]. It is in experimental arthritis that microprobe experiments showed that substance P is present over the whole of the dorsal horn following a severe stimulus to an inflamed joint [45]. Thus the contrasting wide presence of ir substance P following stimulation of an inflamed joint and discrete presence following punching a normal digital pad (which is shown in Figure 2) could result from a protection of substance P released from joint afferents through coreleased calcitonin gene-related peptide.

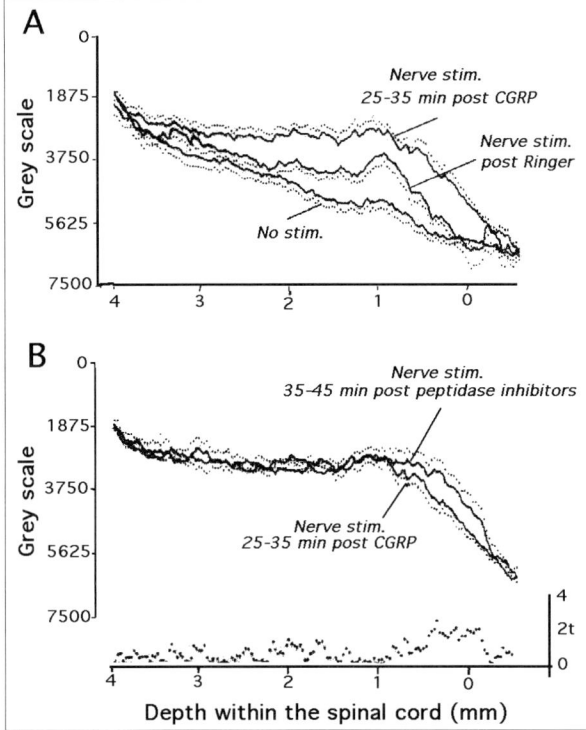

Figure 3. The effects of microinjection of Ringer's solution, a solution of CGRP (10-3M) and of a mixture of the peptidase inhibitors enalaprilat and kelatorphan on the distribution of evoked release of ir substance P in the spinal cord. A :The mean image analyses of three groups of microprobes are shown : those present in the spinal cord in the absence of nerve stimulation (no stim), those present in the spinal cord during electrical stimulation of the ipsilateral tibial nerve but following microinjection of Ringer's solution in the upper dorsal horn (nerve stim post Ringer) and those present with nerve stimulation but following microinjection of CGRP, 10⁻³M (nerve stim 25-35 min post CGRP). B :The similar patterns of ir substance P following microinjection of CGRP or peptidase inhibitors.

These experiments on tachykinin release do permit limited conclusions on the roles that tachykinins may play in the dorsal horn. Firstly, neurokinin A cannot function as an excitatory transmitter signalling the onset, offset and intensity of a peripheral noxious stimulus. Its persistence and lack of somatotopic distribution militate against such a role. Substance P could subserve such a role. If, however, the action of calcitonin gene-related peptide in inhibiting SP degradation is a physiological control and, for example, comes into play with inflammation, then it would be anticipated that perceived pain would outlast the duration of the peripheral stimulus and be poorly localised when inflammation develops. As regards to the fiber types releasing these peptides both tachykinins could be released from the central terminals of polymodal nociceptors. The release of neurokinin A by relatively non-damaging noxious stimuli when compared with substance P may simply reflect the more rapid degradation of substance P following release rather than their release from different fiber types. It is possible, however, that substance P and calacitonin gene-related peptide are relatively enriched in the population of silent nociceptors which require sensitization during inflammation to be excited by a peripheral stimulus [46].

Somatostatin

Somatostatin has been localized by immunoreactive techniques to small diameter dorsal root ganglion neurones and to the superficial laminae of the dorsal horn of several species [14, 21, 31]. Fewer dorsal root ganglion cells contain ir somatostatin than contain ir substance P : in the cat about 5% of these neurones contain ir somatostatin [31]. Studies *in vivo* have examined release of somatostatin by means of push-pull cannulae and antibody microprobes.

Kuraishi *et al.* [30] have measured ir somatostatin release in the rabbit spinal cord in response to cutaneous stimuli using push-pull cannulae. The noxious thermal stimulation employed evoked ir somatostatin release within the ipsilateral dorsal horn, but noxious mechanical stimulation was ineffective.

Antibody microprobes have been used in the lumbar dorsal horn of anaesthetized cats. Such microprobes have revealed a basal presence of ir somatostatin in the absence of peripheral stimulation in the region of the substantia gelatinosa 40. There was also a presence of ir somatostatin at the surface of the cord. The basal presence of ir somatostatin in the substantia gelatinosa region was readily detected on microprobes placed in the cord for only 5 min [40], and was much more prominent than that observed for ir substance P in the same spinal region under similar conditions [11]. It was considered that this release of ir somatostatin might result from continuous firing of thermoreceptors. With microprobes, however, it was found that following immersing the hind limbs into water of temperatures between 15°-31°C, the ir somatostatin presence in the substantia gelatinosa region was similar to basal levels. Release of ir somatostatin was produced when the stimulus temperature was noxious. With a stimulus temperature of 52°C this release of ir somatostatin was very apparent [40] and is illustrated in Figure 4.

Although both ir substance P and ir somatostatin were released by noxious skin heating, the release patterns of these 2 peptides differed for mechanical stimulation. Thus, using the noxious mechanical stimulation previously found adequate to evoke ir substance P release (alligator clips to the digital pads), no release of ir somatostatin in the substantia gelatinosa region was recorded [40].

The specificity of ir somatostatin release in relation to the type of noxious stimulus evoking release makes it unlikely that this peptide is released from polymodal nociceptors. A more probable source is from some form of specialized thermal nociceptor such as those described in the hind paw skin of the cat [25]. It is not known if such nociceptors contain somatostatin. The interpretation of these findings is complicated not only by the coexistence of other peptides such as substance P and cholecystokinin in these cells, but by species differences. In the rat, ir somatostatin and ir substance P occur in separate populations of dorsal root ganglion neurones [21, 31] while in the cat, most of the ir somatostatin-containing cells also contain ir substance P but not *vice versa* [31]. Thus in the cat, it is tempting to speculate that the subset of dorsal root ganglion neurones containing both ir somatostatin and ir substance P might be specialized heat nociceptors.

While a proportion of the ir somatostatin in laminae I and II is of primary afferent origin, experiments examining the results of dorsal rhizotomy and capsaicin treatment have shown that intrinsic spinal neurones contribute significantly to the intraspinal pool of ir somatostatin [17, 42]. The results of the microprobe experiments with noxious heat would still require that these intrinsic spinal neurones be selectively excited by noxious thermal, but not mechanical afferent input.

Possibly favouring a release predominantly from intraspinal neurones as opposed to primary afferent fibers are experiments which find somatostatin to inhibit the firing of neurones of the spinal cord [5, 43]. It is thus improbable that somatostatin is an excitatory transmitter released from the central terminals of thermal nociceptors although it could be co-released with an excitatory compound and subserve an as yet undefined function.

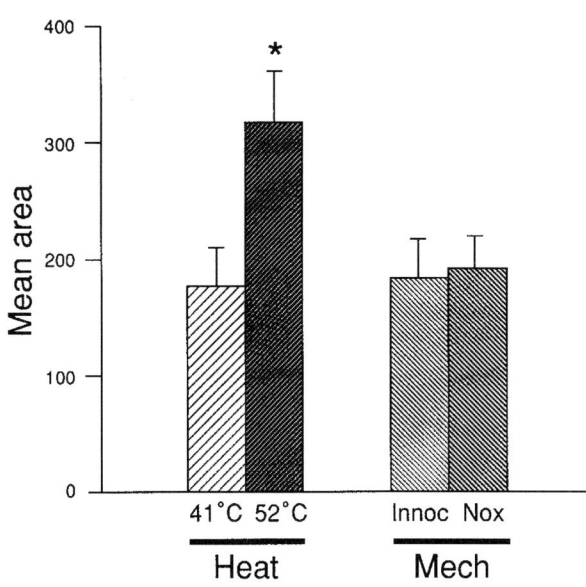

Figure 4. Release of ir somatostatin by noxious thermal but not noxious mechanical stimulation. The results are derived from antibody microprobes inserted with the spinal cord. With the analysed image of the autoradiograph of each microprobe, a computer program determined the area of the zone of inhibition of binding corresponding to laminae I and II. The mean area together with the standard error of the mean is plotted for the four illustrated groups of microprobes. The noxious thermal stimulus (52°C) significantly increased the area of reduced binding of 125I-somatostatin to microprobes compared to the group with a stimulus temperature of 41°C. There was no such difference when noxious and non-noxious mechanical stimuli were used. (Reproduced with permission from [40].)

Calcitonin gene-related peptide (CGRP)

CGRP is contained within a high proportion of dorsal root ganglion neurones including both small and large diameter cell bodies [4, 18, 26]. Within the spinal cord, CGRP is found in motoneurones but in no other intrinsic neurone [6]. Thus in a spinal animal the release of CGRP within the dorsal horn can confidently be attributed to release from the central terminals of primary afferents.

Release of CGRP under *in vivo* conditions has been studied with antibody microprobes [39]. In the anaesthetized cat a basal presence of irCGRP was found in the region of the substantia gelatinosa and this was significantly increased by noxious mechanical and thermal stimulation of the skin. It is unknown if the release of CGRP is enhanced *in vivo* during inflammation but an *in vitro* study of the spinal cord of animals with peripheral inflammation did show enhanced release of CGRP [2]. An interesting result is that of Klein *et al.* [27] who observed that electrical stimulation of small diameter afferents of the sciatic nerve of the rat resulted in depletion of CGRP demonstrated by immunocytochemistry of sections of the spinal cord. Such a depletion is consistent with stimulus-evoked release. Although CGRP is present in some large diameter dorsal root ganglion cells, non-noxious cutaneous stimulation did not evoke spinal release in the study of Morton and Hutchison [39].

Since CGRP is present in so many dorsal root ganglion cells, it seems improbable that it is associated with a particular functional type. Thus CRGP probably does not function as a simple transmitter of information. The role of CGRP in inhibiting degradation of SP has been discussed earlier in this paper. The receptor mediated effects of CGRP on spinal processing of sensory information are little understood, but given the abundance of this neuropeptide it is an important area for future research.

Galanin

Although galanin was originally reported as occurring in a small proportion of dorsal root ganglion neurones [37, 48], a subsequent study found galanin to occur in a higher proportion of such cells in the normal rat than CGRP [28.] The reasons for these differences are not apparent.

Morton and Hutchison [39] detected a basal presence of galanin in the substantia gelatinosa of the cat but these were not altered by peripheral nerve stimulation or noxious cutaneous stimuli. More recently galanin release has been examined in arthritic rats (Hope *et al.* unpublished). These animals had a basal presence of galanin diffusely in the spinal cord which was reduced when a severe stimulus was applied to the inflamed joint. The reason for this apparent inhibition of release is unclear. Galanin levels rise dramatically in the dorsal horn after peripheral adotomy [48] but the stimulus to the release of this newly synthesized peptide has not been examined.

Concluding remarks

One of the surprises of studies of neuropeptide release is the ability of some of these compounds to resist rapid degradation and to access sites relatively remote from sites of release. If degradation of neuropeptides is subject to physiological controls, then a highly plastic situation emerges. It is difficult to predict the consequences for spinal processing of afferent information but it appears that widespread and long lasting alterations in the excitability of spinal neurones and of the pathways to such cells can follow spinal release of neuropeptides.

References

1. Battaglia G, Rustioni A. Co-existence of glutamate and substance P in dorsal root ganglia neurons of the rat and monkey. *J Comp Neurol* 1988 ; 277 : 302-12.
2. Beck-Sickinger AG, Grouzmann E, Hoffmann E, Gaida W, Van Meir EG, Waeber B, Jung G. A novel cyclic analog of neuropeptide Y specific for the Y2 receptor. *Eur J Biochem* 1992 ; 206 : 957-64.
3. Cameron AA, Leah JD, Snow PJ. The coexistence of neuropeptides in feline sensory neurons. *Neuroscience* 1988 ; 27 : 969-79.
4. Carlton SM, McNeill DL, Chung K, Coggeshall RE. Organization of calcitonin gene-related peptide immunoreactive terminals in the primate dorsal horn. *J Comp Neurol* 1988 ; 276 : 527-36.
5. Christenson J, Alford S, Grillner S, Hôkfelt T. Co-localized GABA and somatostatin use different ionic mechanisms to hyperpolarize target neurons in the lamprey spinal cord. *Neurosci Lett* 1991 ; 134 : 93-7.
6. Chung K, Lee WT, Carlton SM. The effects of dorsal rhizotomy and spinal cord isolation on calcitonin gene-related peptide-labeled terminals in the rat lumbar dorsal horn. *Neurosci Lett* 1988 ; 90 : 17-32.
7. Dalsgaard CJ, Haegerstrand A, Theodorsson-Norheim E, Brodin E, Hokfelt T. Neurokinin-A like immunoreactivity in rat primary sensory neurons : coexistence with substance P. *Histochemistry* 1985 ; 83 : 37-40.
8. Difiglia M, Aronin N, Leeman SE. Light microscopic and ultrastructural localisation of immunoreactive substance P in the dorsal horn of monkey spinal cord. *Neuroscience* 1982 ; 7 : 1127-40.
9. Duggan AW, Hendry IA. Laminar localization of the sites of release of immunoreactive substance P in the dorsal horn with antibody coated microelectrodes. *Neurosci Lett* 1986 ; 68 : 134-40.
10. Duggan AW, Hendry IA, Green JL, Morton CR, Hutchison WD. The preparation and use of antibody microprobes. *J Neurosci Methods* 1988 ; 23 : 241-7.
11. Duggan AW, Hendry IA, Green JL, Morton CR, Hutchison WD. Cutaneous stimuli releasing immunoreactive substance P in the dorsal horn of the cat. *Brain Res* 1988 ; 451 : 261-73.
12. Duggan AW, Hope PJ, Jarrott B, Schaible HG, Fleetwood-Walker SM. Release spread and persistence of immunoreactive neurokinin A in the dorsal horn of the cat following noxious cutaneous stimulation. Studies with antibody microprobes. *Neuroscience* 1990 ; 35 : 195-202.
13. Duggan AW, Schaible HG, Hope PJ, Lang CW. Effect of peptidase inhibition on the pattern of intraspinally released immunoreactive substance P detected with antibody microprobes. *Brain Res* 1992 ; 579 : 261-9.
14. Forssmann WG. A new somatostatinergic system in the mammalian spinal cord. *Neurosci Lett* 1978 ; 10 : 293-7.
15. Gibbins IL, Furness JB, Costa M, MacIntyre I, Hillyard CJ, Girgis S. Colocalization of calcitonin gene-related peptide-like immunoreactivity with substance P in cutaneous vascular and visceral sensory neurons of guinea pigs. *Neurosci Lett* 1985 ; 57 : 125-30.

16. Gibson SJ, McCrossan MV, Polak JM. A sub-population of calcitonin gene-related peptide (CGRP)- immunoreactive neurons in the dorsal root ganglia also display substance P somatostatin or gelanin immunoreactivity. Proc XII Int Anatom Congress, 1985 : 232.
17. Gibson SJ, McGregor G, Bloom SR, Polak JM, Wall PD. Local application of capsaicin to one sciatic nerve of the adult rat induces a marked depletion in the peptide content of the lumbar dorsal horn. *Neuroscience* 1982 ; 7 : 3153-62.
18. Gibson SJ, Polak JM, Bloom SR, Sabate IM, Mulderry PM, Ghatei MA, McGregor GP, Morrison JF, Kelly JS, Evans RM, Rosenfeld MG. Calcitonin gene-related peptide immunoreactivity in the spinal cord of man and eight other species. *Neuroscience* 1984 ; 4 : 3101-11.
19. Go VLW, Yaksh TL. Release of substance P from the cat spinal cord. *J. Physiol* 1987 ; 391 : 141-67.
20. Gu XH, Casley DJ, Nayler WG. The inhibitory effect of [D-Arg^{1}D-Phe D-Try^{7,9} Leu11] substance P on endothelin-1 binding sites in rat cardiac membranes. *Biochem Biophys Res Commun* 1991 ; 179 : 130-3.
21. Hokfelt T, Elde R, Johansson O, Luft R, Nilsson G, Arimura A. Immunohistochemical evidence for separate populations of somatostatin-containing and substance P- containing primary afferent neurons in the rat. *Neuroscience* 1976 ; 1 : 131-6.
22. Hokfelt T, Ljungdahl A, Terenius L, Elde R, Nilsson G. Immunohistochemical analysis of peptide pathways possibly related to pain and analgesia : enkephalin and substance P. *Proc Natl Acad Sci USA* 1977 ; 74 : 3081-5.
23. Hope PJ, Jarrott B, Schaible HG, Clarke RW, Duggan AW. Release and spread of immunoreactive neurokinin A in the cat spinal cord in a model of acute arthritis. *Brain Res* 1990 ; 533 : 292-9.
24. Hope PJ, Lang CW, Duggan AW. Persistence of immunoreactive neurokinins in the dorsal horn of barbiturate anaesthetised and spinal cats following release by tibial nerve stimulation. *Neurosci Lett* 1990 ; 118 : 25-8.
25. Iggo A. Cutaneous heat and cold receptors with slowly-conducting (C) afferent fibers. *Q J Exp Physiol* 1959 ; 44 : 362-70.
26. Ju G, Hokfelt T, Brodin E, Fahrenkrug J, Fischer JA, Frey P, Elde RP, Brown JC. Primary sensory neurons of the rat showing calcitonin gene-related peptide immunoreactivity and their relation to substance P somatostatin- galanin- vasoactive intestinal polypeptide- and cholecystokinin-immunoreactive ganglion cells. *Cell Tissue Res* 1987 ; 247 : 417-31.
27. Klein CM, Coggeshall RE, Carlton SM, Westlund KN, Sorkin LS. Changes in calcitonin gene-rated peptide immunoreactivity in the rat dorsal horn following electrical stimulation of the sciatic nerve. *Neurosci Lett* 1990 ; 115 : 149-54.
28. Klein CM, Westlund KN, Coggeshall RE. Percentages of dorsal root axons immunoreactive for galanin are higher than those immunoreactive for calcitonin gene-related peptide. *Brain Res* 1990 ; 519 : 97-101.
29. Kuraishi Y, Hirota N, Sato Y, Hanashima N. Stimulus specificity of peripherally evoked substance P release from rabbit dorsal horn *in situ*. *Neuroscience* 1989 ; 30 : 241-50.
30. Kuraishi Y, Hirota N, Sato Y, Hino Y, Satoh M, Takagi H. Evidence that substance P and somatostatin transmit separate information related to pain in the spinal dorsal horn. *Brain Res* 1985 ; 325 : 294-8.
31. Leah JD, Cameron AA, Kelly WL, Snow PJ. Coexistence of peptide immunoreactivity in sensory neurons of the cat. *Neuroscience* 1985 ; 16 : 683-90.
32. Leah JD, Cameron AA, Snow PJ. Neuropeptides in physiologically identified mammalian sensory neurones. *Neurosci Lett* 1985 ; 56 : 257-64.
33. Le Greves P, Nyberg F, Terenius L, Hokfelt T. Calcitonin gene-related peptide is a potent inhibitor of substance P degradation. *Eur J Pharmacol* 1985 ; 115 : 309-11.

34. Lindh B, Lundberg JM, Hokfelt T. NPY- galanin- VIP/PHI-CGRP- and substance P-immunoreactive neuronal subpopulations in cat autonomic and sensory ganglia and their projections. *Cell Tissue Res* 1989 ; 256 : 259-73.
35. Marlier L, Poulat P, Rajaofetra N, Privat A. Modifications of serotonin- substance P- and calcitonin gene-related peptide immunoreactivities in the dorsal horn of the spinal cord of arthritic rats : a quantitative immunocytochemical study. *Exp Brain Re*s 1991 ; 85 : 482-90.
36. McCarson KE, Goldstein BD. Release of substance P into the superficial dorsal horn following nociceptive activation of the hindpaw of the rat. *Brain Res* 1991 ; 568 : 109-15.
37. Melander TT, Hokfelt T, Rokaeus A. Distribution of galanin-like immunoreactivity in the rat central nervous system. *J Comp Neurol* 1986 ; 248 : 475-517.
38. Merighi A, Kar S, Gibson SJ, Ghidella S, Gobetto A, Peirone SM, Polak JM. The immunocytochemical distribution of seven peptides in the spinal cord and dorsal root ganglia of horse and pig. *Anat Embryol (Berl)* 1990 ; 181 : 271-80.
39. Morton CR, Hutchinson WD. Release of sensory neuropeptides in the spinal cord : studies with calcitonin gene-related peptide and galanin. *Neuroscience* 1989 ; 31 : 807-15.
40. Morton CR, Hutchison WD, Hendry IA, Duggan AW. Somatostatin : evidence for a role in thermal nociception. *Brain Res* 1989 ; 488 : 89-96.
41. Nyberg F, Le Greves P, Sundqvist C, Terenius L. Characterization of substance P(1-7) and (1-8) generating enzyme in human cerebrospinal fluid. *Biochem Biophys Res Commun* 1984 ; 125 : 244-50.
42. Priestley JV, Bramwell S, Butcher LL, Cuello AC. Effect of capsaicin on neuropeptides in areas of termination of primary sensory neurones. *Neurochem Int* 1982 ; 4 : 57-65.
43. Sandkuhler J, Fu QG, Helmchen C. Spinal somatostatin superfusion. *In vivo* affects activity of cat nociceptive dorsal horn neurone : comparison with spinal morphine. *Neuroscience* 1990 ; 34 : 565-76.
44. Schaible HG, Hope PJ, Lang CW, Duggan AW. Calcitonin gene-related peptide causes intraspinal spreading of substance P released by peripheral stimulation. *Eur J Neurosci* 1992 ; 4 : 750-7.
45. Schaible HG, Jarrott B, Hope PJ, Duggan AW. Release of immunoreactive substance P in the spinal cord during development of acute arthritis in the knee joint of the cat : a study with antibody microprobes. *Brain Res* 1990 ; 529 : 214-23.
46. Schaible HG, Schmidt RF. Effects of an experimental arthritis on the sensory properties of fine articular afferents. *Neurophysiology* 1985 ; 54 : 1109-22.
47. Toresson G, Carreras de las C, Brodin E, Bertilsson L. Neuropeptide K is present in human cerebrospinal fluid. *Life Sci* 1990 ; 46(23) : 1707-14.
48. Xu XJ, Wiesenfeld-Hallin Z, Villar MJ, Fahrenkrug J, Hokfelt T. On the role of galanin substance P and other neuropeptides in primary sensory neurons of the rat : studies on spinal reflex excitability and peripheral axotomy. *J Neurosci* 1990 ; 2 : 733-43.
49. Yaksh TL, Jessell TM, Gamse R, Mudge AW, Leeman SE. Intrathecal morphine inhibits substance P release from mammalian spinal cord *in vivo*. *Nature* 1980 ; 286 : 155-7.
50. Zimmerman M. *International review of physiology : neurophysiology II*. Baltimore : University Park Press, 1976 : 179-221.

18

Pharmacological and physiological modulations of the release of peptides from nociceptors

F. CESSELIN, E. COLLIN, S. BOURGOIN, M. POHL,
A. MAUBORGNE, J.J. BENOLIEL, M. HAMON

*INSERM U 288, Neurobiologie Cellulaire et Fonctionnelle,
Faculté de Médecine Pitié-Salpêtrière, Paris, France.*

Studies of the possible modulations by GABA, adreno- and 5-HT receptor active drugs of the spinal release of neuropeptides (substance P, neurokinin A, somatostatin, calcitonin gene-related peptide) from primary afferent fibers (PAF) involved in the transfer of nociceptive messages indicate that postsynaptic rather than presynaptic sites, with respect to PAF, are likely involved in the antinociceptive effects of intrathecally administered drugs acting at GABA, adreno- and 5-HT receptors. In contrast, opioids could control presynaptically the activity of PAF, by exerting both inhibitory and facilitatory influences through the stimulation of various opioid receptors. Interestingly, endogenous opioids exert a tonic inhibitory control of the spinal release of substance P and calcitonin gene-related peptide.

Spinally administered drugs known to act upon specific classes of pharmacologically defined receptors can alter the spinal processing of inputs evoked by noxious stimuli. In particular, numerous data indicate that opioid, adrenergic, GABA and serotonin (5-HT) receptor ligands are especially active in affecting pain-related behaviours when injected intrathecally in animals (*see* [23, 76], for reviews). However, to date only opioid agonists have really been shown to produce a powerful analgesia when administered at the spinal level in humans.

In the dorsal horn, opioid, GABA, 5-HT, α_2- and β-adrenergic receptors are apparently located both on neuronal elements intrinsic to the spinal cord and on the nerve terminals of bulbospinal and primary afferent neurones. Thus, agonists of these receptors may exert, at least partly, their antinociceptive effects by modulating presynaptically the activity of primary afferent fibers (PAF) (which convey the nociceptive messages to the spinal cord) *via* the receptors they bear [3, 15, 17, 24, 28, 34, 55]. Besides electrophysiological, pharmacological and behavioural studies, the involvement of particular PAF in the transfer of nociceptive messages has been inferred from experiments showing that nociceptive stimuli are able to enhance the spinal release of substance P (SP), neurokinin A (NKA), calcitonin gene-related peptide (CGRP), somatostatin (SRIF) and glutamate, all known neuroactive substances of PAF (*see* [7, 72], for reviews). Thus, the hypothesis of a presynaptic component in the spinal analgesic action of the drugs cited above supposes that these drugs are capable of reducing the spinal release of some of these putative neurotransmitters.

The purpose of the present review is to summarise the data concerning the modulation of the spinal release of neuropeptides *in vivo* and *in vitro* by drugs acting at opioid, GABA, adreno- and 5-HT receptors.

Effects of opioids on the release of neuropeptides from the spinal cord

That opioids, particularly morphine, exert their analgesic effects at the spinal level, at least in part, by inhibiting presynaptically the nociceptive sensory fibers is widely accepted since the report by Jessell and Iversen in 1977 that morphine (10 µM) and D-Ala^2-Met^5-enkephalinamide (3 µM) were able to reduce the K$^+$-evoked release of SP from trigeminal nucleus slices [30]. In fact, the discovery of the multiplicity of opioid receptors, the three main classes (µ δ and κ) of which seem to be present on the spinal terminals of PAF [3], raised soon the possibility that the opioid control of PAF is not so simple as initially thought [39].

Opioids and the spinal release of SP

All authors agree with the fact that opioids stimulating selectively δ receptors are especially potent to control SP-containing PAF. Indeed, the δ opioid agonists DTLET [78] and DPDPE [46] inhibit both the spontaneous [13] and the depolarisation-evoked [1, 22, 39, 52, 63] release of SP from the spinal cord and trigeminal nucleus *in vitro* as well as *in vivo*. Furthermore, the selective blockade of δ receptors by naltrindole [54] induces an enhancement of the spinal release of SP in the rat *in vivo*, suggesting that endogenous opioids acting at these receptors exert a tonic inhibitory control on SP-containing fibers [13] (Figure 1).

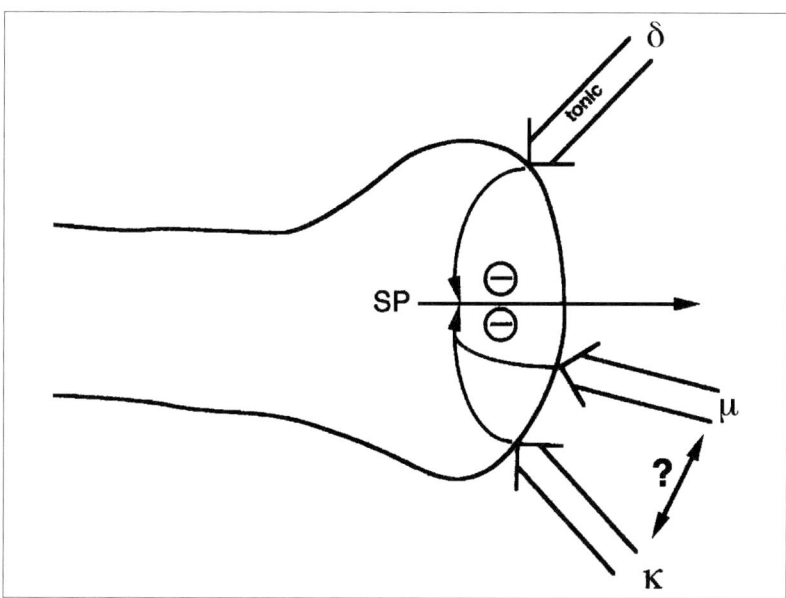

Figure 1. Schematic representation of the opioid control of the spontaneous release of substance P (SP) from the rat spinal cord *in vivo*. The stimulation of δ receptors results in a 256 decrease in SP release. In contrast, the stimulation of μ receptors enhances it, and that of κ receptors is ineffective. However, the simultaneous stimulation of both μ and k receptors leads to a reduction in SP release. The selective blockade of δ receptors (but not that of μ or κ receptors) induces an increase in SP release, indicating that endogenous opioids acting at these receptors exert a tonic inhibitory influence on the peptide release.

In contrast, the possible involvement of other opioid receptor subtypes in the control of SP-containing PAF is still the matter of debate. In the case of κ receptors, most *in vitro* and *in vivo* investigations showed that their selective stimulation by U 50488 H [71] or dynorphin does not exert any effect on the spinal release of SP [1, 14, 22, 39, 52]. However, Chang et al. [8] reported that U 50488 H inhibits SP release from primary sensory neurones, and a biphasic U 50488 H concentration-response curve was recently described by Suarez-Roca and Maixner [64] who observed that 10-30 nM of U 50488 H enhanced, whereas 100 nM reduced the release of SP from rat trigeminal nucleus slices.

Similarly, contradictory data have been reported regarding the modulation of spinal SP release by μ opioid receptors. *In vitro* studies have shown that the selective μ agonists DAGO [21] and PL017 [9] enhance the K^+- or capsaicin-evoked release of SP from rat spinal cord slices [39, 52]. Such an excitatory influence of DAGO was also observed on the spontaneous release of SP *in vivo* in the rat [14]. By contrast, Aimone and Yaksh [1] reported that μ opioid receptor stimulation by the same agonist markedly inhibits the spinal release of SP evoked by intrathecal administration of capsaicin in anaesthetised rats. Interactions between κ and μ receptors in the control of the release of SP from the rat spinal cord could explain the discrepancy between our data [14, 39, 52] and those of Aimone and Yaksh [1]. Indeed, we recently found that κ receptor stimulation, which is inactive on its own to affect the spontaneous release of SP *in vivo*, can alter the effect of μ receptor stimulation on the peptide release [14]. In particular, the stimulatory influence of 10 μM DAGO on SP release is no more apparent in the presence of 10 μM U 50488 H. Moreover, a significant reduction in SP outflow is observed when the artificial cerebrospinal fluid perfusing the subarachnoid space is supplemented with both DAGO and U 50488 H (Figure 1). As indicated by its prevention by either naloxone or nor-binaltorphimine (nBNI), a selective κ receptor antagonist [53], the latter effect requires the stimulation of both μ and κ opioid receptors [14].

Under our experimental conditions, there is apparently no tonic influence of endogenous opioids acting at κ receptors on spinal SP-containing neurones, since 10 μM nBNI do not affect the spontaneous spinal outflow of SP [14]. Accordingly, the stimulation of μ receptors by DAGO is not altered by some κ-dependent control, and an increase in SP outflow is produced by the μ agonist. As the conditions used by Aimone and Yaksh [1] clearly differ from ours (in particular, in their study, SP release was evoked by capsaicin, and animals were anaesthetised with chloralose-urethane - instead of halothane in our laboratory - [14]), it is possible that κ receptors are tonically activated by endogenous opioids in their experiments, so that further stimulation of μ receptors by 10 μM DAGO can induce a decrease in SP release (as found in our laboratory when both κ and μ opioid receptors are stimulated).

These data emphasise the complexity of the opioid control of spinal SP-containing neurones and the difficulties encountered in relevant studies as shown by the contradictory findings reported in the literature (*see* above). Since morphine is able to stimulate μ, δ and κ receptors [10, 37, 67, 75], interactions between them, as illustrated above (*see* Figure 1), can also account for the reported differences in the magnitude and direction of the effects of this alkaloid on spinal SP release. Indeed, morphine-induced changes in SP release under various *in vitro* and *in vivo* conditions have been shown to vary from a complete inhibition [30], to a partial reduction [1, 8, 22, 26, 49], no effect [39, 42] or even a facilitation [52]. These observations make the establishment of full dose-response curves for the effects of opioids on spinal SP release an absolute requirement before any definitive conclusion can be drawn. Such studies are really on the way now as very recently Suarez-Roca *et al.* [61] reported that morphine exerts a concentration-dependent multiphasic effect on the release of SP from rat trigeminal nucleus slices. In the nanomolar range, morphine (1 nM) inhibits the K^+-evoked release of SP, whereas at higher concentrations, 100-300 nM, the alkaloid enhances the peptide release. Furthermore, at 3 μM, morphine again reduces the release of the peptide, and then exerts the opposite effect at 30 μM [61]. These authors provided evidence that the inhibitory effect of 1 nM and 3 μM morphine could be due to the stimulation of high-affinity μ1 and δ receptors, respectively [62]. The stimulatory effects of the drug on the release of SP could result from the stimulation of both μ and δ receptors (in a complexed form) when morphine is used at 100-300 nM, and from that of κ receptors at 30 µM of the drug [62, 64]. Confirmation of these findings and full dose-response curves for the effects of other (selective) opioid agonists on the spinal release of SP are eagerly expected.

Opioids and the spinal release of neurokinin A and somatostatin

Only the effects of morphine on the spinal release of NKA and SRIF have been examined. Thus, Vasko and Harris [69] found no change in the K^+-induced release of SRIF from rat spinal cord slices in the presence of 10 µM morphine, and Lang et al. [35] reported that the alkaloid (5 mg/kg i. v.) does not alter the high-intensity electrical- or noxious stimulation-evoked release of NKA from the spinal cord in cats. Due to the complexity of the action of morphine (as illustrated above), further investigations are obviously needed to allow the definitive conclusion that the spinal release of these two peptides is really not modulated by opioid receptor stimulation.

Opioids and the spinal release of calcitonin gene-related peptide

Studies on CGRP are particularly interesting with regard to the present topic. Indeed, in the dorsal horn, SP, NKA and SRIF are present not only in nerve terminals of PAF but also in other neuronal elements (*see* [72], and references herein), and the released peptides could therefore originate from these various sources. Even direct stimulations of PAF could lead to the release of transmitter(s) which might subsequently excite(s) interneurones to release SP, NKA and/or SRIF. In contrast to the latter peptides, CGRP is almost exclusively located in terminals of PAF ([50] ; *see* also [72]). Consequently, as compared to the spinal release of any other peptide, that of CGRP is probably the best index of PAF activity.

At 10 µM, a concentration which significantly affects the spinal release of SP and met-enkephalin [11, 13, 14], and also at a concentration ten-fold higher, the selective µ opioid receptor agonist, DAGO, exerts no influence on the spontaneous release of CGRP from the rat spinal cord *in vivo* [12]. Since both DAGO and PL017, at 10 µM, were shown to reduce approximately by half the K^+-evoked release of CGRP from rat spinal cord slices [51], this result is rather surprising. There are obviously numerous differences between *in vivo* and *in vitro* conditions, which could lead to such discrepancies. Thus, the inhibitory influence of µ opioid receptor stimulation on the K^+-induced CGRP release under *in vitro* conditions could be masked *in vivo*, due to the activation of some neuronal circuits (disrupted in spinal cord slices) which exert an excitatory action on CGRP-containing PAF. It should also be emphasised that we investigated the effects of DAGO only on the spontaneous outflow of CGRP *in vivo*, and further experiments are needed to assess the possible effects of µ opioid receptor stimulation on noxious stimuli-evoked spinal CGRP release. Finally, it must be pointed out that, depending on their concentrations, opioids can exert opposite effects on a given process (*see* above) and complete dose-response curve for the effect(s) of DAGO on the spinal release of CGRP has also to be established.

The selective stimulation of κ opioid receptors by 10 μM U 50488 H is also devoid of any effect on CGRP release *in vivo* [12]. This is congruent with *in vitro* data showing that another selective κ agonist, U 69593 [33], does not modify the release of CGRP from spinal cord slices [51].

In contrast to DAGO and U 50488 H, the δ opioid agonist DTLET, at 10 μM, significantly increases the spinal release of CGRP *in vivo* [12] (Figure 2). This finding is surprising as it was established that DTLET (and DPDPE) strongly reduce(s) the K^+-evoked release of CGRP from rat spinal cord slices [51]. The same explanations as those proposed for reconciling *in vitro* and *in vivo* data about the modulation by DAGO of CGRP release could also account for the discrepancies between *in vitro* and *in vivo* observations with DTLET. However, it has to be pointed out that only one concentration of DTLET (10 μM) was used in the study by Collin *et al.* [12] and further experiments are needed to establish whether this compound, within a large range of concentrations, regularly exerts a stimulatory influence on spinal CGRP release or may become inhibitory at certain concentrations under *in vivo* conditions. Since naltrindole (10 μM) completely prevents the stimulatory effect of DTLET on CGRP release, it can be concluded that this effect actually involves δ opioid receptors. Electrophysiological studies have already revealed excitatory effects of δ opioid receptor agonists on dorsal horn neurones. Thus, i.t. DSTBULET, a selective δ opioid receptor agonist [16], and iontophoretically applied met-enkephalinamide increase the neuronal responses evoked in the dorsal horn by electrical and thermal cutaneous noxious stimulation [58, 65]. According to Sullivan *et al.* [65], the δ-dependent excitation of these neurones might be indirect, and could thus involve the observed increase in CGRP release. Indeed, CGRP is known to excite dorsal horn neurones [41] and to potentiate the effects of excitatory amino acids on these neurones [47].

The δ opioid antagonist naltrindole (10 μM) does not modify the peptide outflow [12], indicating that there is very likely no tonic excitatory control exerted by endogenous opioids acting at δ receptors on the spontaneous release of CGRP from the rat spinal cord *in vivo*. By contrast, 10 μM naloxone and 10 μM nBNI markedly increase CGRP release. That the effect of naloxone involves μ opioid receptors is supported by the observation that another antagonist with greater selectivity for these receptors, CTOP [25], also leads to a significant enhancement of the peptide release [12].

Thus, whereas experiments with selective agonists did not reveal any change in CGRP release upon the stimulation of μ or κ opioid receptors, investigations using antagonists suggest that endogenous opioids acting at these receptors exert a tonic inhibitory influence on the spinal release of the peptide *in vivo*. These two conclusions appear congruent, rather than contradictory, if the simultaneous stimulation of both μ and κ receptors would be necessary to reduce CGRP release, and the blockade of only one of them, μ or κ, would be sufficient to prevent the inhibitory effect of their concomitant stimulation (Figure 2). Alternatively, it could also be postulated that the μ and κ agonists did not affect CGRP release simply because endogenous opioids were already stimulating these receptors *in vivo*. Effects could thus be expected from

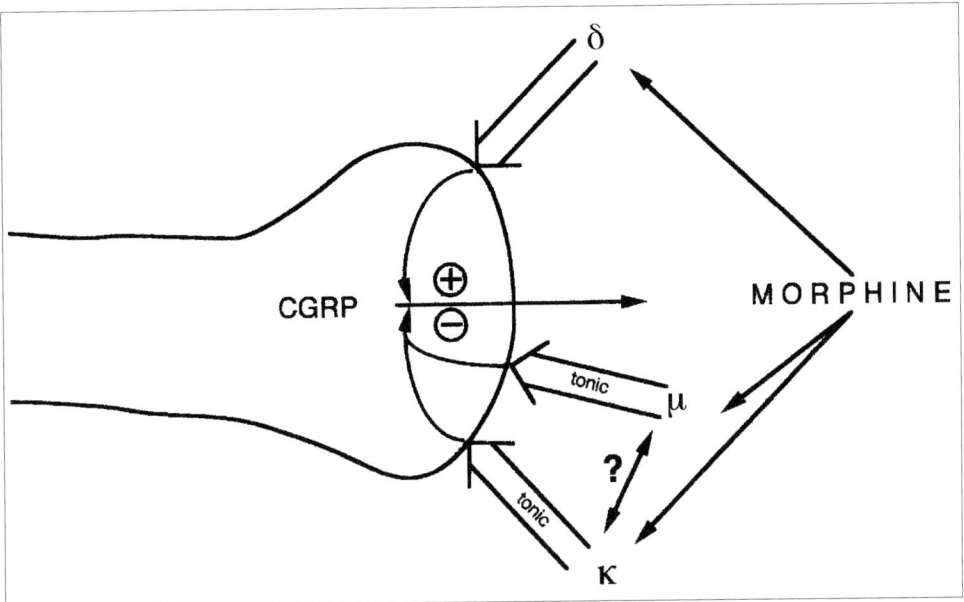

Figure 2. Schematic representation of the opioid control of the spontaneous release of calcitonin gene-related peptide (CGRP) from the rat spinal cord *in vivo*. The selective stimulation of δ receptors provokes an enhancement of the spontaneous release of CGRP. Although the stimulation of either μ or k receptors alone is ineffective, their concomitant stimulation leads to a reduction in the release of CGRP. Whereas the blockade of δ receptors is ineffective, that of either μ or k receptors enhances the spontaneous release of CGRP, suggesting that endogenous opioids acting at both μ and κ receptors tonically reduce the peptide release. Morphine exerts no significant effect on the release of CGRP because it stimulates all μ, δ and κ receptors. Indeed, the inhibitory influence on the peptide release of the simultaneous stimulation of μ and κ receptors is masked by the excitatory effect due to the concomitant stimulation of δ receptors.

antagonists but not from agonists if the tonic control of CGRP-containing neurones by endogenous opioids acting at μ and κ receptors was working at near maximal efficiency.

In line with one of the above hypotheses, we observed that the simultaneous stimulation of both μ and κ opioid receptors by the combined addition of 10 μM DAGO and 10 μM U 50488 H to the perfusing artificial cerebrospinal fluid produces a marked inhibition of the spinal release of CGRP (Figure 2). This effect appears to involve actually the stimulation of both μ and κ receptors, as shown by its prevention by either naloxone or nBNI [12]. Previous studies already emphasised that the stimulation of both μ and κ receptors may be necessary for the action of some opioids. For instance, Tseng and Collins [68] found that the tail-flick inhibition induced by i. t. β-endorphin could be blocked by either μ or κ receptor antagonists. In addition, a synergy in the antinociceptive effects of DAGO and U 50488 H has been demonstrated upon the combined i. t. administration of these two drugs [40, 66].

Neither 20 mg/kg i.v. nor 10-100 μM i.t. morphine affect the spontaneous release of CGRP from the spinal cord in halothane-anaesthetized rats [12]. Similarly, Morton and Hutchison [42] showed that 5-15 mg/kg i.v. of morphine in cats did not reduce the enhancement of spinal CGRP release elicited by electrical stimulation of the tibial nerve or hindpaw immersion in water at 52°C. Although morphine alone is inactive, it becomes inhibitory on the spinal release of the peptide when δ receptors are blocked by naltrindole [12]. Accordingly, it can be proposed that the stimulation of δ receptors by morphine prevents this drug to inhibit CGRP release through the stimulation of both μ and κ receptors (Figure 2). This interpretation agrees with the fact that either naloxone or nBNI is able to prevent the morphine-induced decrease in CGRP release in the presence of naltrindole [12].

If our results [12], together with those of Morton and Hutchison [42] and Morton et al. [44], suggest that the antinociceptive action of i.v. or i.t. morphine does not probably involve a presynaptic inhibition of CGRP-containing PAF, they do not exclude that endogenous opioids could act through this mechanism to reduce nociception. Indeed, our data support the existence of a tonic inhibitory control of the spinal release of CGRP by endogenous opioids acting simultaneously at both μ and κ receptors. Further investigations are needed to examine which endogenous peptides could be involved in this process. However, as the effects of opioid receptor agonists and antagonists were investigated on the "spontaneous" release of CGRP, it remains to be established whether the release of the peptide elicited by noxious stimulations could also be modulated through such mechanisms.

Effects of drugs acting at GABA receptors on the release of neuropeptides from the spinal cord

Contradictory results have been reported regarding the ability of GABA and related agonists to modulate the spinal release of SRIF. Whereas Sawynok et al. [60] and Kuraishi et al. [32] reported that GABA at 100 - 200 μM does not affect the release of SRIF elicited by K^+-depolarisation or capsaicin from rat spinal cord slices, Vasko and Harris [69] found that the amino acid, in a slightly lower concentration range : 10 - 100 μM, is able to reduce the K^+-induced release of the peptide from the same preparation. This inhibitory effect of GABA on the spinal release of SRIF could be blocked by 10 μM bicuculline, suggesting that GABA exerts its action through the stimulation of $GABA_A$ receptors. That $GABA_B$ receptors are not involved in the possible inhibitory influence of GABA on the spinal release of SRIF seems to be confirmed by the fact that a selective agonist of these receptors, baclofen (10 - 500 μM), does not affect the K^+-evoked release of the peptide from rat spinal cord slices [60, 69].

In conclusive results that have also been published regarding the effects of GABA on the spinal release of SP. At 0.1 - 100 μM, the amino acid was shown to exert no effect on the K^+-evoked release of the peptide from rat spinal cord slices [4, 49]. However, at higher concentrations : 0.1 - 1 mM, GABA can reduce slightly the spinal release of SP elicited by high-intensity electrical stimulation of the sciatic nerves in the cat [22]. Similarly, a slight decrease in electrically induced-SP release has been reported in cultured chick dorsal root ganglion cells exposed to 0.1 - 1mM GABA [27]. This inhibitory effect of GABA on SP release could be mimicked, at least partly, by muscimol (1 - 100 µM, [22, 27]) suggesting that it could result from the stimulation of $GABA_A$ receptors. With the exception of Holz et al. [27], who found that 10 µM baclofen reduces the electrically-induced release of SP from chicken dorsal root ganglion cells in culture, all other investigators reported that the stimulation of $GABA_B$ receptors by this drug does not modify the spinal release of SP evoked either by K^+ depolarisation of rat tissues in vitro [4, 60] or by stimulation of the sciatic nerve [22] or the tibial nerve [45] in anaesthetised cats.

GABA (1 - 100 µM) has also been shown to inhibit the release of CGRP from rat spinal cord slices [4]. $GABA_B$ receptors are very likely not involved in the inhibitory effects of GABA since baclofen (1 - 10 µM) is inactive on the K^+-evoked release of the peptide [4]. Furthermore, i. v. injection of 2-10 mg/kg of baclofen does not alter the release of CGRP evoked by electrical or noxious stimulation of a tibial nerve in cats [45]. By contrast, an inhibition of the K^+-evoked CGRP release can be observed with muscimol (10 - 100 µM), and this effect is preventable by bicuculline as expected from the involvement of $GABA_A$ receptors [4].

As summarised above, most investigations [4, 49, 60] have led to the conclusion that the release of SP is very unlikely controlled by GABA-containing interneurones within the rat spinal cord. However, in contrast to CGRP which is located exclusively in PAF, SP is also present in other neuronal elements within the spinal cord (see above). Therefore, one cannot exclude that some inhibitory influence of GABA on the release of SP from PAF could be masked by a persistent outflow of the peptide from the other neuronal elements.

To date, most evidence in the literature suggests that the antinociceptive effects of GABA at the level of the spinal cord are mediated by bicuculline-insensitive $GABA_B$ receptors (see [76] for review). In contrast, GABA-induced inhibition of spinal CGRP (and perhaps SP) release appears to involve bicuculline-sensitive $GABA_A$ receptors [4]. Therefore, this effect is probably unrelated to the antinociceptive action of GABA via the intrathecal route, and postsynaptic rather than presynaptic mechanisms should account for this action [2].

Effects of drugs acting at adrenoreceptors on the release of neuropeptides from the spinal cord

Whereas the K^+- or capsaicin-evoked release of SRIF from slices of rat spinal cord is not affected by norepinephrine [32, 69], this monoamine, clonidine and other α_2-

adrenoreceptor agonists inhibit the K^+- or veratridine-evoked release of SP from the same tissue preparation [5, 48, 49] and chick dorsal root ganglion cells in culture [27]. In vivo, α_2-adrenoreceptor agonists also reduce the spinal release of SP in the rabbit [32] and that evoked by high-intensity electrical stimulation of the sciatic nerves in the cat [22]. In contrast, selective agonists acting at α_1 or β adrenoreceptors do not affect the peptide release in vivo in the cat [22] and the rabbit [31] and in vitro in the rat [5]. The inhibitory effects of both norepinephrine and clonidine can be blocked not only by idazoxan, a selective α_2-adrenoreceptor antagonist [56] but also by prazosin [5, 31, 48]. Although prazosin was initially considered as a selective α_1-antagonist [56], it is also presently known as a high affinity antagonist of the α_{2b} adrenoreceptor subtype [6]. Thus, α_{2b}-adrenoreceptors are likely involved in the norepinephrine- and clonidine-induced decrease in spinal SP release.

Neither β- nor α-adrenoreceptor agonists, including norepinephrine and clonidine, affect the release of CGRP from rat spinal cord slices [5], or guinea pig spinal ganglia in culture [19]. Thus, as previously noted for the effects of GABA on the spinal release of both peptides, there is a dissociation between the effect of α_2-adrenoreceptor stimulation on K^+-induced CGRP and SP release. Whatever the reasons for that, the lack of effect of norepinephrine and clonidine on spinal CGRP release suggests that the antinociceptive action of intrathecally administered α_2-adrenoreceptor agonists does not involve a presynaptic control of the activity of (CGRP-containing) PAF. In agreement with this conclusion, Satoh et al. [59] detected no axo-axonic contacts between noradrenergic fibers and primary afferent nerve terminals in the rat spinal cord. Furthermore, the presynaptic location on PAF of about 20% of spinal α_2-adrenoreceptors that was reported by Howe et al. [28] was not confirmed by Wikberg and Hajos [73] who found that all α_2-adrenoreceptors within the dorsal horn are located on capsaicin-insensitive neurones. Therefore, in line with electrophysiological data [18, 70, 74], it can be concluded that the antinociceptive action of α_2-adrenergic agonists is very probably due to the stimulation of postsynaptic receptors with respect to PAF.

Effects of drugs acting at serotonin receptors on the release of neuropeptides from the spinal cord

Kuraishi et al. [32] recently observed that 5-HT (30-100 µM) reduces the capsaicin-evoked release of SRIF from rat spinal cord slices. In our laboratory, we have examined the possible modulation of spinal SP and CGRP release by drugs acting at 5-HT_{1A}, 5-HT_{1B} and 5-HT_3 receptors. The choice of these 5-HT receptor subtypes was directed by their established presence on nerve terminals of PAF in the rat dorsal horn [15, 24, 36]. Neither 5-HT, selective agonists of 5-HT_{1A} and 5-HT_3 receptors [5], nor 0.1 nM - 10 µM sumatriptan (which acts at 5-HT_{1B} receptors in the rat, [29]) affect the K^+-evoked release of SP and CGRP from rat spinal cord slices (Table I).

Table I. Lack of effect of sumatriptan on the K+-evoked release of SP and CGRP from the dorsal part of the lumbar enlargement of the rat spinal cord. Slices of the dorsal half of the lumbar enlargement were depolarized twice (K1, K2) by 30 mM K+ (for 8 min each) in the course of superfusion with artificial CSF (1 ml/4 min). The first K+ pulse was applied without drug, whereas the 2nd K+ pulse occurred while tissues were exposed to various concentrations of sumatriptan (0 - 10 µM added to the artificial CSF). SP and CGRP were measured in each collected fraction (1 ml), and the ratios K_2/K_1 of K+-evoked SP and CGRP overflow due to the 2nd K+ pulse over that due to the 1st one were calculated. In the absence of sumatriptan ("none"), these ratios were 0.37 ± 0.04 and 0.37 ± 0.02 (means ± S. E. M., $n = 20$), respectively. Each value, expressed as a percentage of the ratio K_2/K_1 in the absence of sumatriptan, is the mean ± S. E. M. of at least 8 independent determinations.

Addition	SP	CGRP
None	100.0 ± 10.8	100.0 ± 5.4
Sumatriptan 0.1 nM	110.4 ± 3.8	98.2 ± 5.4
1 nM	102.1 ± 4.1	94.6 ± 9.4
10 nM	121.6 ± 11.1	91.9 ± 14.7
100 nM	124.3 ± 8.7	94.5 ± 8.6
1 µM	113,5 ± 7.1	91.9 ± 17.6
10 µM	100.0 ± 10.8	100.0 ± 16.2

Similarly, Pang and Vasko [49] in the rat and Go and Yaksh [22] in the cat reported that 5-HT exerts no influence on the spinal release of SP. At variance with these findings, Yonehara et al. [77] observed that 5-HT reduces the release of SP in the trigeminal nucleus of the rabbit. The latter effect can be antagonised by methysergide [77], which blocks indifferently the 5-HT_1 and 5-HT_2, but not 5-HT_3, receptor subtypes [29]. As 5-HT_{1A} and 5-HT_{1B} receptor subtypes do not seem to be involved in a possible control of SP release, one can propose that 5-HT_{1C}, 5-HT_2 or other 5-HT receptors among the numerous types which have been cloned during the recent past (see [38]) mediate the action on the indoleamine.

In contrast to Saria et al. [57] who concluded that 5-HT_3 receptor stimulation exerts a facilitatory influence on the spinal release of CGRP, we did not find any modulatory effect of the potent 5-HT_3 agonist 2-methyl-5-HT on this process [5]. As 5-HT_3 receptors may desensitise rapidly [29], it can be speculated that the discrepancy between our results and those of Saria et al. [57] originates in possible differences between the desensitisation rate of 5-HT_3 receptor in the two studies.

In any case, our data [5] do not support that 5-HT exerts its antinociceptive effect at the spinal level (see [23]) through a presynaptic control of PAF containing SP and/or CGRP. Instead, electrophysiological studies have led to the conclusion that the 5-HT action on spinal neurones located postsynaptically with respect to PAF very probably accounts for the inhibitory influence of the indoleamine on the transfer of nociceptive messages [2, 20].

Conclusion

Although the studies in this field began 16 years ago, with the pioneer work of Jessell and Iversen [30], little is still known with absolute certainty about the possible presynaptic control of PAF by neuroactive molecules. Data remain inconclusive notably because the putative neurotransmitters the release of which can be affected by these drugs cannot generally be ascribed to originate solely from the terminals of PAF. The only exception is CGRP as this peptide is (almost) exclusively located in PAF within the dorsal horn [50].

Assuming that the spinal release of CGRP is therefore a more reliable index of the activity of PAF than the release of other neuroactive substances, available data suggest that the antinociceptive effects of intrathecally administered adreno-, 5-HT and GABA receptor agonists do not involve presynaptic mechanisms. Indeed, neither adrenoreceptor nor 5-HT receptor agonists affect the release of CGRP from the spinal cord. Furthermore, the inhibitory effect of GABA on the peptide release appears to depend exclusively on the stimulation of $GABA_A$ receptors, whereas $GABA_B$ receptors have been shown to mediate the antinociceptive action of i.t. GABA. These data, together with other findings summarised in this review, indirectly support that postsynaptic sites are in fact involved in the antinociceptive effects of intrathecally administered drugs acting at GABA, adreno- and 5-HT receptors.

By contrast, opioids can presynaptically control the activity of CGRP-containing PAF. However, this control appears to be rather complex since the stimulation of δ receptors enhances the spinal release of CGRP *in vivo* in the rat, whereas those of both μ and κ receptors reduce it. These opposite effects probably explain why morphine which acts at μ, δ and κ receptors does not modify the spinal release of CGRP (Figure 2).

Besides these pharmacological data, recent observations gave insights into the functional aspects of the opioid control of nociception. Thus, evidence has been reported that endogenous opioids are involved in the physiological control of PAF by exerting a tonic inhibitory influence, through the stimulation of μ and κ receptors, on the spinal release of CGRP, and through that of δ receptors, on the spinal release of SP.

References

1. Aimone LD, Yaksh TL. Opioid modulation of capsaicin-evoked release of substance P from rat spinal cord *in vivo*. *Peptides* 1989 ; 10 : 1127-31.
2. Alhaider AA, Lei SZ, Wilcox GL. Spinal 5-HT_3 receptor-mediated antinociception : possible release of GABA. *J Neurosci* 1991 ; 11 : 1881-8.
3. Besse D, Lombard MC, Zajac JM, Roques BP, Besson JM. Pre- and post-synaptic distribution of μ, δ and κ opioid receptors in the superficial layers of the cervical dorsal horn of the rat spinal cord. *Brain Res* 1990 ; 521 : 15-22.

4. Bourgoin S, Pohl M, Benoliel JJ, Mauborgne A, Collin E, Hamon M, Cesselin F. γ-aminobutyric acid, through $GABA_A$ receptors, inhibits the potassium-stimulated release of calcitonin gene-related peptide but not that of substance P-like material from rat spinal cord slices. *Brain Res* 1992 ; 583 : 344-8.
5. Bourgoin S, Pohl M, Mauborgne A, Benoliel JJ, Collin E, Hamon M, Cesselin F. Monoaminergic control of the release of calcitonin gene-related peptide- and substance P-like materials from rat spinal cord slices. *Neuropharmacology* 1993 ; 32 : 633-40.
6. Bylund DB, Ray-Prenger C, Murphy TJ. Alpha-2A and alpha-2B adrenergic receptor subtypes : antagonist binding in tissues and cell lines containing only one subtype. *J Pharmacol Exp Ther* 1988 ; 245 : 600-7.
7. Cesselin F, Pohl M, Collin E, Bourgoin S, Le Bars D, Hamon M. In vivo release of sensory putative neurotransmitters from the spinal cord. Effects of electrical and noxious stimulations. In : Hökfelt T, Schaible HG, Schmidt RF, eds. *Neuropeptides, nociception and pain.* Mainz : Akademie der Wissenschaften und der Litteratur, 1994 : in press.
8. Chang HM, Berde CB, Holz GG, Steward GF, Kream RM. Sufentanil, morphine, met-enkephalin, and κ-agonist (U-50, 488H) inhibit substance P release from primary sensory neurons : a model for presynaptic spinal opioid actions. *Anesthesiology* 1989 ; 70 : 672-7.
9. Chang KJ, Wei ET, Killian A , Chang JK. Potent morphiceptin analogs : structure-activity relationships and morphine-like activities. *J Pharmacol Exp Ther* 1983 ; 237 : 325-38.
10. Clark MJ, Carter BD, Medzihradsky F. Selectivity of ligand binding to opioid receptors in brain membranes from the rat, monkey, and guinea pig. *Eur J Pharmacol* 1988 ; 148 : 343-51.
11. Collin E, Bourgoin S, Mantelet S, Hamon M, Cesselin F. Feedback inhibition of met-enkephalin release from the rat spinal cord *in vivo. Synapse* 1992 ; 11 : 76-84.
12. Collin E, Frechilla D, Pohl M, Bourgoin S, Le Bars D, Hamon M, Cesselin F. Opioid control of the release of calcitonin gene-related peptide like-material from the rat spinal cord *in vivo. Brain Res* 1993 ; 609 : 211-22.
13. Collin E, Mauborgne A, Bourgoin S, Chantrel D, Hamon M, Cesselin F. In vivo tonic inhibition of spinal substance P (like material) release by endogenous opioid(s) acting at δ receptors. *Neuroscience* 1991 ; 44 : 725-31.
14. Collin E, Mauborgne A, Bourgoin S, Mantelet S, Ferhat L, Hamon M, Cesselin F. Kappa-/mu-receptor interactions in the opioid control of the *in vivo* release of substance P-like material from the rat spinal cord. *Neuroscience* 1992 ; 332 : 347-55.
15. Daval G, Vergé D, Basbaum AI, Bourgoin S, Hamon M. Autoradiographic evidence of serotonin1 binding sites on primary afferent fibers in the dorsal horn of the rat spinal cord. *Neurosci Lett* 1987 ; 83 : 71-6.
16. Delay-Goyet P, Sequin C, Daugé V, Calenco G, Morgat JL, Gacel G, Roques BP. ^{3}H DSTBULET, a new linear hexapeptide with both an improved selectivity and a high affinity for δ-opioid receptors. *NIDA Res Monogr Ser* 1987 ; 75 : 197-200.
17. Desarmenien M, Feltz P, Occhipinti G, Santangelo F, Schlichter R. Coexistence of $GABA_A$ and $GABA_B$ receptors on A and C primary afferents. *Br J Pharmacol* 1984 ; 81 : 327-33.
18. Fleetwood-Walker SM, Mitchell R, Hope PJ, Molony V, Iggo A. An α_2 receptor mediates the selective inhibition by noradrenaline of nociceptive responses of identified dorsal horn neurones. *Brain Res* 1985 ; 334 : 243-54.
19. Franco-Cereceda A, Rydh M, Dalsgaard C. Nicotine- and capsaicin-, but not potassium evoked CGRP-release from cultured guinea-pig spinal ganglia is inhibited by Ruthenium red. *Neurosci Lett* 1992 ; 137 : 72-4.
20. Giesler GJ, Gerhat KD, Yezierski RP, Wilcox TK, Willis WD. Postsynaptic inhibition of primate spinothalamic neurons by stimulation in nucleus raphe magnus. *Brain Res* 1981 ; 204 : 184-8.
21. Gillan MGC, Kosterlitz HW. Spectrum of the μ-, δ- and κ-binding sites in homogenates of rat brain. *Br J Pharmacol* 1982 ; 77 : 461-9.

22. Go VLW, Yaksh TL. Release of substance P from the cat spinal cord. *J Physiol (Lond)* 1987 ; 391 : 141-67.
23. Hamon MD, Collin E, Chantrel D, Vergé D, Bourgoin S. The contribution of monoamines and their receptors to pain control. In : Basbaum AI, Besson JM, eds. *Towards a new pharmacology of pain*. Chichester : John Wiley and Sons Ltd, 1991 : 83-102.
24. Hamon M, Gallissot MC, Ménard F, Gozlan H, Bourgoin S, Vergé D. 5-HT$_3$ receptor binding sites are on capsaicin-sensitive fibers in the rat spinal cord. *Eur J Pharmacol* 1989 ; 164 : 315-22.
25. Hawkins KN, Knapp RJ, Lui GK, Gukya K, Kazmierski W, Wan YP, Pelton JT, Hruby VJ, Yamamura HI. [^{3}H]-[H-D-Phe-Cys-Tyr-D-Trp-Orn-Thr-Pen-Thr-NH$_2$] ([^{3}H]CTOP), a potent and highly selective peptide for mu opioid receptors in rat brain. *J Pharmacol Exp Ther* 1989 ; 248 : 73-80.
26. Hirota N, Kuraishi Y, Hino Y, Sato Y, Satoh M, Takagi H. Met-enkephalin and morphine but not dynorphin inhibit noxious stimuli-induced release of substance P from rabbit dorsal horn *in situ*. *Neuropharmacology* 1985 ; 24 : 567-70.
27. Holz IV GG, Kream RM, Spiegel A, Dunlap K. G proteins couple a-adrenergic and GABA receptors to inhibition of peptide secretion from peripheral sensory neurons. *J Neurosci* 1989 ; 9 : 657-66.
28. Howe JR, Yaksh TL, Go VL. The effect of unilateral dorsal root ganglionectomies or ventral rhizotomies on α$_2$-adrenoreceptor binding to, and the substance P, enkephalin, and neurotensin content of, the cat lumbar spinal cord. *Neuroscience* 1987 ; 21 : 385-94.
29. Hoyer D. The 5-HT receptor family : ligands, distribution and receptor-effector coupling. In : Rodgers RJ, Cooper SJ, eds. *5-HT$_{1A}$ agonists, 5-HT$_3$ antagonists and benzodiazepines : their comparative behavioural pharmacology*. Chichester : John Wileys and Sons, 1991 : 31-57.
30. Jessell TM, Iversen LL. Opiate analgesics inhibit substance P release from rat trigeminal nucleus. *Nature* 1977 ; 268 : 549-51.
31. Kuraishi Y, Hirota N, Sato Y, Kaneko S, Satoh M, Takagi H. Noradrenergic inhibition of the release of substance P from the primary afferents in the rabbit spinal cord dorsal horn. *Brain Res* 1985 ; 359 : 177-82.
32. Kuraishi Y, Minami M, Satoh M. Serotonin, but neither noradrenaline nor GABA, inhibits capsaicin-evoked release of immunoreactive somatostatin from slices of rat spinal cord. *Neurosci Res* 1991 ; 9 : 238-45.
33. Lahti AR, Mickelson MM, McCall JM, von Voigtlander PF. [^{3}H]U69593, a highly selective ligand for the opioid κ receptor. *Eur J Pharmacol* 1985 ; 109 : 281-4.
34. Lamotte C, Pert CB, Snyder SH. Opiate receptor binding in primate spinal cord. Distribution and changes after dorsal root section. *Brain Res* 1976 ; 112 : 407-12.
35. Lang CW, Duggan AW, Hope PJ. Analgesic doses of morphine do not reduce noxious stimulus-evoked release of immunoreactive neurokinins in the dorsal horn of the spinal cat. *Br J Pharmacol* 1991 ; 103 : 1871-6.
36. Laporte AM, Kidd EJ, Vergé D, Gozlan H, Hamon M. Autoradiographic mapping of central 5-HT$_3$ receptors. In : Hamon M, ed. *Central and peripheral 5-HT$_3$ receptors*. London : Academic Press, 1992 : 157-87.
37. Magnan J, Paterson SJ, Tavani A, Kosterlitz HW. The binding spectrum of narcotic analgesic drugs with different agonist and antagonist properties. *Naunyn-Schmiedeberg's Arch Pharmacol* 1982 ; 319 : 197-205.
38. Matthes H, Boschert U, Amlaiky N, Grailhe R, Plassat JL, Muscatelli F, Mattei MG, Hen R. The mouse 5-HT$_{5A}$ and 5-HT$_{5B}$ receptors define a new family of serotonin receptors : cloning, functional expression and chromosomal localization. *Mol Pharmacol* 1993 ; 43 : 313-9.
39. Mauborgne A, Lutz O, Legrand JC, Hamon M, Cesselin F. Opposite effects of δ and μ opioid

receptor agonists on the *in vitro* release of substance P-like material from the rat spinal cord. *J Neurochem* 1987 ; 48 : 529-37.
40. Miaskowski C, Sutters KA, Taiwo YO, Levine JD. Antinociceptive and motor effects of delta/mu and kappa/mu combinations of intrathecal opioid agonists. *Pain* 1992 ; 49 : 137-44.
41. Miletic Y, Tan H. Iontophoretic application of calcitonin gene-related peptide produces a slow and prolonged excitation of neurons in the cat lumbar dorsal horn. *Brain Res* 1988 ; 446 : 169-72.
42. Morton CR, Hutchison WD. Morphine does not reduce the intraspinal release of calcitonin gene-related peptide in the cat. *Neurosci Lett* 1990 ; 117 : 319-24.
43. Morton CR, Hutchison WD, Duggan AW, Hendry IA. Morphine and substance P release in the spinal cord. *Exp Brain Res* 1990 ; 82 : 89-96.
44. Morton CR, Hutchison WD, Hendry IA. Intraspinal release of substance P and calcitonin gene-related peptide during opiate dependence and withdrawal. *Neuroscience* 1991 ; 43 : 593-600.
45. Morton CR, Hutchison WD, Lacey G. Baclofen and the release of neuropeptides in the cat spinal cord. *Eur J Neurosci* 1992 ; 4 : 243-50.
46. Mosberg HI, Hurtz R, Hruby VJ, Gee K, Yamamura HI, Galligan JJ, Burks TF. Bis-penicillamine enkephalins possess high specificity toward δ opioid receptors. *Proc Natl Acad Sci USA* 1983 ; 80 : 5871-4.
47. Murase K, Ryu PD, Randic M. Excitatory and inhibitory amino acids and peptide-induced responses in acutely isolated rat spinal dorsal horn neurons. *Neurosci Lett* 1989 ; 103 : 56-63.
48. Ono H, Mishima A, Ono S, Fukuda H, Vasko MR. Inhibitory effects of clonidine and tizanidine on release of substance P from slices of rat spinal cord and antagonism by α-adrenergic receptor antagonists. *Neuropharmacology* 1991 ; 30 : 585-9.
49. Pang IH, Vasko MR. Morphine and norepinephrine but not 5-hydroxytryptamine and γ-aminobutyric acid inhibit the potassium-stimulated release of substance P from rat spinal cord slices. *Brain Res* 1986 ; 376 : 268-79.
50. Pohl M, Benoliel JJ, Bourgoin S, Lombard MC, Mauborgne A, Taquet H, Carayon A, Besson JM, Cesselin F, Hamon M. Regional distribution of calcitonin gene-related peptide-, substance P-, cholecystokinin-, Met$_5$-enkephalin-, and dynorphin A(1-8)-like materials in the spinal cord and dorsal root ganglia of adult rats : effects of dorsal rhizotomy and neonatal capsaicin. *J Neurochem* 1990 ; 55 : 1122-30.
51. Pohl M, Lombard MC, Bourgoin S, Carayon A, Benoliel JJ, Mauborgne A, Besson JM, Hamon M, Cesselin F. Opioid control of the *in vitro* release of calcitonin gene-related peptide from primary afferent fibers projecting in the rat cervical cord. *Neuropeptides* 1989 ; 14 : 151-9.
52. Pohl M, Mauborgne A, Bourgoin S, Benoliel JJ, Hamon M, Cesselin F. Neonatal capsaicin treatment abolishes the modulations by opioids of substance P release from rat spinal cord slices. *Neurosci Lett* 1989 ; 96 : 102-7.
53. Portoghese PS, Lipkowski AW, Takemori AE. Binaltorphimine and nor-binaltorphimine, potent and selective κ-opioid receptor antagonists. *Life Sci* 1987 ; 40 : 1287-92.
54. Portoghese PS, Sultana M, Takemori AE. Naltrindole, a highly selective and potent non-peptide δ opioid receptor antagonist. *Eur J Pharmacol* 1988 ; 146 : 185-6.
55. Price GW, Wilkin GP, Turnbull MJ, Bowery NG. Are baclofen-sensitive GABA$_B$ receptors present on primary afferent terminals of the spinal cord ? *Nature* 1984 ; 307 : 71-4.
56. Ruffolo RR, Nichols AJ, Stadel JM, Hieble JP. Structure and function of α-adrenoreceptors. *Pharmacol Rev* 1991 ; 43 : 475-505.
57. Saria A, Javorsky F, Humpel C, Gamse R. 5-HT$_3$ receptor antagonists inhibit sensory neuropeptide release from the rat spinal cord. *Neuroreport* 1990 ; 1 : 104-6.
58. Sastry BR, Goh JW. Actions of morphine and met-enkephalin-amide on nociceptor driven neurones in substantia gelatinosa and deeper dorsal horn. *Neuropharmacology* 1983 ; 22 : 119-22.

59. Satoh K, Kashiba A, Kimura H, Maeda T. Noradrenergic axon terminals in the substantia gelatinosa of the rat spinal cord. An electron-microscopic study using glyoxylic acid-potassium permanganate fixation. *Cell Tissue Res* 1982 ; 222 : 359-78.
60. Sawynok J, Kato N, Havlicek V, LaBella FS. Lack of effect of baclofen on substance P and somatostatin release from the spinal cord *in vitro*. *Naunyn-Schmiedeberg's Arch Pharmacol* 1982 ; 319 : 78-81.
61. Suarez-Roca H, Abdullah L, Zuniga J, Madison S, Maixner W. Multiphasic effect of morphine on the release of substance P from trigeminal nucleus slices. *Brain Res* 1992 ; 579 : 187-94.
62. Suarez-Roca H, Maixner W. Morphine produces a multiphasic effect on the release of substance P from rat trigeminal nucleus slices by activating different opioid receptor subtypes. *Brain Res* 1992 ; 579 : 195-203.
63. Suarez-Roca H, Maixner W. δ-opioid-receptor activation by [D-Pen^2,D-Pen^5]enkephalin and morphine inhibits substance P release from trigeminal nucleus slices. *Eur J Pharmacol* 1992 ; 229 : 1-7.
64. Suarez-Roca H, Maixner W. Activation of kappa opioid receptors by U50488H and morphine enhances the release of substance P from rat trigeminal nucleus slices. *J Pharmacol Exp Ther* 1993 ; 264 : 648-53.
65. Sullivan AF, Dickenson AH, Roques BP. δ-opioid mediated inhibitions of acute and prolonged noxious-evoked responses in rat dorsal horn neurones. *Br J Pharmacol* 1989 ; 98 : 1039-49.
66. Sutters KA, Miaskowski C, Taiwo YO, Levine JD. Analgesic synergy and improved motor function produced by combinations of μ-δ- and μ-—opioids. *Brain Res* 1990 ; 530 : 290-4.
67. Takemori AE, Ikeda M, Portoghese PS. The mu, kappa, and delta properties of various opioid agonists. *Eur J Pharmacol* 1986 ; 123 : 357-61.
68. Tseng LF, Collins KA. The tail-flick inhibition induced by β-endorphin administered intrathecally is mediated by activation of κ- and μ-opioid receptors in the mouse. *Eur J Pharmacol* 1992 ; 214 : 59-65.
69. Vasko MR, Harris V. γ-aminobutyric acid inhibits the potassium-stimulated release of somatostatin from rat spinal cord slices. *Brain Res* 1990 ; 507 : 129-37.
70. Villanueva L, Chitour D, Le Bars D. Effects of tizanidine (DS 103-282) on dorsal horn convergent neurones in the rat. *Pain* 1988 ; 35 : 187-97.
71. Von Voigtlander PF, Lahti RA, Lundens JH. A selective and structurally novel non-mu (kappa) opioid agonist. *J Pharmacol Exp Ther* 1983 ; 224 : 7-12.
72. Weihe E. Neurochemical anatomy of the mammalian spinal cord : functional implications. *Ann Anat* 1992 ; 174 : 89-118.
73. Wikberg JES, Hajos M. Spinal cord α_2-adrenoreceptors may be located postsynaptically with respect to primary sensory neurons : destruction of primary C-afferents with neonatal capsaicin does not affect the number of [^{3}H]clonidine binding sites in mice. *Neurosci Lett* 1987 ; 76 : 63-8.
74. Willcockson WS, Chung JM, Hori Y, Lee KH, Willis WD. Effects of iontophoretically released amino acids and amines on primate spinothalamic tract cells. *J Neurosci* 1984 ; 4 : 732-40.
75. Wood PL, Charleson S, Lane D, Hudgin RL. Multiple opiate receptors : differential binding of mu, kappa, and delta agonists. *Neuropharmacology* 1981 ; 20 : 1215-20.
76. Yaksh TL, Stevens CW. Properties of the modulation of spinal nociceptive transmission by receptor-selective agents. In : Dubner R, Gebhart GF, Bond MR, eds. Proceedings of the Vth World Congress on Pain, Elsevier 1988 : 417-35.
77. Yonehara N, Shibutani T, Imai Y, Ooi Y, Sawada T, Inoki R. Serotonin inhibits release of substance P evoked by tooth pulp stimulation in trigeminal nucleus caudalis in rabbits. *Neuropharmacology* 1991 ; 30 : 5-13.
78. Zajac JM, Gacel G, Petit F, Dodey P, Rossignol P, Roques BP. Deltakephalin, Tyr-D-Thr-Gly-

Phe-Leu-Thr, a new highly potent and fully specific agonist for opiate δ receptors. *Biochem Biophys Res Comm* 1983 ; 111 : 390-7.

Achevé d'imprimer par Corlet, Imprimeur, S.A.
14110 Condé-sur-Noireau (France)
N° d'Imprimeur : 7903 - Dépôt légal : décembre 1994

Imprimé en C.E.E.